Fashion Apparel, Accessories, & Home Furnishings

Fashion Apparel, Accessories, & Home Furnishings

JAY DIAMOND

ELLEN DIAMOND

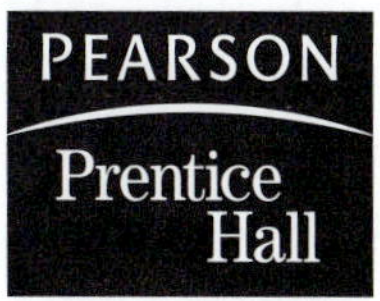

Upper Saddle River, New Jersey 07458

Library of Congress Cataloging-in-Publication Data
Diamond, Jay.
Fashion apparel, accessories, & home furnishings / Jay Diamond, Ellen Diamond. — 1st. ed.
p. cm.
Includes index.
ISBN 0-13-177686-X
1. Clothing trade. 2. Clothing and dress. 3. Dress accessories. 4. House furnishings.
I. Diamond, Ellen. II. Title.
TT497.D477 2007
746.9'2—dc22 2005028974

Editor-in-Chief: Vernon R. Anthony
Senior Acquisitions Editor: Eileen McClay
Assistant Editor: Maria Rego
Director of Manufacturing and Production: Bruce Johnson
Managing Editor: Mary Carnis
Production Liaison: Janice Stangel
Manufacturing Manager: Ilene Sanford
Manufacturing Buyer: Cathleen Petersen
Production Editor: Heather Willison, Carlisle Publishing Services
Executive Marketing Manager: Ryan DeGrote
Senior Marketing Assistant: Les Roberts
Senior Marketing Coordinator: Elizabeth Farrell
Director, Image Resource Center: Melinda Reo
Manager, Rights and Permissions: Zina Arabia
Manager, Visual Research: Beth Brenzel
Manager, Cover Visual Research & Permissions: Karen Sanatar
Image Permission Coordinator: Richard Rodrigues
Printer/Binder: Command Web
Cover Printer: Phoenix Color
Cover Design Coordinator: Miguel Ortiz
Cover Designer: Ruta Fiurino, Fruti Design
Cover Image: © Uripos; eStock Photo

Pearson Education LTD.
Pearson Education Singapore, Ptc. Ltd
Pearson Education, Cananda, Ltd
Pearson Education–Japan
Pearson Education Australia PTY, Limited
Pearson Education North Asia Ltd
Pearson Educación de Mexico, S.A. de C.V.
Pearson Education Malaysia, Ptc. Ltd
Pearson Education. Upper Saddle River, NJ

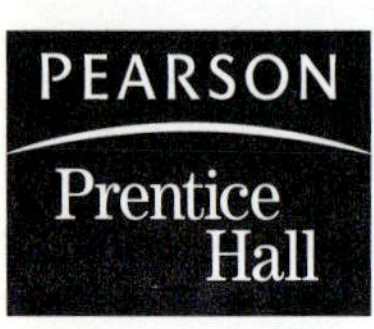

10 9 8 7 6 5 4 3 2 1
ISBN 0-13-177686-X

Brief Contents

Contents

Preface

For those entering the fashion industry as designers, manufacturers, sales professionals, retail buyers and merchandisers, fashion directors, advertisers, and a host of other professions, a complete knowledge of its technical and creative aspects is essential for a successful career. *Fashion Apparel, Accessories, & Home Furnishings* provides essential, up-to-the-minute details that are imperative to understand the raw materials used in fashion product manufacturing, the apparel classifications and their product lines, the numerous different wearable accessories and enhancements, and the host of home furnishings that deliver pizzazz in interior design.

The book is divided into five sections that cover the general nature of the fashion industry as well as its more specialized segments. In the Introduction to the Fashion Industry section, the discussion centers on the industry's nature and scope, careers, and the ways in which product information may be mastered. The Materials of Fashion Merchandise section focuses on the various raw materials used in the production of fashion-oriented products. The Apparel Classifications section carefully examines the industries of women's, men's, and children's clothing and their design, manufacturing processes and merchandising. A host of different products that serve both practical needs and fashion sense, including footwear, handbags, luggage, belts, jewelry, watches, gloves, hats, hosiery, scarves, umbrellas, cosmetics, and fragrances makes up the section on Wearable Accessories and Enhancements. Rounding out the merchandise information is the final section, Home Accessories and Decorative Enhancements, which covers tableware, furniture, lighting, wall art, decorative frames, decorative accessories, flooring, wall furnishings, linens, and bedding.

For those interested in making in-depth studies of a particular product, each chapter provides a section called Internet Resources for Additional Research that lists pertinent Web sites and the information they provide.

Each chapter features a wealth of drawings and photographs designed to help readers visually understand the text. In addition to the technical information provided, each chapter features learning objectives, review questions, and exercises.

An instructor's manual, complete with answers to the chapter-end questions, and a test bank and answer key are available.

Acknowledgments

We wish to thank the following people and companies for their generosity in making contributions to this edition of *Fashion Apparel, Accessories, & Home Furnishings:*

Alan Flusser, Alan Flusser Custom Shop; Mark Rykken, Alan Flusser Custom Shop; Heather Cohen, Fur Information Council of America; Brandee Dallow, The Julius Klein Group; Mikimoto; Julius Klein Diamonds; Ritani; James T. Murray Photography; Charles Rosner; Arthur Armstrong, CEO Merle Norman Cosmetics; Prof. Angel Bruno, Nassau Community College; Amy Meadows, Visual Marketing Manager, Marshall Field's; Pearson Asset Library; Associate Dean, Sheri Litt, Florida Community College at Jacksonville; Stanley Ulecki, Merle Norman Cosmetic Studio; Jack Slaughter, Fairfax Gallery; Linda Fain, Fain's Carpet; Sam Jacobson, Dixie Carpet Company; Alan Ellinger, Marketing Management Group.

Special thanks to Thomas Long, a highly regarded glassblower, for his invitation to photograph him at work on his premises, Creative Studios in St. Augustine, Florida.

A special thanks also goes to the reviewers of this text: Farrell D. Doss, Radford University; Cynthia R. Gentzel, Wade College; Ellen R. Goldstein-Lynch, Fashion Institute of Technology; Dianne Hendy, Bauder College; Darlene Kness, University of Central Oklahoma; and Theresa Mastianni, Kinsborough Community College.

We would also like to acknowledge the Pearson Imaging Centers at Pearson Education for their work in scanning all of the wonderful photographs in the book.

SECTION ONE

Introduction to the Fashion Industry

CHAPTER 1

The Nature and Scope of the Fashion Industries

After reading this chapter, you should be able to:

- Discuss why industry professionals should master fashion merchandise information.
- List the fashion industry's major careers and the merchandise information required for success in each of them.
- Assess the different ways in which one might master product information.
- Have a better understanding of the language of fashion.
- Understand the fashion cycle and its effect on the life of different products.
- Discuss the fashion capitals of the world.

The glamour associated with the fashion industry makes it a career goal for many people. Millions watch fashion show extravaganzas such as the events staged on television by Victoria's Secret. Awards ceremonies such as the Oscars and Golden Globes feature celebrity presenters in fashionable ensembles. People all over the world read the multitude of fashion magazines now published in record numbers. This high visibility has attracted many individuals who want to make fashion their life's work.

Unlike many industries that are restricted to certain geographic regions, fashion is a global business. A study of the world of fashion shows that production now takes place in areas that were once considered inaccessible; designs come from arenas that include more than the typical venues of Paris, Rome, and New York City; and retailers of fashion are housed all over the world in brick-and-mortar facilities and more innovative outlets. This business provides opportunities for future practitioners no matter where they might be located or where they would eventually like to live.

This ever-growing industry is also attractive because it provides a host of different components in which many specialties are available. Textile mills create fibers and fabrics; tanneries manipulate leather into supple, attractive materials; fur processors transform pelts and hides into workable materials; lapidaries enhance stones with masterful cuts; and metal workers alloy and shape the raw materials into pliable products. Thus, the stage is set for designers to create striking designs that will motivate consumer purchasing, retailers to select those products that will capture the attention of their markets, and the editorial press to promote the designs and their creators most likely to rise above all that is being offered to the public.

While many areas of expertise are required for success in the world of fashion, product knowledge is one of the more important requisites. Savvy professionals understand the basics of design, materials used in each product classification, and manufacturing processes. Mastering this knowledge base enhances their value as professionals in the fashion industry.

THE SCOPE OF THE INDUSTRY

Fashion apparel, wearable accessories and enhancements, and home products make up a multibillion dollar industry. Although the United States is still a leading player in the fashion arena, its importance has started to decline in terms of global production and distribution. More and more American manufacturers have relocated their production facilities offshore to lower their costs and make them more competitive. With Mexican workers averaging one dollar per hour and Chinese labor costing even less, with one dollar a day as typical pay, the domestic market is in a state of manufacturing decline. However, design facilities are still plentiful in the United States as are the showrooms that sell the goods, trade shows that bring buyers together from all over the world, fashion consultants, fashion publications, and various services such as resident buying offices that provide advisory information to retailers.

Of course, **fashion retailing** is still an enormous business in America, with an ever-growing number of brick-and-mortar operations and off-site fashion ventures such as catalogs, Web sites, and home shopping channels. Traditional retailers include department stores that are either generalists or fashion specialists, chain operations, merchants with brand name recognition, discounters, off-pricers, warehouses, and small entrepreneurships such as boutiques and specialty stores. These companies, coupled with the off-site ventures that continue to increase in volume, make the United States a major fashion retail player.

Licensing agreements continue to play an important role in the fashion industry, as apparel designers sign on with shoe, jewelry, handbag, eyeglass, cosmetics and fragrance, and home furnishing manufacturers to produce lines that bear their marquee signatures. Typically, the involvement is one in which the designer "sells" his or her name to another company in exchange for a fee or commission.

It should be noted that the department store, once a leading force in fashion retailing, has lost some of its consumer appeal. While it still accounts for a great deal of fashion merchandise distribution, its overall volume has significantly diminished. Some merchants are currently trying to ignite the spark in their companies by involving themselves in different types of arrangements. Marshall Field's, for example, has entered a "partnering" program that allows for well-established shops from all over the world, such as the United Kingdom's Thomas Pink, to occupy a portion of its selling floors and hopefully attract new customers to its stores.

In general, the fashion industry is thriving all over the world, making it an excellent arena for employment.

FASHION CAREERS AND MERCHANDISE INFORMATION

Within the fashion industry is a wealth of careers that contributes to the production of raw materials, product design, and marketing. Each component of the field, and the jobs within it, requires knowledge of the merchandise with which the practitioners are involved. Familiarity with product information cuts across each of the industry's components, such as the knowledge of fibers and fabrics. Other skill sets and knowledge bases are required for certain careers, such as an understanding of design elements for designers and product developers.

Let's consider some of the merchandise information that must be mastered in major fashion industry segments.

Materials Producers

Many materials go into the manufacture of apparel, wearable accessories, fashion enhancements, and home furnishings. The most common **raw materials** are textiles, leather, fur, metals, stones, ceramics, wood, and glass.

TABLE 1.1 Selected Textiles Job Titles

Job Title	*Minimum Required Product Knowledge*
Designer	Elements of design, color theory, computer design programs, natural and man-made fiber properties, fabric uses
Colorist	Color theory, dyeing techniques
Converter	Functional and decorative finishes, dyeing techniques, printing procedures
Grapher	Techniques to transfer designer's patterns onto graphs, computer pattern programs, knitting construction
Stylist	Color trends, yarn innovation, fashion forecasting
Fabric Supervisor	Quality control, production, color, dyeing, printing processes, finishing, computer operation
Production Manager	Weaving, printing, dyeing, knitting, finishing, computer operation
Salesperson	Fiber and fabric properties, finishes, color, product uses, knitting and weaving techniques

TEXTILES

A variety of job titles comprises the textiles industry. Each has its own duties and responsibilities to perform and requires different product knowledge necessary for satisfactory performance.

Some of the jobs and the essential product information expertise required for each are presented in Table 1.1.

LEATHER

Those engaged in the production of leather are more concerned with transforming animal hides and skins into usable materials than in the actual design of the garments and accessories (Figure 1.1). The creative uses are relegated to the apparel, accessories, and furniture designers.

Table 1.2 lists the three major positions in the leather industry.

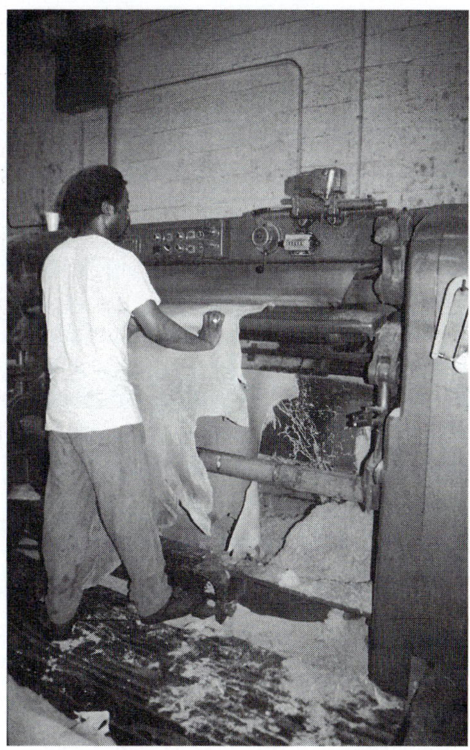

Figure 1.1 Many people are involved in transforming animal hides into usable material.
(Courtesy of Ellen Diamond.)

TABLE 1.2 Selected Positions in the Leather Industry

Job Title	*Minimum Required Product Knowledge*
Tanner	Technical education in terms of transforming raw hides and skins into usable materials, including all tanning methods
Dyer	Knowledge of dyes, dyeing procedures
Finisher	Application of functional and decorative finishes

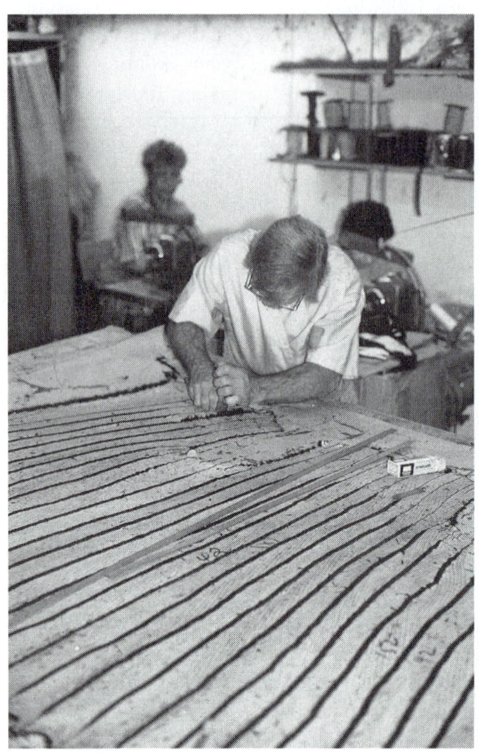

Figure 1.2 A cutter engages in "letting out" a mink pelt, a highly skilled procedure.
(Courtesy of Ellen Diamond.)

FURS

Careers in the fur industry include purchasing pelts; cutting, manipulating, and coloration (Figure 1.2); and selling the finished garments. Table 1.3 lists those jobs and their product information needs.

METALS

Many metals are used in both wearable accessories and home furnishings, from the **precious metals** such as gold to **base metals** such as chromium and iron. Those involved in the manufacture and marketing of metals and metallic merchandise require a wealth of product knowledge to successfully perform their jobs. Some of these positions and the type of knowledge needed in their performance are shown in Table 1.4.

TABLE 1.3 Selected Positions in the Fur Industry

Job Title	*Minimum Required Product Knowledge*
Purchasing Agent	Auction bidding, quality judgment in terms of fur density, color uniformity, and skin matching
Colorist	Dyeing and bleaching agents, techniques
Cutter	Letting out, skin on skin joining
Sales Associate	Construction, coloring techniques, quality, benefits

TABLE 1.4 Selected Positions in the Metals Industry

Jobs	*Minimum Required Product Knowledge*
Purchaser	Market price structure, metal characteristics
Processor	Annealing, rolling, forging, welding, casting, engraving, etching
Enhancer	Florentining, antiquing, embossing
Plater	Precious and base metal characteristics, bonding techniques
Sales Associate	Metal characteristics, qualities, performance

TABLE 1.5 Positions Involved in the Production or Distribution of Precious and Semiprecious Stones

Jobs	*Minimum Required Product Knowledge*
Raw Materials Purchasing Agent	Evaluation of precious and semiprecious stones in terms of quality
Cutter	Various cutting techniques, faceting
Stone Setter	Placement of stones in finished settings
Sales Associate	Quality, stone characteristics
Appraiser	Quality, stone characteristics, "loupe" use, gemological rating systems

STONES

A wealth of stones, natural and man-made, is used in jewelry and as enhancements in apparel products. Each type of stone has specific properties that make it important. Those who are involved in either their production or distribution must have specific knowledge so that they can most satisfactorily perform their job responsibilities (Table 1.5).

CERAMICS

The different types of ceramic products available today have increased tremendously. They include fine art and utilitarian pieces such as dinnerware. The people in the ceramics trade are either in the creative aspect of the business or are involved in selling (Table 1.6).

WOOD

One of the most widely used materials in home furnishings is wood. It is used extensively for flooring, walls, serving pieces, and home accessories. Many different types of wood are used both functionally and decoratively, making these materials essential for those in the field to have a complete understanding of the characteristics of various woods. Table 1.7 describes some of those positions.

GLASS

Used both as functional and decorative products in home furnishings and jewelry, glass has become a popular product for consumer use. Its uses include drinking vessels, dinnerware,

TABLE 1.6 Selected Positions in the Ceramics Industry

Jobs	*Minimum Required Product Knowledge*
Designer-Artist	Elements of design, methods of production such as throwing, use of wheel, color
Colorist	Knowledge of color harmonies, color wheel
Buyer	Assessment of raw materials

TABLE 1.7 Selected Positions in the Wood Industry

Jobs	*Minimum Required Product Knowledge*
Designer	Principles and elements of design
Finisher	Finishing applications such as dye classifications, dye applications, sanding
Carpenter	Use of tools, installations (such as for floors and walls), wood characteristics
Purchasing Agent	Wood characteristics, global markets

TABLE 1.8 Selected Positions in the Glass Industry

Jobs	*Minimum Required Product Knowledge*
Designer	Understanding of design principles and elements
Colorist	Knowledge of color harmonies
Chemist	Knowledge of chemical properties
Purchasing Agent	Ability to distinguish among the different glass properties
Sales Associate	Properties of glass types

tabletops, mirrors, and fashion jewelry. The price points range from modest to expensive, depending on the quality and styling. Table 1.8 lists fashion-related jobs in the glass industry.

Manufacturers

From apparel and accessories to home furnishings, the manufacturing industry offers numerous careers related to fashion. Critical functions involve design, production, merchandising, and distribution. Included are positions as designers, pattern makers, product managers, merchandisers, stylists, production managers, sample makers, purchasing agents, quality controllers, customer servicers, and sales associates.

DESIGNER

Large companies employ a creative team that is directed by a head designer and might include a variety of assistants with varying responsibilities. In these large fashion operations, the head designer generally establishes the collection's direction and directs assistants to develop individual styles for his or her consideration. The head designer has the final say about which styles will make it into the **collection** and which will be discarded. Of course, many head designers create some of the silhouettes themselves. The manner in which the designer operates depends on his or her overall duties, such as fabric design and selection and trimmings selection (Figure 1.3). In smaller companies, the design task is generally the responsibility of one individual who wears many hats.

Whether one is the head of the design team, an assistant, or a one-person "department" who has complete responsibility for design, today's creators must be technically trained. Where yesteryear required only the ability to drape and draw, those involved in design must be adept at the various **computer-aided design (CAD) programs** used in the development of a style.

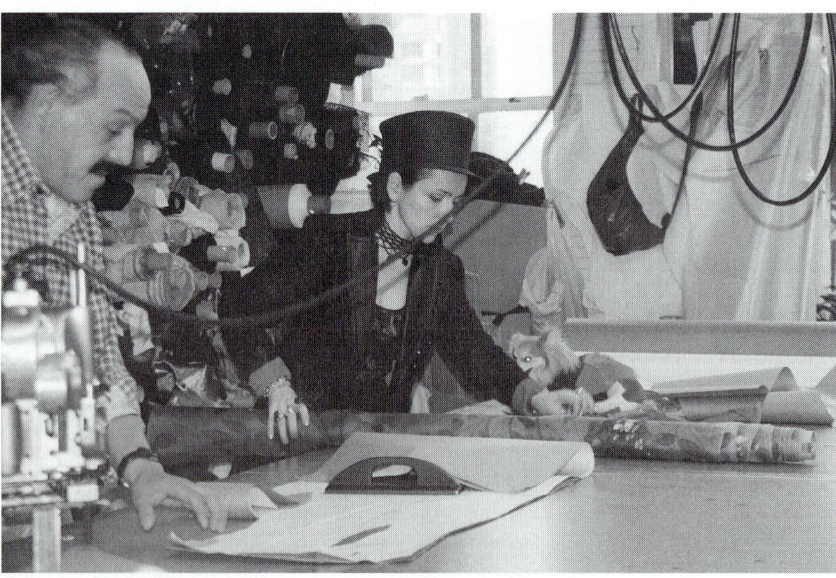

Figure 1.3 A fashion designer and cutter select the fabric best suited for a design. *(Courtesy of Ellen Diamond.)*

Of course, a complete knowledge of design theory, pattern making, and sewing must be mastered in addition to sketching, draping, and rendering. Schools across the country, such as Pratt Institute, Parsons, FIDM, and FIT, offer complete programs in which this preparation takes place.

In addition to their technical competency, professional designers must possess significant artistic ability, which is at the core of every design. They must be able to translate into salable styles their inspirations from any number of sources, such as travel to foreign countries, a new movie, a famous period in art, a previous decade in which fashion reigned, popular ethnic cultures, or a theatrical production. The comprehension of color and how to use it to enhance design are also musts for success in the field.

Although creative abilities are of paramount importance, the able designer must also have a sense of the target market so that the designs will serve specific needs. The ability to produce exciting products with viable sales potential is imperative to the success of any company.

Look at any fashion print advertisement or special events and you can see immediately the importance of the designer to the company. Many designer names and company names are one and the same. That name must capture the consumer's attention. A great many, such as Donna Karan, Ralph Lauren, Calvin Klein, and Tommy Hilfiger, are principals of their companies and have significant influence over many of those organizations' operations.

The designer—be it the head or an assistant—provides the lifeblood to the company through his or her ability to create appealing products.

PATTERN MAKER

The unsung hero of the back room is the pattern maker. He or she must transform the original designs into patterns that will be used in the production of the merchandise. A complete knowledge of sewing, production techniques, efficient fabric use, and grading is necessary to perform this job. Today's pattern maker must be proficient with the technology used in this industry. Knowledge of the various CAD systems is a must to be prepared for the challenges of this career. Although pattern making is a vital part of the production process, most entrants in the fashion field are generally focused on design, merchandising, and sales as their career choices. There always seems to be a shortage of these technically trained people who command significantly high salaries.

PRODUCT MANAGER

Working closely with the design team, the product manager's role is a coupling of creativity and merchandising skills. The specific tasks performed include handling purchase orders for materials and trim, costing each style, planning for the necessary yardage for each apparel product, determining the number of individual items needed to be sold before a style goes into production (known in the trade as a **cutting ticket**), scheduling distribution, and assisting with presentations to major retail accounts.

Those best suited for such positions should possess experience in merchandising, operations, sales, and retailing, as well as the ability to communicate verbally and in writing. Formal education in marketing, manufacturing, or merchandising is generally required of those seeking careers as product managers.

MERCHANDISER

For the designer's creations to become salable items, there must be a sense of which market the line will serve; how many different styles will comprise the collection; which types of fabrics will best enhance the projected styles in terms of fiber, construction, and cost; which mills will best provide these materials; and how much the final product will cost.

In some small companies, especially those that specialize in adaptations or **knock-offs** of popular styles, the merchandiser also takes on the task of designer. He or she must, in addition to performing all of the typical merchandising tasks, scan the market for higher-priced items that can be translated into styles that would have a life at his or her company (Figure 1.4). Often, the merchandiser selects such components as silhouettes, sleeves, and necklines from various apparel styles and reassembles them into new models.

Merchandisers for the major companies command high salaries, with those who perform as product developers being paid even more.

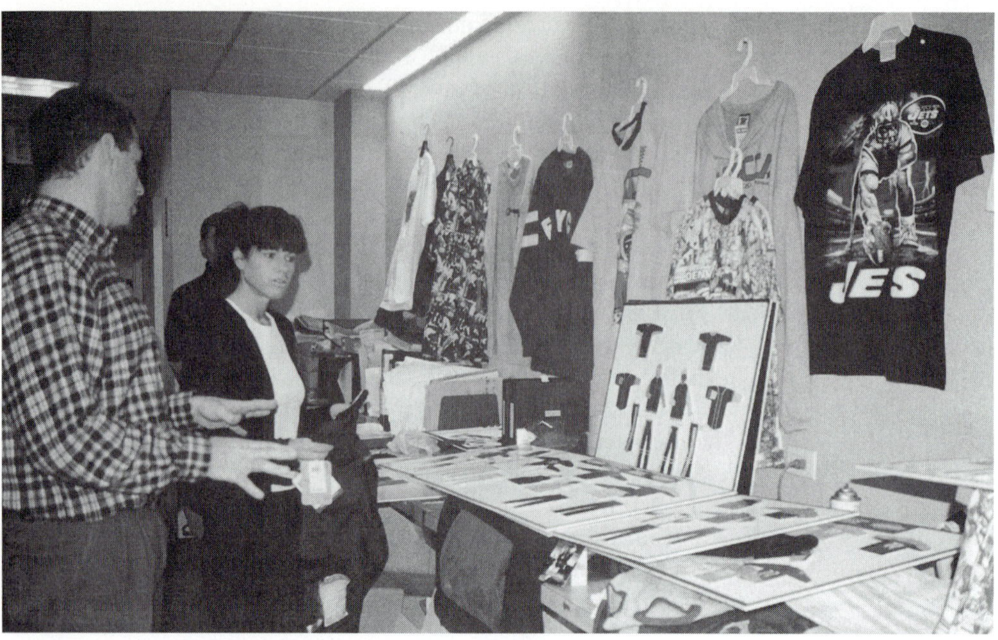

Figure 1.4 Merchandisers select styles that will become part of the line.
(Courtesy of Ellen Diamond.)

STYLIST

Some companies use stylists exclusively instead of designers for the creation of their fashion product lines. Where designers have the technical and artistic ability to create original models, the stylist is an individual with good taste who can recognize the various components that make up a good style, line, or collection.

By visiting textile mills, trimmings companies, fashion forecasters, market consultants, and retailers, the stylist can determine the pulse of the market for the next season and assemble lines that will satisfy the customer's needs and preferences (Figure 1.5).

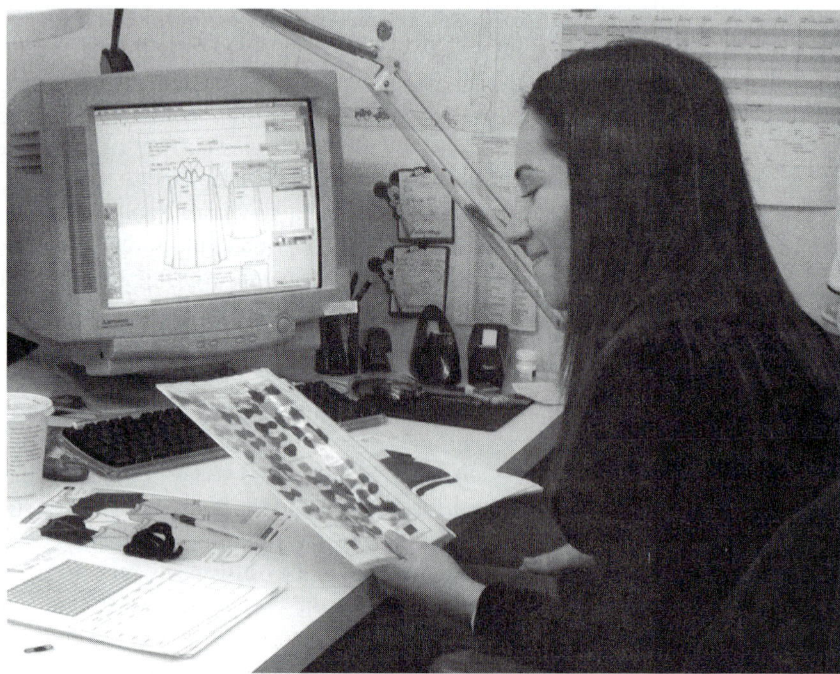

Figure 1.5 A stylist examines colored yarns for use in individual designs.
(Courtesy of Ellen Diamond.)

The job is research oriented and often takes individuals anywhere around the globe where fashion is at its forefront. Places such as Hong Kong, Paris, Milan, and London are typical stops where the stylist may research elements that will be needed for his or her company's line. Oftentimes, mere observation of people on the street offers ideas to the stylist.

In companies that employ designers, a stylist might work as a design assistant, providing the information gathered from researching the market.

PRODUCTION MANAGER

To make certain the manufacturing process is carried out efficiently and on schedule, such areas as actual production, delivery of materials and trimmings, and quality control must be addressed. In short, a skilled production manager must be in charge.

The manufacturing process may be vertically integrated—that is, all of the operations are performed in house by the company or employ outside companies, known as *contractors*, for some of the operations. In this case, the production manager must coordinate the efforts of his or her own factory with the outside agency. To further complicate matters, the vast majority of fashion manufacturers are using off-shore plants to perform some of the manufacturing processes, requiring the production manager to make numerous trips to these off-shore venues.

The individual concerned with production management must have a full understanding of the technology involved in fabric cutting and assembling, the workings of the equipment used in the procedures, CAD systems, the abilities of the people in the plants, the complexity of the different materials used, and anything else that might impede or improve production. Although the designer's styles or models might be considered the backbone of the company, poor-quality production can seriously affect the company's profitability. Production managers are therefore among the highest-paid performers in the fashion industry.

SAMPLE MAKER

After the original design has been hand-rendered, created with the use of a CAD system, or draped on a mannequin, a number of samples must be completed. One might be used for pattern making and others for production purposes and used in the company's showrooms where the lines are offered to the buyers. Specialists in this field must be capable of hand and machine sewing and be competent in the translation of the designer's work into models.

PURCHASING AGENT

The materials used in the production of apparel, wearable accessories, and home furnishings include textiles, leather, furs, metals, stones, plastics, Lucite, vinyls, glass, wood, ceramics, and a variety of trimmings and findings (functional trims such as zippers). In small companies, a jack-of-all-trades performs the purchasing duties, whereas in the larger companies, the chores may be split among a few people. Whatever the situation, those responsible for buying the material must have knowledge of the various materials' resources, the products and their characteristics, and their role in the designer's creations.

Purchasing agents are also concerned with production schedules, price points, and any role that the materials will play in the development of the line. To satisfactorily plan the purchases, these agents must be proficient in mathematics so that yardage can be assessed and sufficiently competent to negotiate the terms and write the orders.

QUALITY CONTROLLER

With the enormous amount of competition in the apparel, accessories, and home furnishings market, each company must be concerned with quality. Such attention will bring greater profits to the company and encourage repeat business from the retailers season after season.

The individual responsible for keeping quality at a level prescribed by management must be aware of production at every point and be able to catch manufacturing errors. Whether it is ill-matching buttons, zippers that have been improperly sewn, or stripes that do not properly align, any error, no matter how slight, must be corrected. The quality controller must be meticulously responsible and capable of recognizing potential problems during production. This position requires continuous presence on the job, regularly examining the products for flaws. When little attention is paid to quality control, merchandise returns and cancellations are possible, reducing the company's ability to make a profit.

CUSTOMER SERVICER

More and more fashion manufacturers are making certain that customer satisfaction is guaranteed. Customer servicers interface with retailers in person and via phone hotlines and Web sites through which customers may air their complaints or merely obtain information about product care. By providing this service, these employees make repeat business more likely.

People in customer service must be both knowledgeable about the company's lines and willing to help correct any problems associated with purchases. They might be dealing with an irate customer whose swimsuit ran during use in a pool or whose garment shrunk after laundering or a retail buyer complaining about shoddy construction. Whatever the situation or origin of the complaint, it is the responsibility of those in customer service to be cordial and to help make any necessary adjustments.

Those best suited for this career must have excellent communications skills, a pleasant attitude, and the ability to solve problems.

SALESPERSON

It is the seller, more than most others in the industry, whose competency determines whether or not the company's products will reach the retailer. Sales people who work for apparel, wearable accessories, and home furnishings manufacturers are among the highest paid in the industry. With monetary rewards based on commission, straight salary, or a combination of both, they are capable of substantial incomes.

Selling for the manufacturer involves two different groups of purchasers: those who work as retail buyers and those who represent resident buying offices and often act as agents for the retailer. Whether it is the small fashion operation, major department store, chain organization, or resident buying office, the job calls for the same involvement.

The professional seller must be able to generate business for the company by establishing positive rapport with the customer (Figure 1.6). Once a trust has been

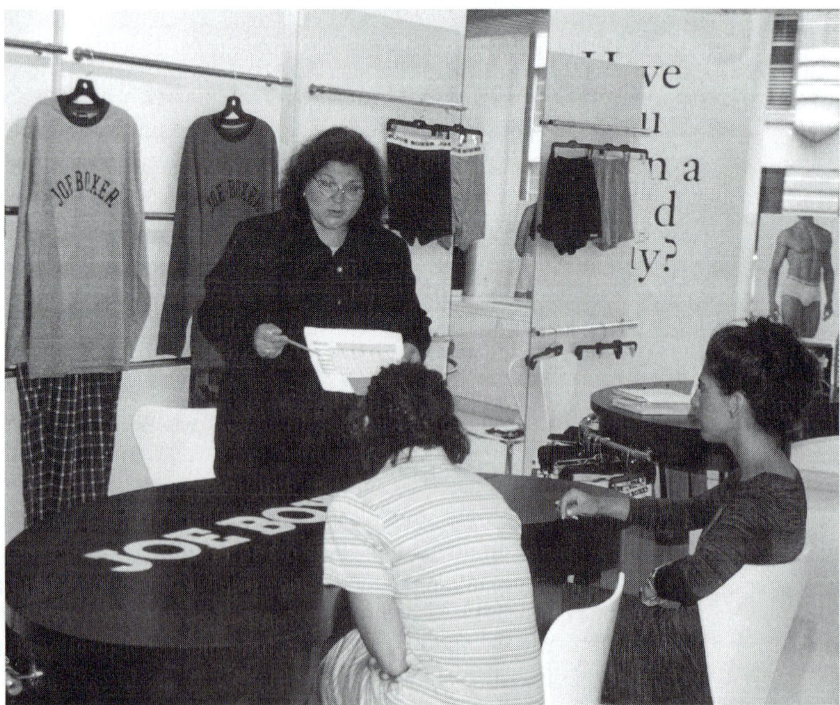

Figure 1.6 The professional seller is the lifeblood of the manufacturer.
(Courtesy of Ellen Diamond.)

TABLE 1.9 Selected Fashion Manufacturing Positions

Jobs	*Minimum Required Product Knowledge*
Designer	CAD programs, drawing, draping, color harmony, design principles and elements, textiles
Pattern Maker	CAD programs, sewing, construction techniques, fitting, textiles
Product Manager	Merchandising, distribution techniques, quality, sales, communication
Merchandiser	Mathematics, textiles, trimmings, silhouettes, design principles, color
Stylist	Textiles, design principles, research fundamentals, drawing, CAD programs
Production Manager	Textiles, trimmings, manufacturing techniques, production programs, quality features, design
Sample Maker	Sewing, textiles, construction techniques, draping, CAD
Purchasing Agent	Textiles and other materials, trimmings, merchandising, mathematics, negotiating
Quality Controller	Product construction, textiles and other materials, fit, color, design elements
Customer Servicer	Product expertise, sales, construction techniques
Salesperson	Fundamentals of selling, textiles and other materials, design elements and principles, trimmings and findings

established and the recommended items of the past season sold, the seller's job is simplified and repeat business is easier to maintain. Those who sell fashion and have established a regular clientele often find that customers follow them even if they move on to new companies.

The seller must have good verbal skills and be able to take the customer through the various stages of the sales presentation. Helping the buyer with merchandising plans, promotional endeavors, and visual presentations are just some of the other duties salespeople perform. Of course, understanding the product, including everything from production to design, is extremely helpful in making a sale.

Manufacturers also provide a host of other fashion careers as fit models, who are at the designer's service to make certain that the original sample is appropriately crafted; cutters; sewers; finishers; inventory expeditors; those responsible distributing the finished goods; and order processors.

Table 1.9 summarizes selected positions available at the manufacturer and the minimum amount of product knowledge needed for each.

Retailers

Through a vast network of on-site and off-site operations, those who wish to serve the ultimate consumer's needs with apparel, wearable accessories, and home furnishings may establish careers in management, merchandising, promotion, and store operations. With employment opportunities all over the world, participants need only to find the geographic location in which they would like to live and begin to practice what they have learned about the field.

Retailing, more than any other industry component, offers formal training for those interested in pursuing management-level careers. Through executive development programs or executive training, qualified individuals, primarily college graduates, set out on a path that will eventually lead to the specific career for which they are best suited. The goal might be that of buying fashion apparel or accessories, working as a fashion director, or managing a unit of a chain organization. Most companies that offer such programs combine classroom instruction with on-the-job training. In this way, theoretical practices can be learned and applied to both on-site and off-site situations.

Those who prove themselves with their initial retailing assignments generally find that upward mobility is easy to achieve. Assistant buyers become buyers, and department managers usually are offered the reins as group or store managers. Although initial salaries are sometimes considered low in comparison with other industries, those who reach the higher levels of employment easily catch up in compensation. A good liring, coupled with the excitement generated by the ever-changing fashion business, makes retailing a great place to use one's abilities.

MERCHANDISE MANAGERS

Those who make the ultimate decisions concerning buying and merchandising practices in the retail environment are the merchandisers. They are among the highest-paid individuals in retailing. Most organizations use a plan that involves both a general and several divisional merchandise managers.

The *general merchandise manager* (GMM) is the company's ultimate decision maker in terms of product mix, acquisition, and fashion direction. He or she sets goals and determines merchandise budgets, price points, and the merchandising policy. Since there is only one GMM, this is the plum merchandising position. Formal education and a wealth of experience in the merchandising realm are the basic requirements for the position.

The *divisional merchandise manager* (DMM) is subordinate to the GMM. Most fashion retail operations, other than small businesses such as boutiques, employ several DMMs. Each is charged with the responsibility of managing one specific fashion classification such as menswear, accessories, and home furnishings. They work closely with the general merchandise manager to determine the budgets for their respective classifications and fashion direction for the company. Each DMM supervises a number of buyers, providing guidance and expertise to each for merchandise acquisition and the general fashion direction of their departments. They also regularly interface with other upper-level managers such as those in advertising and promotion, to make certain that their divisions are adequately represented.

BUYERS

Two levels of buyers are typical in retailing operations. The one with major responsibility is simply known as the *buyer*. His or her subordinate is the assistant buyer. Each has specific duties and responsibilities to perform, with the buyer's determined by the DMM and the assistant's by the buyer.

The *buyer* is responsible for the acquisition of merchandise that will be offered for sale to the customer (Figure 1.7). Decisions in terms of domestic and offshore resourcing, merchandise selection, merchandise placement on the selling floors, pricing, and markdowns are just some of his or her responsibilities. With the enormous movement to offshore product purchasing, the buyer's job requires a great deal of travel to markets around the world. Because of the need to travel, less time is spent in the company's headquarters, leaving a

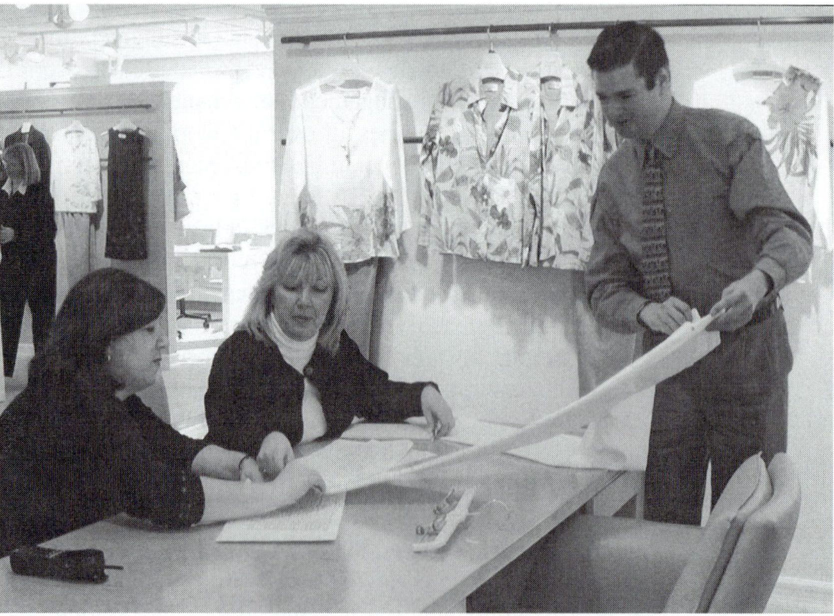

Figure 1.7 Buyers view collections and select the products most suited for their clientele. *(Courtesy of Ellen Diamond.)*

great deal of the buyer's once-required participation to others, such as assistant buyers and department managers. To carry out the requirements of the position, the buyer must be computer literate, have a good knowledge of mathematics, and be able to communicate verbally, in traditional writing, and in the proper use of e-mails.

The *assistant buyer* is generally chosen from those who have completed their stints in an executive training program. Typically, he or she is there to help the buyer with selecting resources, prescreening collections, following up on orders, interfacing with managers in other company divisions, determining customer's wants and needs, and working on the selling floor during peak sales periods. Those who have successfully completed their tenures as assistant buyers, typically in four years, are often promoted to the rank of buyer.

MANAGERS

Depending on the size of the company, management positions may be limited to one for a boutique or other small operation to significant numbers as in department stores. Those in the fashion segment of retailing may serve as a department manager, group manager, or store manager.

Department managers, in the case of major brick-and-mortar stores, serve specific areas of the store such as menswear, shoes, and accessories. They are middle managers, carrying out the policies and procedures established by the company's executive team. Working within specific guidelines, they may hire sales associates, prepare work schedules, handle customer complaints, act as liaison with the buyer to relay customer requests, physically arrange merchandise displays, and sell on the floor.

These individuals generally come from the ranks of executive training programs or are promoted from the selling floor.

In large retail brick-and-mortar operations, *group managers* are in charge of a number of individual department managers. They are responsible for making certain that the individual managers carry out their duties; they plan staff needs, screen and hire department managers, and make recommendations, where appropriate, to each manager.

Becoming *store manager* is the goal most lower-level managers hope to achieve. Although the appointment to this level is difficult in department stores since the number of branches are relatively few, it is more easily reachable in the chain store organization with dozens, even hundreds of units. The Gap, for example, operates 3,000 stores across the country, the potential for increasing store management positions.

FASHION DIRECTOR

Primarily serving in an advisory capacity, the fashion director provides fashion information to the retail operation's buyers and merchandisers before they make their purchases. Not only do they supply the individual buyers with specific fashion product information for their individual departments, fashion directors provide an overview of the market so that each buyer's purchases will coordinate and blend with those of the other buyers in the company. For example, if the fashion director alerts the dress buyer that red will be the season's "hot color," the shoe buyer can order the same color shoes, enabling consumers to satisfy both needs. Without such forecasting assistance, each purchaser would act independently, resulting in the lack of unifying elements in the company's merchandise mix.

Aside from the advisory function, most fashion directors assist the retailer's product developers who create private label goods of the market's design trends, which might inspire them in their merchandise development. Other duties include producing and directing fashion shows, interfacing with the visual merchandising department to suggest displays that might enhance certain merchandise, traveling to the mills to learn about fabric trends, visiting fashion forecasters, and keeping top management informed of potential changes in the industry's direction for apparel, wearable accessories, and home furnishings.

The job provides the individual with a role for developing the retailer's fashion image and offers monetary rewards and exciting environments in which to work.

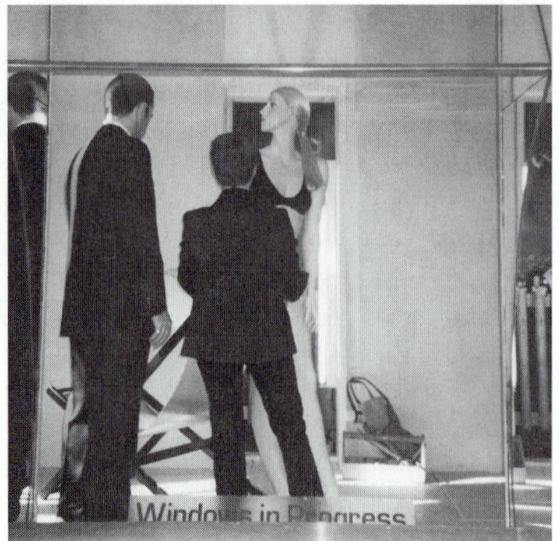

Figure 1.8 Visual merchandisers discuss the installation of a window display.
(Courtesy of Ellen Diamond.)

VISUAL MERCHANDISER

Those whose responsibility centers on the presentation of the merchandise on the selling floors and in window displays are collectively known as *visual merchandisers*. The level of visual involvement depends on the store's location, size, and design; the manner in which business is conducted; and the dollar investment management is wiling to make.

Typically, department stores provide the vast majority of careers in visual merchandising. With a traditional dedication to featuring interesting, eye-appealing displays, this retail segment spends more in this area than any other type of retailer. The "majors" such as Lord & Taylor, Macy's, Bloomingdale's, and Marshall Field's have large visual merchandising staffs. Individuals in these companies perform such duties as background design construction, sign making, and trimming.

At the head of the visual team is a director or, to indicate the importance of the position to the company, a vice president who manages a team that includes prop and theme designers, lighting experts, installers, sign makers, and carpenters.

Many department store branches use a small nucleus of visual merchandisers who work at the retailer's headquarters and develop displays and other visual concepts used in the various units (Figure 1.8). Some companies employ teams of trimmers who rotate through the stores and install displays. Small retailers often use independent freelancers who work either on contract or individual installation, providing everything from the background materials to the actual trim.

Whatever the level of visual merchandising, this area demands artistic training and excellence. Although the beginning salaries are generally low at the entry-level positions, those who achieve the higher levels of employment are handsomely rewarded.

SPECIAL EVENTS DIRECTOR

The major department stores regularly feature special events that focus on designers, collections from foreign countries, fashion shows, and other programs that emphasize their position as fashion leaders and innovators. Personal appearances by such luminaries as Ralph Lauren and Donna Karan are commonplace.

The special events director develops these concepts and brings them to fruition. Those with special creative talents are best suited for the job. With the same merchandise and services found in many of today's department store environments, the special events director must design programs that will distinguish the company from the competition.

To carry out these events successfully, the director must be able to coordinate long-range planning and effectively communicate with the outside sources necessary for such endeavors.

PUBLIC RELATIONS DIRECTOR

For any retailer to be successful, as many customers as possible must be attracted to the company. One of the ways in which this is accomplished is through the use of positive public relations. By informing the public of programs and events that might motivate them to visit a store, order from a catalog, or shop online, the retailer can expect sales to rise.

It is one thing for a company to offer a special event and quite another to sufficiently capture customers' attention to make them participate. The public relations director interacts with the media in hope that they will provide coverage in their newspapers or news broadcasts of the company and its merchandise. When a new fragrance is being promoted, for example, and a celebrity makes a personal appearance in the store to promote it, the company benefits from the event if it is featured in local television spots on local television. In this way, the retailer's name is mentioned along with the personality appearance, often stimulating the consumer to attend. When Tommy Hilfiger made the rounds and appeared in Jacksonville's Belk stores to promote his new fragrance, the crowds came in record numbers.

The public relations director must have excellent communication skills. He or she is required to regularly write concise press releases that are earmarked for the media's attention and eventual placement in print or on the air. If those releases are well written, the media is more likely to use them than make major changes.

ADVERTISING MANAGER

One look at any newspaper immediately reveals the significant role advertising plays to bring shoppers to the store and off-site outlets. With the enormity of the advertising expenditure and the highly competitive nature of the retail environment, it is necessary to develop a program that will uniquely present each company to the public.

With creative expertise, advertising directors can provide a particular look or image to their programs. By developing a certain character in their ads through such devises as stylized fashion figures, retailers allow customers to quickly differentiate their advertising from others.

Those interested in such careers should have formal education in advertising and be capable of writing copy, preparing artwork, and creating layouts. Those who work for fashion-oriented retailers would also benefit from taking courses on the different products and materials used in fashion merchandise production.

Table 1.10 represents many of the retail positions and the minimum amount of product knowledge necessary for success in these positions.

Market Consultants

In the fashion industry, the chance for success for manufacturers, designers, materials producers, and retailers is generally enhanced when outside organizations are used to provide information that will help with merchandise planning. Several types of companies provide the information and skills for fashion operations to be successful. They are resident buying offices, fashion forecasters, and reporting services.

TABLE 1.10 Selected Retail Positions

Jobs	*Minimum Required Product Knowledge*
Merchandise Manager	Fashion terminology, styles, colors, construction techniques, textiles and other materials
Buyer	Silhouettes, patterns, fabrications, construction, color harmonies
Manager	Fashion silhouettes, textiles and other materials, construction, color arrangements
Fashion Director	Styles, silhouettes, color, fabrics, patterns, construction techniques, quality differences
Visual Merchandiser	Textiles, color, silhouettes
Special Events Director	Styles, textiles and other materials, color harmonies
Public Relations Director	Trends, silhouettes, fashion terminology, color theories
Advertising Manager	Silhouettes, styles, fashion terminology, color, fabrics

RESIDENT BUYING OFFICES

These teams of market consultants serve manufacturers, designers, and retailers by providing a range of different services. Manufacturers and designers need a venue where their collections can be featured and shown to retailers. Retailers need a place where a multitude of lines may be seen for purchase consideration.

Within the resident buying office, numerous positions make up their rosters. Of primary importance are the buyers and assistant buyers who scour the market for new collections, preview the next season's offerings, assess fashion trends, and make general plans for their recommendations to retail operation buyers and merchandisers.

To be prepared to properly execute their duties and responsibilities, the resident buying office buyers must be fully versed in the terminology of the trade and have the ability to make fashion-purchasing decision that best serve the needs of their clients. Through the successful completion of a college degree, preferably one that concentrates on business and more specifically fashion merchandising, these buyers and their assistants are best prepared to handle the challenges of their demanding work.

FASHION FORECASTERS

In the ever-changing field of fashion where style acceptance comes and goes rapidly, retailers, manufacturers, and designers generally try to investigate fashion products and their potential popularity. The forecaster helps those responsible for making fashion decisions by researching market trends through visits to materials producers and design capitals all over the world.

The primary function of those who work as forecasters is to provide such information as color trends, fabric uses, silhouette preferences, and price points as early as one year before the information is needed to make manufacturing and purchasing decisions.

An understanding of the fashion industry, the ability to assess trends and perform other research, a knowledge of textiles and other materials, and the skills necessary to communicate this information to clients are required for those wishing to enter the field.

REPORTING SERVICES

Some companies specialize in providing information on the status of the fashion market through written visual reporting. Unlike the resident buying office that is directly involved in purchasing, the reporting services are solely in business to provide information to retailers that includes citing best sellers and potentially hot items for their consideration.

MASTERING PRODUCT INFORMATION

To play a significant role in the world of fashion in any of the aforementioned industry segments and to move to the highest levels of employment, a complete understanding of the merchandise offered for sales is essential. The designer who creates the collections needs to know the details of the fabrics he or she is considering. The manufacturer who translates the designs into usable products must be aware of any pitfalls that might hamper production. The salesperson must be able to highlight the items' salient features while attempting to close the sale. The retail buyer must be able to assess the marketplace and bring the right merchandise mix to his or her company. For everyone involved in creating and distributing fashion merchandise, the more product savvy he or she is, the better customer relations and sales will be.

The key to acquiring the appropriate product information and sufficiently mastering it is to find the right learning vehicle. Merchandise information can be acquired in many ways. Some of the resources that enable individuals to fortify themselves with fashion-oriented product knowledge are discussed in the following sections.

Formal Courses

Many colleges and universities offer courses that deal specifically with product information. These include a wealth of textile offerings that feature basic and advanced applications. Fiber analysis, construction techniques, and methods of dyeing, printing, and finishing are covered. Fashion apparel courses on women's, men's, and children's wear focus on manufacturing procedures, computerized design, fabrication selection, and construction. For those interested in learning about wearable accessories such as shoes, jewelry, handbags, scarves, belts, and other small items, courses in fashion accessories are provided. With growing sales in fashion for the home, a wealth of interior design and home furnishings courses feature information on furniture, housewares, flooring, and other accessories.

These learning offerings are available as either courses in regular degree programs or in continuing education offerings. Some educational institutions, in addition to their on-campus offerings, are presenting courses online for those unable to fit conventional courses into their schedules.

Videos and DVDs

More and more ancillary materials are being produced that focus on the various product classifications. In particular, many videos and DVDs focus on the nature of each merchandise classification and on the manufacturing processes and their characteristics. They are used in classroom instruction in colleges and universities around the globe and by many fashion manufacturers and retailers to help their staffs learn the fine points of each product.

Company Literature

Many components of the fashion industry prepare literature that deals specifically with merchandise information. The major fiber producers such as Dupont, for example, prepare a host of different publications that offer the most detailed information regarding the manufacture, uses, and care of their fibers. Apparel and accessories manufacturers also publish and disseminate information on their offerings to the retail community to familiarize their buyers, merchandisers, managers, and sales associates on the points that will help them successfully market products to consumers. These pamphlets, brochures, and other materials run the gamut from one-time offerings to regular publications produced as often as once a month.

Textbooks

Some textbooks, such as this one, cover the entire fashion industry, while others focus on just one segment, such as textiles. They offer a wealth of information to help students master the various products. Textbooks often begin with the history of fashion and conclude with today's offerings.

Online Sources

The Internet continues to be a resource for a wide range of merchandise information to professionals and consumers alike. Web sites on textiles, for example, feature everything from the latest fiber innovations to the basics of fiber and fabric offerings. You may begin at a specific Web site or conduct a general inquiry on a search engine by entering a keyword, such as *leather*, to locate a host of different Web sites that should provide a great deal of product information on the subject. The amount of information provided via the Internet continues to grow. The Internet as a fashion merchandise resource tool is excellent to keep abreast of the latest innovations in the field.

PRODUCT INFORMATION ESSENTIALS

Using one or more of the aforementioned methods for mastering product information is imperative in understanding and assessing fashion's different components. The better the understanding of fashion and its different product classifications, the more likely one will succeed in the field.

Throughout this text, pertinent information is presented regarding each of the categories, with a wealth of definitions and concept explorations. For example, Chapter 2 focuses on fiber classifications, manufacturing processes, uses, and characteristics. Other chapters present detailed information on different apparel groupings to enable those in the fashion industry with a keen knowledge of how each may be characterized. In the home furnishings sections, each product class is carefully addressed so those who must make professional decisions regarding their manufacture, purchase, and sale will be better prepared for those aspects of the job.

THE LANGUAGE OF THE FASHION INDUSTRY

In addition to mastering the specifics of fashion-oriented merchandise information, an understanding of the industry is essential to achieve success.

Like many industries, the fashion arena has a language all its own. Let's consider a few common terms.

Style. The characteristics that distinguish one apparel, accessories, or home furnishings design from another. Styles do not change, although their acceptance by consumers may vary widely. For example, bell-bottoms is a style featuring pant legs that flair at the bottom. The style does not change, but its popularity does.

Fashion. The style that is popular or prevails at the time. Miniskirts and platform shoes are both styles that may be in fashion, depending on their current acceptance by consumers.

Silhouette. The shape or outline of a design. There are basically three silhouettes in fashion apparel: (1) tubular, or falling in a straight line, (2) the bustle that features interest in the back of the garment, and (3) the bouffant that characteristically flares out in fullness.

Fad. A fashion that is short-lived. When a style gains quick acceptance from the public but disappears almost as quickly, it is a fad.

Classic. A style that is a basic, integral part of a wardrobe. A strand of pearls, blazer jacket, and pair of loafers are considered to be classics.

Couturier(e). A French term used to describe the most original fashion designers.

Haute couture. The fashion houses of Paris that belong to the Chambre Syndicale de la Couture Parisienne.

Prêt-a-porter. A French term used to describe ready-to-wear.

Knock-off. A copy of a higher-priced design.

Custom made. Merchandise that is specifically tailored to fit a customer's measurements or requirements.

Resource. A term used by the retailer to describe the manufacturers or wholesalers from whom they purchase.

Fashion cycle. The stages through which fashions pass, from introduction to decline.

Trend. The direction in which fashion is moving.

Hot item. A best-selling item that is reordered again and again.

Price point. A specific price at which a line is offered for sale.

Off-price. A price that is lower than the original wholesale price.

Offshore production. When a manufacturer creates a line in one country and has it produced in another.

THE FASHION CYCLE

When a particular style embraced by the consumer is worn for at least one season, it is called a *fashion*. When the period of acceptance is extremely brief, it is called a *fad*. There is no specific period of time necessary to be called one or the other. Styles pass through four different phases from their inception to demise, better known as the *fashion cycle*.

The cycle (Figure 1.9) begins with the introduction stage, moves into a growth period, proceeds to a maturity stage, and falls from favor in a period of decline.

Introduction Stage

Generally, when a style is introduced into the marketplace, it is at the highest price points. It might be a new silhouette featured in a couturier's collection or one that is part of a distinctive manufacturer's line. At this point, there is no way of knowing if the style will be popular with retail buyers and the consumer public. Thus, the introduction stage is costly to the producer who has spent considerable money on fabrics, trim, and creation of the items. This being the case, the newest styles are usually expensive to purchase. If the garments, accessories, or home furnishings are successful sellers, the knock-offs are readied for distribution at lower price points.

Growth Stage

If the style is generally accepted, a variety of adaptations at many different prices are in the marketplace. The original design generally has significant success, but so do the copies marketed at a fraction of the price. When Tod shoes first introduced its signature design that bore the identifiable little leather accents at the back of the shoe, the original sold, and still does, for around $400. The copies, on the other hand, sold for a fraction of the price at $100 or less.

Maturity Stage

At this point, the style achieves its greatest sales volume. The time of maturity might be one season, or many. Although the industry tries to motivate the consumer to buy at least one item in the style, the purchase of many gives the style a longer life. In the case of designer jeans in the early 1970s, consumers were so taken with the fashion that wardrobes all over the

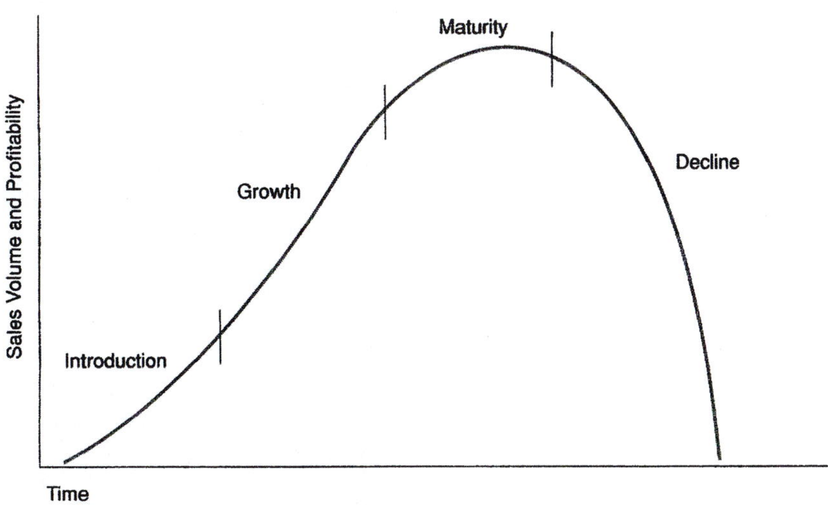

The stages of the fashion cycle.

Figure 1.9 The fashion cycle encompasses four stages.

country featured numerous pairs. The difficulty with this period in the fashion cycle for manufacturers and retailers is their ability to determine when popularity will decrease. All too often, the decline comes quickly, leaving the industry with merchandise that the public no longer considers fashionable.

Decline Stage

At the point when it appears the style is losing popularity, the original designer or manufacturer has abandoned the item, readying something new for the marketplace. During this period, left-over pieces are drastically reduced to prices that will sell quickly. It is urgent to rid the inventory of such items before they are no longer desired at any price.

Many manufacturers have opened their own stores in outlet centers from coast to coast so that they may dispose of the merchandise heading for decline. Others use off-price merchants or closeout Web sites that buy at prices that are far below the original wholesale, for disposal.

GLOBAL FASHION CAPITALS

Although it was once an industry concentrated in just a few domestic and foreign markets, today's fashion arena is globally based. While New York City still reigns as America's fashion capital, and Paris, Milan, and London are still foreign arenas for innovative style, the depth and breadth of the fashion industry spreads into other regions across the globe.

Domestically, in addition to New York City, regional fashion markets are dominant forces in Los Angeles, San Francisco, and Chicago, with international venues in Hong Kong, Singapore, Spain, Germany, Scandinavia, Brazil, South Korea, Japan, and Canada.

The American Fashion Capitals

With its significant design presence and wholesale concentration, New York City remains the primary locale for America's fashion industry. While this area has the major concentration, others in regional markets continue to make progress in their quest to become fashion innovators and suppliers.

SEVENTH AVENUE

Fashion professionals that include the creative forces, manufacturers, retail operations, and market consultants generally rely upon the pulse of Seventh Avenue to determine what will be the next trend to take the country by storm (Figure 1.10). While the term *Seventh Avenue*

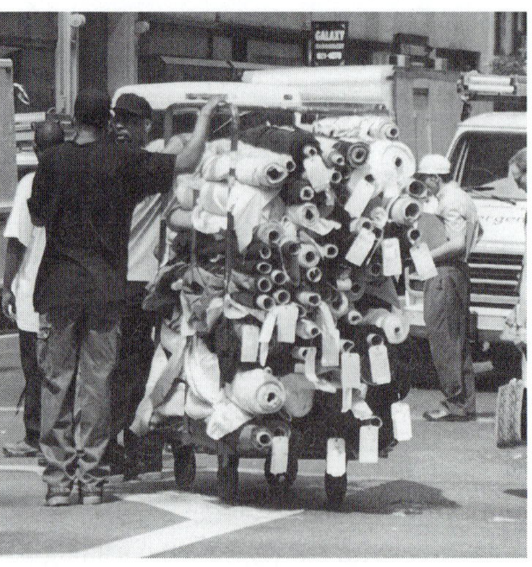

Figure 1.10 Rolls of fabric make their way to Seventh Avenue designers.
(Courtesy of Ellen Diamond.)

is technically a geographical location, it isn't meant to describe a specific street. In practice, it refers to the *garment center*, an area that includes Seventh Avenue, but also the surrounding areas from Broadway to Ninth Avenue, and the side streets that begin at West 35th Street and continue on to West 41st Street.

While these are the heart and soul of the New York City fashion center, its borders continue to expand to other Manhattan neighborhoods such as Soho, Greenwich Village, and the upper west side.

Today's garment center, or Seventh Avenue, while still the driving force of America's fashion industry, no longer holds a monopoly. Although fashion is still created in these areas and showrooms are aplenty for buyers to visit to purchase the collections, production has for the most part moved offshore. Through the use of joint ventures and wholly owned subsidiaries, companies have opted to manufacture their lines in many countries where the cost of production is a fraction of what it is in the United States.

Regional Wholesale Markets

Fashion designers and marketers also have a presence in other areas in the United States. Some companies are based in these arenas, while others that are based in New York City maintain showrooms to enable their retail clients to fulfill their merchandise needs.

Heading the list is Los Angeles. Popular companies such as Karen Kan and Carole Little are headquartered there, as are upscale designers such as Bob Mackie and James Galanos. Following LA's West coast lead is San Francisco where the Gap, Banana Republic, and Jessica McClintock are based.

Other high-profile regional markets include Chicago, with the Chicago Apparel Mart housing the majority of fashion wholesale showrooms; Dallas, with the Dallas Apparel Mart being the primary fashion destination for retail buyers; and Atlanta, where the Atlanta Apparel Mart is home to more than 2,000 showrooms.

Overseas Fashion Capitals

In Europe and Asia, fashion is alive and well. Fashion companies on these continents create original designs and manufacture their own products as well as those that have been created in the United States.

PARIS

Although a great deal of couture design has found homes in other parts of the globe, Paris still reigns as one of the premier fashion capitals of the world. Names like Lagerfeld, Lacroix, and Chanel still call Paris their home and continue to stun fashion's editorial press and consumers with collections that reveal uniqueness and excitement. Coupled with the original couture designs, prêt-a-porter (ready-to-wear) has made this fashion capital even more important. This latter classification has saved many a couture house from shutting its doors because of the shrinking consumer market for more extravagant offerings.

MILAN, ITALY

With the vast collections of silk produced in nearby Como and a wealth of other fine fabrics found in the Milanese mills, Milan continues to be an enormously successful fashion capital (Figure 1.11). With Armani leading the way and Missoni and Ferre following his lead, this Italian center continues to make headlines in both couture and ready-to-wear.

LONDON

Once a staid fashion city where fine custom tailoring was its most striking asset, London's offerings today have joined Europe's creative elite. Buyers from all over the world flock to London for cutting-edge apparel and accessories that have been designed by such talents as Vivienne Westwood, Zandra Rhodes, and Betty Jackson. Of course, men's wear still reigns in London with Savile Row the leading purveyor of fine men's wear.

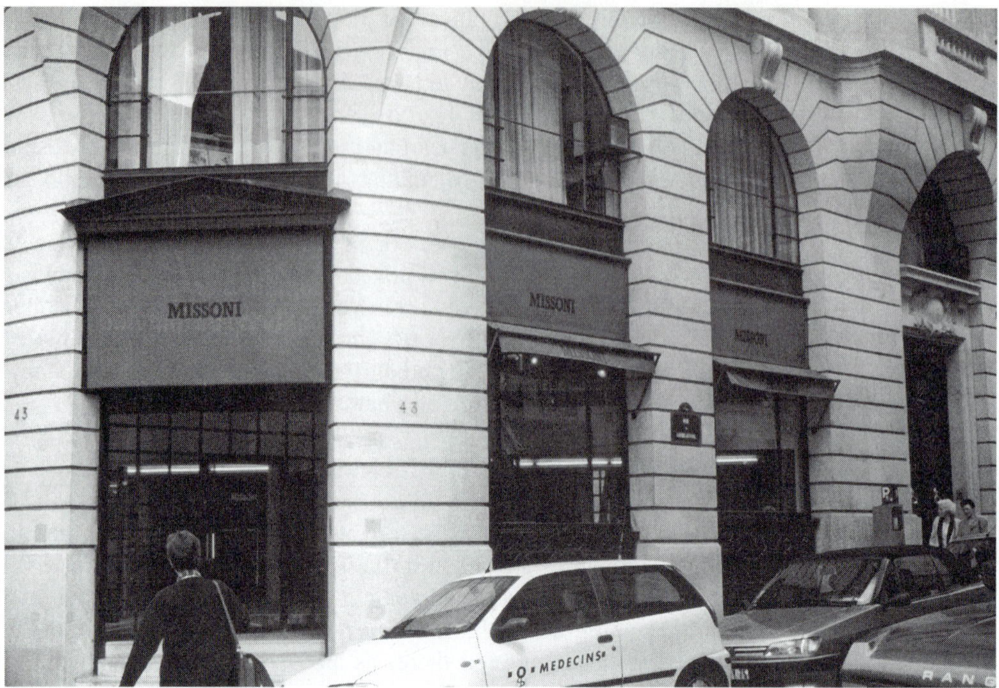

Figure 1.11 Milan with couturier fashion houses like Missoni, leads the way in innovative styling. *(Courtesy of Ellen Diamond.)*

SPAIN

While its forte is not fashion-forward design recognition as is some of its European neighbors, Spain has achieved global recognition with fine leather products. Apparel and footwear in particular have made Spain the country where buyers flock to place orders for leather merchandise.

GERMANY

Fashion has become a major industry in Germany with designers such as Hugo Boss being recognized globally for men's apparel and Jil Sander for her collection of upscale women's apparel. Each of these companies has expanded its horizons with boutiques bearing those names in places like New York City, Cannes, Florence, and other fashionable locations.

SCANDINAVIA

The world of fashion has seen an increase in the manufacturing community of the Scandinavian countries. Leading the pack with name recognition is Finland's Marimekko with a vast assortment of fabrics and home furnishings. Sweden has also emerged as a fashion resource with its increase in glass shipments to other parts of the world. Copenhagen, known for its own glass production, has taken newer initiatives by becoming the producer of a wealth of "Venetian" glass. In the apparel arena, Norway has become a leader in moderately priced fashion.

EASTERN BLOC COUNTRIES

With a lesser-known, but nonetheless important, role in the fashion industry, Poland and Hungary are becoming more well-known. Their part has been as manufacturing partners of such retailers as Federated, for whom they produce much of the company's private label brands. They also are the production arms of design operations throughout the rest of the fashion world. With the cost of production significantly lower in these countries than in many others, Poland and Hungary offer the potential for greater profitability.

JAPAN

With its already established reputation as one of the world's premier silk producers, Japan has become a leader in yet another part of the fashion industry, with its fashion-forward designs and manufacturing operations for overseas companies. Acclaimed designers such as Hanae Mori, Kenzo, Rei Kawakubo, and Issey Miyake have catapulted Japanese design to new heights. In addition, many factories are involved in producing the designs of famous American designers such as Donna Karan.

HONG KONG

While original design takes a back seat to manufacturing for other global fashion operations, China has started to gain recognition with its own creative endeavors with such companies as Toppy and Episode. More and more young designers are joining the fray with original creations that are taking the fashion industry by storm.

CANADA

As a partner in the North American Free Trade Agreement (NAFTA) along with the United States and Mexico, Canada has begun to successfully export its men's and women's apparel abroad. In fact, it has become the second most important exporter of better-quality men's wear to the United States, right after Italy.

MEXICO

The Mexican role in fashion has been primarily as a manufacturer for overseas companies. While it does produce a great deal of apparel and accessories, Mexico's home furnishings have been most important to the fashion world.

Internet Resources for Additional Research

www.fashion-careers.biz offers information on every type of fashion career from design to marketing.

www.FashionSchools.com features a wealth of different fashion schools and programs in the United States and abroad.

www.fashioninformation.com provides up-to-the-minute information on fashion trends.

Merchandise Information Terminology

Fashion retailing
Licensing agreements
Raw materials
Precious metals
Base metals
Collection
Computer-aided design (CAD) program
Cutting ticket
Knock-offs
Style
Fashion
Silhouette
Fad
Classic
Couturier(e)
Haute couture
Prêt-a-porter
Custom made
Resource
Fashion cycle
Trend
Hot item
Price point
Off-price
Offshore production

EXERCISES

1. Log on to such search engines as *www.google.com* to determine the size of today's fashion industry in terms of manufacturers, people employed, and geographic importance. Using this information, prepare a written report on the industry.

2. Contact an association that deals specifically with one sector of the fashion industry to determine its depth and breadth. By entering the keyword for that industry, such as *textiles*, on a search engine, a wealth of information can be found. The data should then be assembled into a report that addresses that industry's current status.
3. Select a particular fashion career and report on the basic requirements one needs to achieve success in it. You might contact a retail buyer, fashion designer, or manufacturer for your information.

Review Questions

1. Why have American-based fashion designers and manufacturers outsourced their production to other countries?
2. With the recent decline in sales, how have some department stores tried to recapture their importance in the retail arena?
3. What is some basic product knowledge needed by a "converter" in the textile industry to make him or her sufficiently prepared to enter the field?
4. In what areas must a purchasing agent in the fur industry be proficient to satisfactorily carry out a successful career?
5. How different is today's fashion designer's preparation from those that preceded them twenty years ago?
6. Which two areas of competence are necessary for the product manager to achieve success in the apparel manufacturing classification?
7. Why has customer service become more important than ever before to the fashion industry?
8. Contrast the differences between a major retailer's general merchandise manager and the divisional merchandise managers.
9. How does the assistant buyer serve the needs of the head buyer?
10. How important is the role of fashion director to a retail organization?
11. What is the major role played by a public relations director in a fashion retailing operation?
12. In what way does the resident buyer assist the retail buyer?
13. How does the fashion forecaster help the designer, manufacturer, and retailer make better judgments?
14. If one is unable to find the time to attend formal classes, how can he or she acquire product knowledge so necessary for success in a fashion career?
15. Differentiate between the terms *fashion* and *style*.
16. What is meant by the term *prêt-a-porter*?
17. Why is it important for the fashion manufacturer to be able to assess the potential for decline of a style?
18. Although Seventh Avenue is used to describe New York City's garment center, where is it actually geographically based?
19. What phenomenon has saved Paris from becoming extinct in the fashion world?
20. What role do the eastern bloc nations play in fashion?

SECTION TWO

The Materials of Fashion Merchandise

CHAPTER 2

Textiles

After reading this chapter, you should be able to:

- Discuss the various techniques used in fiber production.
- Explain the numerous types of methods used in the transformation of fiber into fabric.
- Prepare a natural fibers table that includes the characteristics inherent in each.
- Develop a list of natural and manufactured fiber fabrics and their uses as wearable products.
- Differentiate among the different methods of printing and dyeing used in textile production.
- List several finishes applied to fabrics and the advantages afforded by each.

The distinctive rustling sound made by the movement of taffeta; the intricately detailed jacquard designs embellished in spectacular brocades; the quiet, elegant feel of furlike cashmere; and the bold, colorful patterns inherent in exciting stripes and prints all bring the fashion designer's creations to life. The excitement generated by the parade of collections on the world's fashion runways is heightened by the fabric choices used in the apparel. It is not a chance marriage that couples the fabric and silhouette. The blending of these two elements makes each piece into an individual style.

Aesthetics alone are not sufficient when fabrics are being produced. Although appearance is certainly an essential ingredient, function must be considered as well. The business traveler who must make a fresh entrance immediately after a long journey should arrive looking as freshly and impeccably dressed as though he or she had just traveled across town. The fabrics used in the garments worn for this purpose must resist unwanted wrinkles and unsightly creases. The pleasure traveler's tightly packed wardrobe must be removed from the garment bag, unruffled, ready to use in many areas where freshening facilities might be difficult to find. In the coverings used for upholstered furniture, consideration must be given to the ease with which stains are removed.

The textile industry is a highly sophisticated network of specialists who apply their technological knowledge to the needs of the apparel, wearable accessories, and home furnishings world. The constant interaction of these fashion segments assures that the end product, the needs of the consumer, will be served.

Manufacturers and designers search all the domestic markets and offshore producers around the globe for fibers and fabrics they can use in the production of their collections. Some fibers, such as silk, are not domestically available and must be secured overseas. Linen, with its unique characteristics, while available in several venues, is often purchased in Belgium, if high quality is demanded. When hand-loomed woolens are required, as is the case in quality menswear, then Italy is generally the choice. Other fibers, notably the manufactured types, have broad areas of domestic production, allowing product manufacturers greater latitude in their procurement.

The clothing designer must assess the fabric's characteristics in terms of drapability, eye appeal, and function. The buyer must recognize various fabrics and fibers and their inherent qualities. Sales associates must assist the consumer by making the right fabric choices for special needs. In all of these cases, a working knowledge of textiles is imperative.

TEXTILE FIBERS

Dating back to ancient times, Egyptians wore garments made of cotton, flax, and wool. Cotton fabrics, woven 5,000 years ago, have been discovered in India. From that time until the beginning of the twentieth century, our forefathers' needs were limited to those same natural fibers as well as silk. Although they were able to satisfy their clothing requirements with these basic fibers, certain limitations in terms of their availability restricted their use. Cotton, for example, could not withstand the cold climates of Europe's northernmost regions, and silk, found primarily in Asia, was in short supply. They were severely limited to a modest variety of fabrics made from natural fibers. Not until a chemist's curiosity about how silkworms made silk led to the discovery of the first manufactured fiber, rayon, did the industry's horizons expand.

A **fiber** is any substance, natural or manufactured, that comes in single hairlike strands. These very small parts are then made into yarns and ultimately into fabric. **Natural fibers** come from a variety of plants and animals. Manufactured, or man-made, is the generic term that includes all chemically made **textile fibers,** including rayon, acetate, polyester, acrylic, metallic, saran glass, olefin rubber, and modacrylic. Each of the natural and man-made fibers has characteristics that make them suitable for various uses.

Natural Fibers

Cotton and flax are the major natural plant or vegetable fibers used in the creation of apparel, wearable accessories, and furnishings for the home. Others such as hemp, ramie, and jute are also found in these products, but to lesser extents. Wool, cashmere, alpaca, vicuna, camel's hair, angora, and mohair are animal fibers, of which wool is the most widely used. Silk, although taken from the shell or cocoon of the silkworm, is also classified as an animal fiber because it is primarily made up of the secretions of the worm.

COTTON

Cotton grows in warm climates, with the bulk of it grown in the United States, the People's Republic of China, India, Brazil, Egypt, Mexico, Pakistan, and Turkey.

The planting process generally begins in the spring, but some areas of Texas begin as early as February 1 and others, such as Missouri, as late as June 1. The seeding is accomplished with mechanical planters that open trenches, drop the seeds inside, and cover them. Fertilizers are used to enhance growth, and chemicals keep weeds and insects from impairing the crops. Once the crops have ripened and the leaves have been removed, they are harvested by machines that work fifty times faster than people who were once hired to do the job.

The cotton is next transported to the gin where it is cleaned and ginned, a process that separates the seed from the fiber. The ginned fiber, called *lint* at this stage, is pressed into bales that weigh about 480 pounds. Because cotton is a natural fiber, it is available in a number of different grades. At this point in the process, each bale is examined to determine its grade in terms of length of the fiber, known as the **staple,** and its color and cleanliness. The fiber now heads for the textile industry with the linters, small, fuzzy, downlike substances, and the seeds head for other industrial use. The staples run anywhere from $1/2$ to $2\,1/2$ inches in length and are considered for their final fabric use.

All cotton must be carded, which is a detangling procedure. Cotton that requires a silkier, smoother appearance is also combed (Table 2.1). Cotton that is combed drapes better than that which has been only carded. Wool, as we will see later, also uses carding and combing.

Cotton affords the wearer numerous advantages. Among them are:

Softness. The natural textured surface cushions itself against the skin and feels more comfortable.

Breathability. Cotton removes body moisture by absorbing it and transmitting it into the air, thus making the wearer cooler and lighter.

TABLE 2.1 US Imports of Combed Cotton Yarns
Value in US$, Volume in Kilos, Unit Value in US$/Kilo
Sorted Out by Jan–May 04 Volume

		Jan–May 04 Volume	*2003 Volume Change*	*Jan–May 04 Volume Change*	*2001 Volume Share*	*Jan–May 04 Volume Share*
	World	28,157,399	26.47%	45.96%	100.00%	100.00%
F	Mexico	8,074,247	29.27%	18.89%	39.43%	28.68%
F	Pakistan	5,509,336	−3.14%	181.39%	10.25%	19.57%
Q	Brazil	2,999,057	32.65%	65.75%	0.66%	10.65%
Q	Indonesia	2,707,121	75.71%	350.03%	4.91%	9.61%
F	Canada	2,111,813	376.29%	3975.05%	0.29%	7.50%
Q	Malaysia	1,145,220	16.59%	−3.96%	2.45%	4.07%
Q	Korea	1,110,149	145.18%	61.09%	1.77%	3.94%
Q	Egypt	928,955	414.55%	−37.73%	3.60%	3.30%
Q	Thailand	869,581	1.14%	36.19%	4.36%	3.09%
Q	China	853,544	55.12%	38.84%	4.60%	3.03%
F	EI Salvador	376,387	32.19%	26.46%	1.14%	1.34%
F	Uzbekistan	334,718	−25.01%	−74.03%	8.27%	1.19%
Q	Turkey	223,456	−55.23%	2665.54%	7.19%	0.79%
F	Switzerland	216,914	48.20%	−15.47%	0.00%	0.77%
Q	Vietnam	183,525	58.44%	−56.22%	0.00%	0.65%
F	Argentina	150,186	−33.34%	50.54%	0.02%	0.53%
F	Bahrain	88,943	−15.75%	−80.30%	0.48%	0.32%
F	Peru	16,809	−24.68%	−49.94%	0.88%	0.06%
F	Bulgaria	14,563	-	-	0.00%	0.05%
F	Spain	2,166	100.00%	-	0.00%	0.01%
F	Germany	1,993	−83.97%	530.70%	0.04%	0.01%
F	Italy	1,950	42.82%	−99.58%	5.84%	0.01%
Q	Taiwan	1,110	−94.52%	96.81%	1.96%	0.00%

F: Quota-free, Q: Quota applied on imports

Compiled data from U.S. Department of Commerce / OTEXA ©EmergingTextiles.com (1998–2004)

Absorbency. Because the fiber absorbs so much moisture, drawing it up through its interior walls, it is perfect for terry cloth apparel such as beach coats that require immediate water absorption.

Temperature control. This year-round fiber protects against the wind without trapping body moisture in cold weather and helps to keep the body cool and dry in warm weather. Its versatility makes it one of the most widely used fibers.

Performance. It is static free, hypoallergenic, and pill free. It is simple to care for, washes with no trouble, and easily retains its original feel and color.

As do all fibers, cotton has some unfavorable characteristics. Most, however, can be corrected with properly applied finishes. It has little luster, poor elasticity and resiliency, and a tendency to mildew. It also has a tendency, if not pretreated, to shrink considerably when laundered. The finishes used for cotton and other fibers are addressed later in the chapter.

Some of the cotton fabrics that are found in apparel, accessories, and home furnishing include:

Broadcloth. A plain-weave, smooth, flat fabric that is used extensively in shirts, blouses, and sportswear.

Chambray. A plain-weave fabric that uses a set of white yarns, used for dresses, sportswear, children's wear, pajamas, and some table linens.

Corduroy. A ribbed, pile fabric that comes in a variety of patterns and weights and is used for trousers, jackets, casual wear, and upholstery.

Denim. A rugged fabric constructed with the twill weave. It was used initially for work clothes but has become a fashion favorite for jeans and other leisure wear (Figure 2.1); also used for upholstered furniture.

which is explored later, is based on a small opening in the silkworm's jaw called a spinneret. Scientists have expanded on this opening to produce filament yarns in the lab.

When the cocoons have achieved their desired size, they are first sorted according to color, shape, and texture, all of which affect the final silk product. After they have been sorted, the sericin, a gummy substance, is softened and removed so that the silk can be unwound. The unwinding process is called **reeling,** which takes place in a hot water basin. Because one silk filament is too fine to unreel by itself, approximately ten are unwound at the same time and drawn together into one filament. Any remaining sericin is boiled off either at this point or after weaving to uncover the fiber's natural beauty.

Some of silk's advantages are:

Strength. Because it is the strongest of the natural fibers, it resists abrasion and gives the wearer many years of service.

Comfort. It is extremely soft to the touch and on the skin. It is elastic and retains its original shape. As it readily absorbs moisture, it is comfortable in a warm atmosphere.

Care. It may be dry cleaned or washed. Washing, however, should be done by hand, unless the garment has been processed for machine laundering.

Shrinkage. The amount of shrinkage is minimal. If shrinking occurs after washing, the garment can be put back into its original size though pressing.

Appearance. It is the most luxurious of all fibers, with a unique natural luster (Figure 2.5).

On the negative side, silk tends to water spot. Exposure to perspiration can damage the fabric, and it will weaken if continuously exposed to sunlight.

Silk is used extensively for wearable products, draperies, and upholstered furniture in a variety of weights and textures. Some silk fabrics used in fashion apparel, wearable accessories, and home furnishings include:

Alpaca. A fine-textured, slightly lustrous fabric that is woven to resemble cloth made from South American alpacas.

Broadcloth. A spun silk, woven with a firm yet soft feel.

Boucle. A nubby, textured fabric, woven of yarn that has been twisted to produce a loopy thread.

Chiffon. An airy, gossamer sheer that has a floating quality in motion.

Crepe de Chine. A lustrous, light crepe with a soft, rippled effect.

Georgette. A soft, sheer fabric with a crepelike texture.

Honan. The best grade of Chinese silk, similar to pongee, but more finely woven.

Point d' esprit. Silk net that is woven with a raised dot.

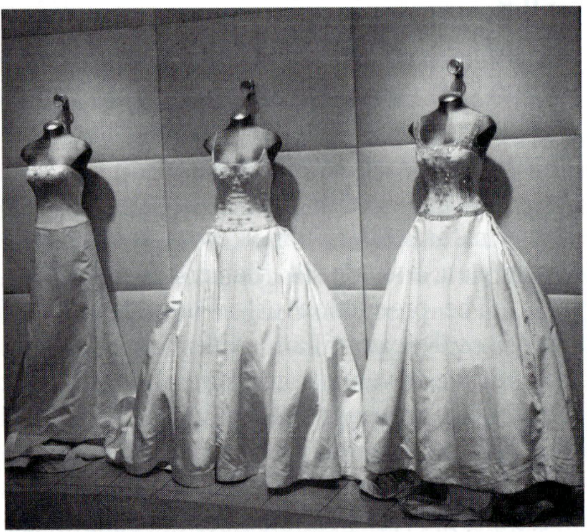

Figure 2.5 Silk is the fabric of choice for elegant wedding gowns because of its luxurious appearance. *(Courtesy of Ellen Diamond.)*

Poult de soie. A rich, soft fabric with a faint rib.

Pongee. A light- or medium-weight Chinese silk fabric made from tussah silk.

Satin. A smooth, shiny fabric.

Shantung. A soft, lustrous fabric with sparse, irregular ridges in the texture.

Surah. A soft, silk fabric with a pronounced diagonal rib.

Taffeta. A fine, lustrous fabric that is characterized by both its crispness and sound made through movement.

Tussah. A springy silk with sparse, irregular ridges in the texture that has been woven from the silk of uncultivated silkworms in Asia.

MISCELLANEOUS

In addition to the most commonly used natural fibers, designers often choose some that are lesser known to best suit their creative needs. They might be chosen for their naturally inherent textures, unusually soft feel, unique appearance, or an ability to perform better than some of the more commonly used fibers.

Some may be extremely expensive, such as cashmere and vicuna, whereas others may fall into the less costly range, such as ramie. They fall into two distinct classifications, the animal or hair group and the vegetable category.

Hair Fibers

Cashmere. A soft, luxurious fiber that is used in the finest of sweaters and other costly apparel and accessories. It comes from the Asian goat.

Angora rabbit hair. Moderately priced, when compared with cashmere and some of the other specialty hairs, it comes from a French rabbit that is specially raised for its fiber. It is extremely fine and is used primarily for sweaters. One drawback is that it sheds.

Vicuna. One of the costliest of the group, its thin, soft hair comes from the vicuna of South America.

Mohair. A strong, resilient fiber, naturally lustrous, that comes from the Angora goat.

Alpaca. Natural fiber known for its silky appearance and strength. The alpaca's hair is much longer than ordinary sheep's wool. Raised in the Andes, alpacas are shorn of their hair, which is used for fine coats and suits.

Camel's hair. Wool-like texture that is extremely soft and lustrous and comes from Mongolian and Tibetan camels. It is used primarily for coats, suits, and sports coats.

Vegetable Fibers

Ramie. A strong abrasion-resistant fiber used extensively today with cotton for sweaters.

Jute. Medium-quality strength with a rather rigid feel. The fiber is sometimes used for belts and canvas handbags.

Hemp. Coarse and brittle, its uses are limited. It is occasionally used when rough textured materials are needed.

Manufactured Fibers

A chemist's curiosity about how silkworms made silk led to the discovery of the first **manufactured,** or man-made as it was once called, fiber, rayon. The chemist developed his first artificial fibers in about 1850 from a substance he extracted from the inner layers of the trees that produced mulberry leaves, the diet of the silkworm. That substance was cellulose. When a French chemist, Count Hilaire de Chardonnet, displayed a few yards of "artificial silk," the name he used to describe the fiber, at an international exhibition, it created a sensation. In 1891, he built the first commercial artificial silk plant in France. A half century later the fiber was dubbed *rayon*, the "ray" because of its sheen and the "on" to suggest a fiber such as cotton.

Rayon was first produced in the United States in 1910 at a fiber factory in Pennsylvania. In 1924, a second cellulose product known as *acetate* was introduced. Little did the world know that this was just the beginning of a revolution in the textile industry that would produce an array of fibers that could be manufactured in the laboratory.

The two basic types of manufactured fibers are cellulosic and noncellulosic. **Cellulosic fibers,** which include rayon, acetate, and triacetate, are made from fibrous substances found in plants and can be produced with a minimum of chemical steps. The **noncellulose group** is much broader and uses molecules in various combinations of carbon, hydrogen, nitrogen, and oxygen derived from petroleum, natural gas, air, and water.

The Federal Trade Commission has assigned generic names to the twenty noncellulosic fibers, among which are acrylic, nylon, polyester, olefin, and spandex. Numerous manufacturers such as Monsanto, Fiber Industries, Inc., and BASF Corporation produce these fibers under trade names such as Dacron, Acrilan, Trevira, Lycra, and Cantrece. Not all the major fibers can be used as wearable fabrics and are therefore relatively unknown to the consuming public. Only those that are used by the fashion apparel, accessories, and home furnishings industries are addressed in this chapter.

Manufactured fibers, although delivering enormous advantages for textile producers and fashion manufacturers as well as the consumer, have sometimes had less than enthusiastic acceptance from the public. Polyester, for example, with all of its virtues was initially labeled a "tacky" fiber. In 1951 it was considered the miracle fiber of the twentieth century, but then it fell on hard times as a fashion fiber. Its poor image was difficult for the industry to reverse until a "new polyester" started to make headlines in the late 1980s when designers such as Calvin Klein embraced **microfiber** for their upscale collections. Fashion forecaster David Wolfe of the Doneger Group, America's leading resident buying office and market consulting group, referred to it as a "Godsend for the American consumer, a dream come true." So significant are its virtues today and its future potential, with sales at more than $1 billion in the early 2000s, that it deserves special attention as a fashion fiber.

The major microfiber trade names are Koch Industries; Micromattique, originally developed by Dupont; Fiber Industries; MicroSpun; and Hoechst Celanese's Trevira Micronesse.

Among the advantages afforded by this fiber are:

Feel. It can be maneuvered to have the feel of several different fabrics, including washed silk, chamois, taffeta, satin, and velvet.

Drapability. It drapes *extremely* well and can be used to enhance form-fitting designs.

Practicality. It is lightweight, easy to launder, strong, and wrinkle-free.

Versatility. It takes prints with greater clarity than other fibers and is colorfast.

MAJOR GENERIC GROUPS

There are twelve major groups of manufactured fibers, eight of which are found in considerable abundance in fashion apparel, wearable accessories, and home furnishings. Each has specific characteristics that are unique and are available under trade names that belong to their producers. For example, Zafran is nylon that is produced by BASF Corporation, Solara is an acrylic product of Monsanto, and Estron is an acetate owned by Eastman Chemical Products.

The textiles that are achieved with these manufactured fibers come in a wide range of textures, appearances, and feels. They are used to produce fabrics that bear the same names as those produced with natural fibers such as batiste, which is synonymous with cotton; flannel, generally associated with wool; satin, often a silk fabric; shantung, another silk favorite; and crash, a heavyweight linen product. The manner in which they are converted from their fiber state to yarn and then to fabric, dictates the types of fabrics that will eventually be used for wearable items and home furnishings.

Table 2.2 features the eight major generic groups of fashion-oriented manufactured fibers, their characteristics, the types of fabrics they are used to produce, and their apparel and home furnishings uses.

TABLE 2.2 Major Generic Groups of Manufactured Fibers

Fibers	*Characteristics*	*Fabrics*	*Wearable Uses*	*Home Products*
Acetate	Luxurious feel and appearance, wide range of colors and lusters, excellent drapability and softness, relatively fast drying, shrink-resistant	Brocade, crepe, double knit, faille, knitted jersey, lace, satin, taffeta, tricot	Blouses, dresses, foundation garments, lingerie, linings, shirts, slacks, sportswear	Draperies, upholstery
Acrylic	Soft and warm, wool-like, lightweight, retains shape, resilient, quick-drying, moth-resistant, resistant to sunlight, oil, and chemicals	Fleece and pile fabrics, face fabrics in bonded materials, simulated furs, jerseys	Dresses, infant wear, knitted garments, skirts, ski wear, socks, sportswear, sweaters, work clothes	Blankets, carpets, draperies, upholstery
Modacrylic	Soft, resilient, abrasion- and flame-resistant, quick-drying, resists acids and alkalies, retains shape	Fleece fabrics, knit-pile fabric backings, nonwoven fabrics	Deep pile coats, trims, linings, simulated furs, wigs, and hairpieces	Blankets, carpets, flame-resistant draperies and curtains, rugs
Nylon	Exceptionally strong, supple, abrasion-resistant, lustrous, easy to wash, resists damage from oil and many chemicals, resilient, low in moisture absorbency	Knitted and woven fabrics	Blouses, dresses, foundation garments, hosiery, lingerie and innerwear, raincoats, ski and snow apparel, suits, windbreakers	Bedspreads, carpets, draperies, curtains, upholstery
Olefin	Unique wicking properties that make it very comfortable; abrasion-resistant; quick-drying; resistant to deterioration from chemicals, mildew, perspiration, rot, and weather; sensitive to heat; soil-resistant; strong; very lightweight; excellent colorfastness	Knitted and woven fabrics	Pantyhose, underwear, sports shirts, sweaters	Carpet, carpet backing, slipcovers, upholstery
Polyester	Strong, resistant to stretching and shrinking, resistant to most chemicals, quick-drying, crisp and resilient when wet or dry, wrinkle- and abrasion-resistant, retains heat-set pleats and crease, easy to wash	A variety of knitted and woven fabrics	Blouses, shirts, children's wear, dresses, half hose, ties, lingerie, underwear, permanent press garments, slacks, suits	Carpets, curtains, draperies, bedding
Rayon	Highly absorbent, soft and comfortable, easy to dye, versatile, good drapability	Knits, pile fabrics, woven fabrics that simulate flax	Blouses, coats, dresses, jackets, lingerie, linings, millinery, rainwear, slacks, shirts, suits, ties	Bedspreads, blankets, carpets, draperies, sheets, slipcovers, tablecloths, upholstery
Spandex	Can be stretched 500 percent without breaking, lightweight	Elasticized woven and knitted fabrics	Athletic apparel, bathing suits, foundation garments	None

TRANSFORMING FIBER INTO YARN

We have learned that the natural fibers must go through some preliminary processes before they can be considered sufficiently viable to be turned into yarn or continuous threadlike strands. Cotton and flax, for example, must be separated from their plants and wools cleaned after being shorn. The manufactured fibers need no extra processing because they are laboratory produced and ready for transformation into yarn after the appropriate chemicals have been mixed.

Natural fibers are either short or thin and must be condensed in some manner to make them appropriate for use as fabrics. They must undergo spinning at this point. Fibers that are engineered in the laboratory do not generally require spinning, except in cases in which they are meant to resemble fabrics that are usually made of natural fibers.

Spinning

Cotton, flax, and wool have staple sizes that range from approximately 1/2 to 36 inches in length. Their sizes require that they be spun together to form the yarn needed for textile construction. Although silk is naturally produced in long filaments and does not need to be spun, many cocoons are damaged, causing the filaments to break into smaller pieces. These shorter staples then undergo **spinning** much the same as the other natural fibers (Figure 2.6).

Our ancestors used the hand-driven spinning wheel to make yarn. Today, modern textile plants use a variety of machines and numerous spinning techniques to accomplish the same result, but much more quickly and efficiently.

Manufactured fibers are produced as continuous filaments and may be used in fabric production without using the spinning process. To produce some materials that resemble the natural spun varieties, however, these filaments are cut into smaller pieces or staples and then spun in the same manner as their natural fiber counterparts. Rayon, for example, when used to imitate linen, goes through the spinning process.

Various spinning methods are used, with ring spinning the most common in the United States. Open-end spinning is a newer system that is three to five times faster, with air jet the fastest at a rate that is seven to ten times that of the conventional ring technique.

During filament processing, manufacturers use certain additives such as dye before the solution is extruded into yarn. The technique of dyeing is discussed along with other additives in a later section of this chapter.

Filament Production

All manufactured fibers are formed by forcing a thick, syrupy substance through tiny holes in metal plate which resembles a showerhead, called a *spinneret*. The process is known as *extrusion*, from the silkworm who extrudes the strands of silk in the same manner. The size of the filament yarn is determined by the size of the holes in the spinneret. The holes in each device range from one to as many as a thousand.

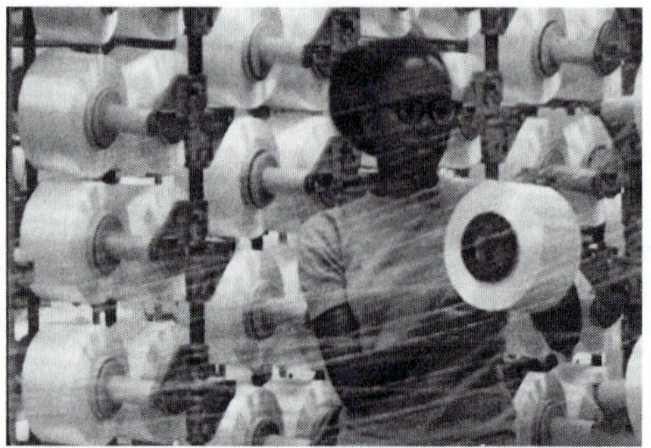

Figure 2.6 Fiber is spun into yarn. *(Courtesy of Ellen Diamond.)*

After the emergence from the spinneret, the fibers are solidified. The extrusion and hardening process is called *spinning*. The three spinning techniques are wet, dry, and melt.

As they are hardening or after they solidified, the fibers are stretched to reduce the diameter. This process increases strength and stabilizes their ability to stretch without breaking.

FABRIC CONSTRUCTION

Several methods are used in the construction of fabric. **Weaving** is the most widely used, followed by knitting. Other techniques used for apparel, accessories, and home furnishings include felting, crocheting, and bonding.

Weaving

Fabrics that are woven are constructed by the interlacing of two or more sets of yarns at right angles (Figure 2.7). The vertical, or lengthwise, yarns are called *warps* and are the stronger of the two. They are placed first on the loom. The horizontal, or crosswise, yarns are *fillings* and are interlaced with the warps. The three basic weaving techniques are plain, twill, and satin (Figure 2.8). Others such as the pile, jacquard, and dobby require more complicated construction.

PLAIN WEAVE

The simplest method, the **plain weave,** is accomplished in a manner that is similar to that of stringing a tennis racket. The filling yarns are interlaced over and under the warp yarns. Both fine and thick fabrics may be manufactured in this manner, the end result determined by the yarns used.

A variation, called the *basket weave*, can be used to achieve a different appearance. It requires the interlacing of two or more sets of yarns as though they were one. Although the end result is a fabric that has a different dimension than that of the traditional plain weave,

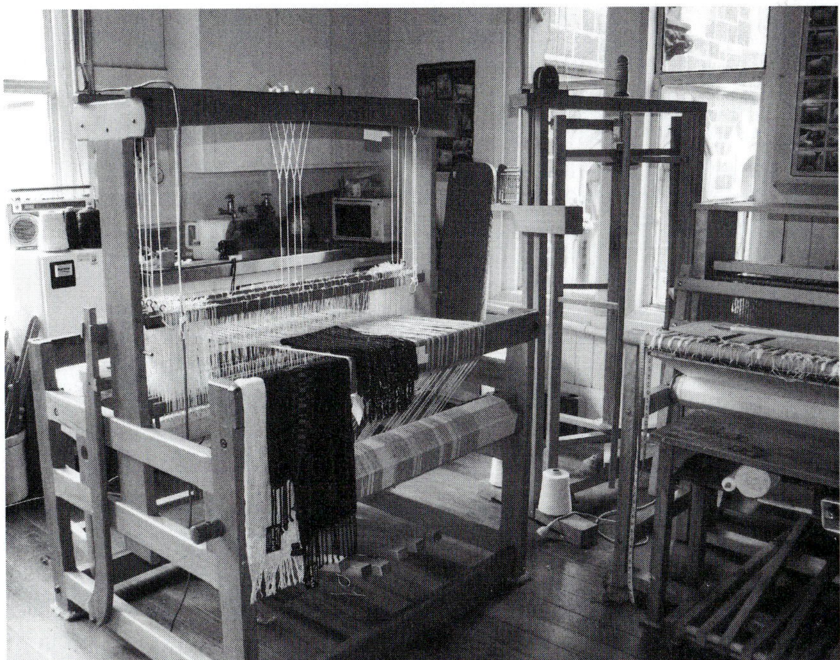

Figure 2.7 The loom is set to produce the desired weave.
(Courtesy of Ellen Diamond.)

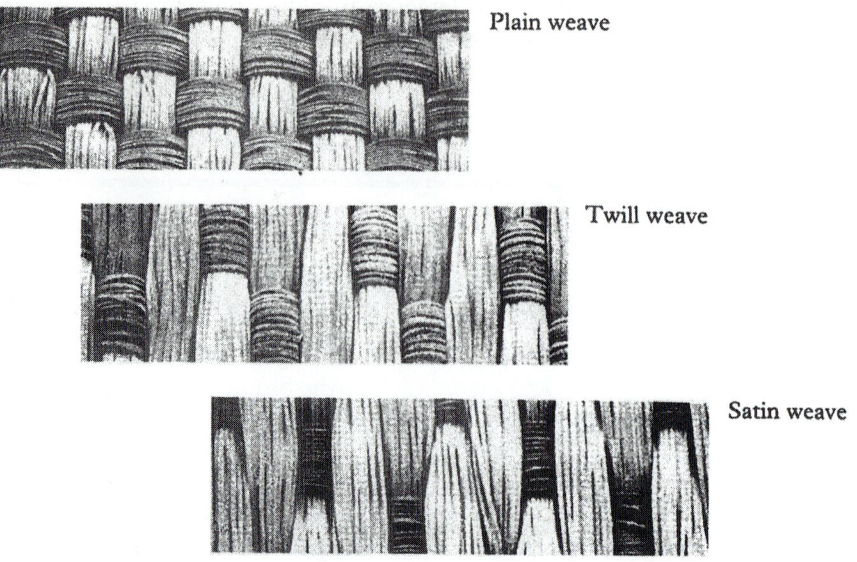

Figure 2.8 Most apparel fabrics are woven using the plain, twill, or satin weaves.

the disadvantage is that the yarns may shift out of place during the final product manufacturing stage or during laundering.

TWILL WEAVE

When durability is desired, the **twill weave,** which produces a diagonal line, is used. The technique involves each filling yarns to follow an over-one, under-two course though the warp yarns. Variations of this weave can create different effects, as in the case of the herringbone pattern. In this fabric, the diagonals run upward to both the right and left side of the fabric. Denim is a prime example of a fabric made with the twill weave.

SATIN WEAVE

When the desired result is a smooth, shiny surface, the **satin weave** is chosen. The yarns are not interlaced at close intervals as in the other basic techniques, but are floated from four to twelve times before interlacing takes place. The floating, or reduction in the number of interlacings, allows for more light on the surface, giving fabrics of this type their natural luster. Although a shiny surface has been accomplished, the fewer interlacings cause the fabric to wear poorly and show abrasion after repeated wearings.

PILE WEAVE

When a furlike, plush surface is desired, the **pile weave** is used. Its production requires three sets of yarns, a regular set of warps, a regular set of fillings, and an additional set that may be either warps or fillings that forms the dimensional surface. The raised surface yarns may then be left alone, as in the case with terry cloth, or cut, as in the case with velvet.

JACQUARD WEAVE

The most complicated of the techniques is the **jacquard weave,** which requires an intricate loom, called the *jacquard loom*, for construction. A series of punched cards that predetermine the design were once used to achieve the most intricate of patterns. Today, the computer aids in the production of jacquard designs, helping to reproduce the patterns in a fraction of the time it once took. Unlike other construction techniques that use one set of warps, the jacquard loom may use as many as 4,000 to achieve the effect. Given the complexity of the production, fabrics made in this manner are costly and are used only for detailed, unusual motifs.

DOBBY WEAVE

A simple geometric pattern may be reproduced with the **dobby weave.** Constructed on a special loom, the technique produces fabrics such as "birdseye pique," used in some women's sportswear and small patterns for men's ties.

Knitting

Fabrics that are knitted are done so by using hooked needles to pull one loop of yarn through another loop and interlocking them. As new loops are formed, they are drawn through those previously shaped. This may be accomplished by hand, when fine, quality garments are the goal, or by machine. Of course, hand-knitted wear is costly and has a limited market.

The two basic types of **knitting** techniques are weft and warp. Goods that are horizontally produced are called *weft*, with the stitches running from side to side for the width of the fabric. *Warp* knitting uses a large number of yarns to make the goods, with each yarn looped around a single needle and vertically attached to the other loops.

The sophistication of the knitting machines enables manufacturers to produce a vast array of goods, using the finest to the thickest fibers. Single jersey, double jersey, ribs, and intricate jacquards are easily manufactured with these specialized machines. The latest technology of the electronic knitting machines enables the industry to turn out goods at unimaginable speeds.

Felting

The production of fibers such as wool into fabric without first transforming them into yarn is known as **felting.** The process requires the mechanical action of agitation, friction, and pressure in the presence of heat and moisture. The scales on the edges of the fiber interlock, preventing them from returning to their original position. The major use of felted fabrics is for hats, with occasional use in casual jackets.

Bonding

The process of **bonding** involves adhering two fabrics together. Each may be first constructed with the same or different methods. The front side or face of the fabric may be woven and the backing knitted. Webs are formed that adhere to the two layers, producing the bonded fabric.

Crocheting

Intricately designed laces may be produced through **crocheting.** It requires the use of threads made with hooks. They are either accomplished by hand or machine, with the former available at considerable expense. Full-crocheted garments and accessories such as hats and gloves are sometimes available, but the majority of crocheted fabric is used for trim.

FINISHING FABRICS

Although the fabrics are somewhat serviceable at this point, most do not have the appearance to arouse customer inspection nor the enhancements that improve their characteristics. Color is a primary finish that gives life to the garments, accessories, or home furnishings and makes them stand out from the rest. Patterned designs may also change the common or ordinary textile into something spectacular. Pucci prints, for example, that are gaining significant popularity once again with their bold, geometric shapes transform the mundane into the sensational.

Delustering. A process to remove the sheen on many manufactured fibers that often makes them less attractive. The process employs a variety of chemicals.

Singeing. Use of heat to even and smooth fabrics that have been constructed with short staples and thus have a fuzziness on the surface. The fabric is quickly passed over a gas flame to burn off the tiny fibers. To eliminate the sparking that often accompanies the singeing, the fabric is immediately placed in a water bath and then dried.

Mercerization. Used on cotton to increase the sheen. The fabric is immersed in a solution of sodium hydroxide for a few minutes. This finish also improves strength and absorbency, making it a functional finish as well as an appearance enhancer.

Schreinerizing. A type of calendering that produces a low-luster appearance on the surface. This is achieved by fine, diagonally engrained rollers that pass over the fabrics.

Plisseing. A crinkly effect gained by using sodium hydroxide, which is pasted on the fabric where shrinkage would take place to produce a puckered look.

Shearing. A process to smooth pile-woven fabric surfaces that are irregular as they come from the loom. Using equipment that is similar to a lawn mower, the pile is uniformly cut.

Functional Finishes

Whereas the previous finishes are used to please the eye, the following group of **functional finishes** renders fabrics more serviceable to users.

Durable press. A finish achieved with resins and heat curing, which helps a garment keep its shape with little or no ironing after washing.

Flame retardency. A term used to describe fabrics that have received a chemical treatment to make them resistant to burning.

Preshrinking. A variety of processes that retards fabric shrinkage. Sanforized is a well-known trade name for a preshrinking process that guarantees treated fabric will not shrink by more than 1 percent.

Sizing. Adding starch or similar materials to fabrics to add strength, body, weight, and stiffness; it can also prevent damage.

Water repellent. Fabrics treated with special finishes to resist water but still permit air to flow through them. Waterproofing, which actually prevents penetration, requires a rubber-coated base.

Wrinkle resistance. Special chemicals used to either prevent fabric wrinkling or to permit them to shake out all at once.

Antistatic. Applying chemicals to the fabrics to keep them from clinging.

Mothproofing. Using chemical sprays to repel moths from wool.

Permanent press. Through heat setting, resins, or liquid ammonia, creating permanent creases or pleats. Although some man-made goods are naturally permanently pressed, other textiles and natural fibers may be required to undergo the finish to improve salability.

Soil release. A finish that is extremely important to fabrics that have been permanently pressed because they tend to hold dirt. Soil release is accomplished by adding special chemicals that release stains more easily from garments and upholstered furniture.

TEXTILE REGULATIONS

The federal government has enacted many pieces of legislation that have helped consumers to properly evaluate the fibers in the products they buy. Some address all fibers and fabrics, whereas others address specific individual fibers.

Some of these have had far-reaching effects, and consumers are more aware of fibers than ever before. The next page briefly outlines the important points of some of these acts.

Textile Fiber Identification Act

Each garment must be labeled to include the generic names of the fibers used, the percent of the individual fibers, and, if imported, the country of origin.

Wool Product's Labeling Act

The percent of wool and its category must be listed. The categories include wool fiber that has never been used before (**new** or **virgin wool** designations are appropriate); fiber that has fallen away during the processes such as carding or combing, or fibers that have been reclaimed from spun yarn or knitted products; **reprocessed wool,** which was made into a wool product that was never used but restructured back into wool fiber; and **reused wool,** fiber that was made into a product that was used by the consumer and then turned back into the fiber state.

Flammable Fabrics Act

This act originally outlawed the use of highly flammable fibers and permitted only those that passed a burning test. It was later amended to include nontextile fibers such as plastics. Some specific tests administered under the provisions of this act are the 45-degree angle test for wearing apparel, which touches a flame to the fabric at that angle, and the vertical test for children's sleepwear, which vertically exposes the garment to flame and records the burning time.

Federal Trade Rule on the Care Labeling of Textile Wearing Apparel

Apparel must have permanent tags affixed that give appropriate care and maintenance instructions.

MARKETING TEXTILES

Few industries use as many approaches to market their products as the textile industry. Fiber producers spend enormous sums trying to get the product into the ultimate consumers' hands.

Promotion does not stop at this level. A great deal of involvement comes from trade associations and organizations that interface with manufacturers. The following is a list of some of these and their endeavors.

The Wool Bureau

Established in 1949, the Wool Bureau is the U.S. branch of the International Wool Secretariat (IWS), which represents major growers in the Southern Hemisphere. Its role is to educate the public on the merits of wool through advertising and promotion and to assist manufacturers and retailers through wool product research and development. The Wool Bureau created the now familiar Woolmark and the Woolblend Mark, which immediately tells the consumer that the product is made of wool. The bureau also maintains laboratories that help to improve wool products; sponsors merchandising programs that initiate cooperative advertising between wool producers and apparel, accessories, and home products designers; and provides information on color, fabric, and fashion trends through its fashion office.

Cotton Incorporated

This organization is responsible for increasing the retail market share of American cotton fiber. Its goal is to enhance U.S. consumer preference for cotton and cotton-containing fabrics.

It accomplishes this by planning and executing a strategic program of research, product development, and market promotion. It operates a Cottonworks library, a vital source of information for the manufacturing industry, which showcases fabrics from hundreds of mills and knitters who manufacture cotton fabrics.

National Cotton Council

This is the unifying force of the U.S. raw cotton industry's seven segments: producers, ginners, warehousers, merchants, cottonseed crushers, cooperatives, and textile manufacturers. The council's mission is to compete effectively and profitably in fiber and oilseed markets at home and abroad. It is involved in the technical aspects of the industry, public relations, and promotion.

Internet Resources for Additional Research

www.textiles.com is a comprehensive Web site that offers a complete overview of the textile industry.
www.emergingtextiles.com features the latest reports on the global textile industry.
www.hometextilestoday.com is an online weekly fashion and business resource that reports on home textiles.

Merchandise Information Terminology

Fiber
Natural fibers
Textile fibers
Cotton
Staple
Broadcloth
Chambray
Corduroy
Denim
Jersey
Oxford
Plisse
Poplin
Sateen
Seersucker
Terry cloth
Velour
Velvet, velveteen
Flax
Retting
Art linen
Cambric
Canvas
Crash
Damask
Handkerchief linen
Lawn
Wool
Grading
Scouring
Woolen
Worsted
Covert
Crepe
Donegal
Felt
Flannel
Gabardine
Herringbone
Loden
Merino
Serge
Shetland
Tweed
Silk
Filament
Sericulture
Reeling
Alpaca
Broadcloth
Boucle
Chiffon
Crepe de Chine
Georgette
Honan
Point d' esprit
Poult de soie
Pongee
Satin
Shantung
Surah
Taffeta
Tussah
Hair fibers
Cashmere
Angora rabbit hair
Vicuna
Mohair
Alpaca
Camel's hair
Vegetable fibers
Ramie
Jute
Hemp
Manufactured fibers
Cellulosic fibers
Noncellulosic fibers
Microfiber
Acetate
Acrylic
Modacrylic
Nylon
Olefin
Polyester
Rayon
Spandex
Spinning
Weaving
Plain weave
Twill weave
Satin weave
Pile weave
Jacquard weave
Dobby weave
Knitting
Felting
Bonding
Crocheting
Gray goods
Finishes
Solution dyeing

Stock dyeing
Yarn dyeing
Piece dyeing
Cross dyeing
Garment dyeing
Acid dyes
Chrome dyes
Basic dyes
Direct dyes
Disperse dyes
Fiber reactive dyes
Napthol dyes
Vat dyes
Screen printing
Roller printing
Hand-transfer printing
Calendering
Flocking
Napping
Embossing
Moireing
Delustering
Singeing
Mercerization
Schreinerizing
Plisseing
Shearing
Functional finishes
Durable press
Flame retardency
Preshrinking
Sizing
Water repellent
Wrinkle resistance
Antistatic
Mothproofing
Permanent press
Soil release
New wool
Virgin wool
Reprocessed wool
Reused wool

EXERCISES

1. Visit the Web site of any major textile trade association featured in this chapter to request materials about its organization. Using the acquired information, prepare a report on the manner in which it serves the textile fiber it represents.
2. Cut narrow strips of paper, eight inches long, and construct "fabrics" that use the basket weave, a six-float satin weave, and a twill weave. Take the constructions to a fabric retailer and locate swatches of material that use the same techniques you have used in your task. Mount them in pairs, side by side on a foam board, so that the class can compare your work with the pieces obtained at the store.
3. Examine a number of issues of fashion apparel and home furnishings magazines for the purpose of collecting designs that reveal their fiber contents. Prepare a presentation on foam board for five designs used and their benefits to the consumer.

Review Questions

1. In addition to the aesthetics of the fabric, what else must be considered before it is used in the manufacture of a garment, accessory, or upholstery?
2. What is the difference between the terms *fiber* and *yarn?*
3. What are the four natural fibers and their characteristics?
4. Why has cotton remained a favorite of the apparel, accessories, and home furnishings industries and the consumer market?
5. Describe the construction used in producing velvet, denim, and sateen.
6. What purpose does the hackling stage in flax production serve?
7. What are the major differences between woolens and worsteds?
8. In what way does the natural silk fiber differ from cotton, flax, and wool?
9. Name four hair fibers and a characteristic of each.
10. What are the two basic types of manufactured fibers?
11. Why is microfiber hailed as one of the greatest fabric innovations to be produced in the last twenty years?
12. What advantages does polyester afford the wearer?
13. Define the terms *spinning* and *filament processing*.
14. What is a spinneret?
15. How does the basket weave differ from the plain weave?
16. Why is it so difficult to produce a jacquard design? How is the process accomplished?
17. In what way is felting different from weaving or knitting?
18. Define the term *gray goods.*
19. Which dyeing technique allows for color sealing?

20. Describe the process that enables a two-colored piece of fabric to receive its colors.
21. What is the most important consideration when choosing a dye that is to be laundered or worn in the water?
22. Briefly discuss the silk screening process.
23. Define *calendaring, embossing,* and *moireing.*
24. What is the difference between water repellency and waterproofing?
25. Discuss the purpose of the Wool Bureau.

CHAPTER **3**

Leather

After reading this chapter, you should be able to:

- Assess the size of the leather industry and discuss its importance in terms of the apparel, accessories, and home furnishings markets.
- Trace the processing stages that turn hides and skins into materials suitable for consumer use.
- Understand the language of leather used by the industry's professionals.
- Learn how leather products should be cared for to maximize their usefulness.
- Discuss some of the programs and services afforded this industry by its trade associations.

A cyclist roars into town on a Harley Davidson, and an anxious job applicant patiently waits to be interviewed at a prestigious law firm. In these snapshots from completely different worlds, each person uses a common element to underscore his or her presence. What single ingredient could these individuals use in these totally different situations? In a word, the answer is leather! The biker, resplendent in his thick leather garb accentuated by heavy zippers and studs, personifies the "macho" image, whereas the fledgling attorney, her apparel discreetly but prominently accessorized with the "right" Coach leather briefcase, exudes an air of confidence and sophistication. What other single fashion ingredient is capable of quickly establishing an indelible impression for its wearer?

Leather offers something for everyone. Men, women, and children from all walks of life seem to have an increasing fascination for the mystique of this raw material and the array of products fabricated from it (Figure 3.1). The motorcycle jacket has made the transition from the standard gear of the biking world to must-have attire for the fashion conscious by coloring it bright orange or silver or acid washing it to make an even more exciting statement. Printed suedes for special-occasion dressing, plaid leather suits, bomber jackets emblazoned with peace symbols, and ski wear that can be washed by either hand or machine are just some of the industry's creations that have extended the use for this material (Figure 3.2).

In the home furnishings arena, the use of leather has been taken to new heights. Not only is it used in informal room settings on sofas and chairs, but also for accents on accessory throw pillows. Designers are choosing a wealth of exciting colors and patterns, in addition to the standard color palette, to lend excitement to these environments.

The days when leather was thought of as merely a serviceable material have long passed. Its functional qualities coupled with its many fashion orientations and uses make it an exceptional material for designers to use to reach many markets.

With significant technological advances that have enabled leather designers to silkscreen colorful prints and patterns and create a variety of soft textures, the industry continues to expand. Today, according to the Leather Apparel Industry, leather boasts sales of more than $3 billion annually. With its continued acceptance in all phases of fashion, the future is even more promising.

The three major world centers of cattle producers for leather are the United Sates, Russia, and Western Europe. Argentina, Brazil, and Mexico also figure prominently in cattle production.

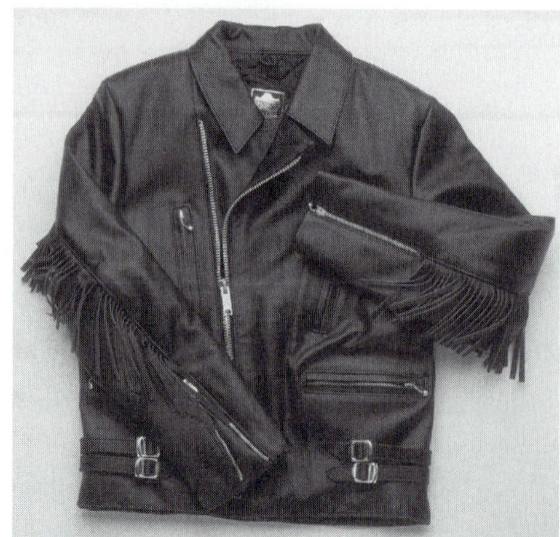

Figure 3.1 Fringe gives this leather jacket a fashionable flair.
(Courtesy of Dorling Kindersley Media Library, Dave King.)

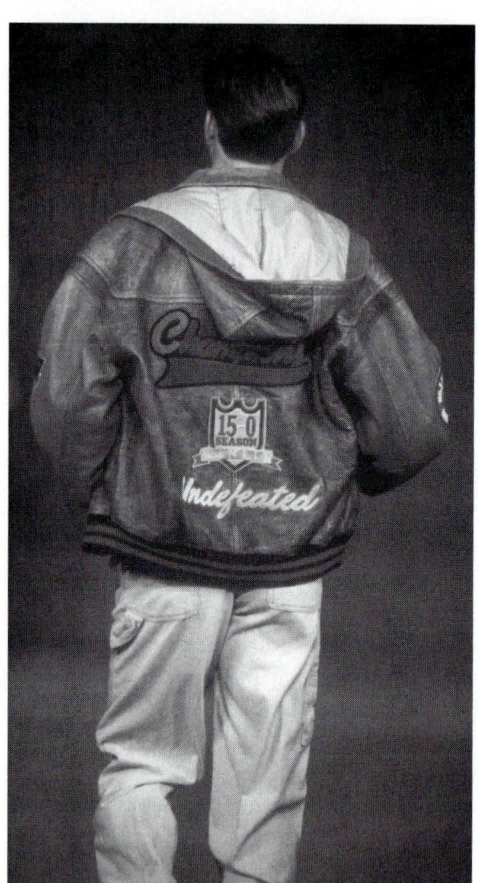

Figure 3.2 This hooded jacket combines fashion and function.
(Courtesy of Ellen Diamond.)

LEATHER CATEGORIES

Leather is the general term for all hides and skins with their original fiber structure more or less left intact. The hair may or may not have been removed from the **hides** (pelts of the larger animals) or **skins** (pelts from smaller animals).

Numerous animal groups are used in the production of leather for apparel, accessories, and home furnishings. They and their specific uses are:

Cattle. Steer, cow, and bull hides are used for shoe and slipper outsoles and heels, briefcases, gloves, garments, handbags, wallets, and furniture upholstery. Large calves or undersized cattle (collectively, the producers of **kipskins** or **kips**) are used to manufacture shoe uppers and linings, gloves, garments, and hats.

Sheep and lamb. The wooled skins, hair skins, and shearlings typical of this group are used for shoes, gloves, garments, pants, handbags, hats, and accent rugs.

Goat and kid. The skins in this classification are used for shoe uppers, fancy leather handbags, gloves, and garments.

Equine. Horse, colt, and zebra produce leather that is primarily for shoe uppers and soles, gloves, and garments.

Buffalo. Both domesticated land and water buffalo hides are used for shoe soles and uppers, fancy leather goods, portfolios, and handbags.

Pig and hog. This group includes the skins from the pig, hog, and boar, but also the peccary and carpincho variety of pigs, characterized by special markings. Collectively, this classification is used for gloves, fancy leather products, and shoe uppers.

Deer. Fallow deer, reindeer, antelope, gazelle, elk, and caribou skins produce leather for shoe uppers, gloves, apparel, fancy leather accessories, and moccasins.

Kangaroo and wallaby. Their use is restricted to shoe uppers.

Exotics and fancies. Frog, seal, shark, walrus, and turtles are the aquatics of the group; camel, elephant, ostrich, and pangolin are the land classification; and alligator, crocodile, lizard, and snake represent the reptiles. Each has distinctive characteristics and markings that make them appropriate for unusual apparel and accessories.

All of these hides and skins must be processed before they can be used in production.

PHYSICAL PROPERTIES OF LEATHER

As we learned in the previous chapter on textiles, different fibers have different characteristics and properties that make many of them unique for specific purposes. The laboratories have engineered man-made fibers that give us an enormous range and variety of colors. With leather, however, the material is natural and, except for certain finishing applications during processing, the inherent properties in all hides and skins are virtually the same. Not only does its beauty enhance any design, but its physical properties make the final products functional as well as fashionable.

Tensile Strength

Leather is extremely high in terms of tensile strength. By definition, it can withstand a significant amount of stress without tearing apart. The material must undergo extensive stretching in initial processing and then later by the manufacturers of shoes, in particular, who must significantly stretch the leather over lasts, or forms on which construction takes place. Therefore, excellent tensile strength is important.

Tear Strength

When compared with textiles, leather is far superior in terms of its ability to resist tearing. When fabrics are used, except for felt, it is necessary to turn the edge of the material and sew it so that it will not fray or tear. With leather, however, this is rarely necessary and, even in the cases necessary for punched holes or slits, stitching is not generally essential for additional tear resistance.

Elongation

Leather is versatile in terms of elongation; it can be stretched to varying lengths without fear of breaking. The elongation property can be controlled, as the need arises, when **tanning**, or preserving, and fat liquoring take place, as we discuss in the next section on "Processing Leather."

Flexibility

The flexibility of leather under a wide range of temperatures is considerable. When properly tanned or preserved, it will usually withstand the problems of brittleness and cracking due to cold and heat. It is also a perfect performer when wet.

Absorption

Leather absorbs water as well as moisture from the air and removes it from other materials with which it comes into contact. This is particularly important for shoes in which perspiration is absorbed from the lining materials and quickly spread throughout the leather uppers for greater foot comfort.

Breathing and Insulating

If you have ever worn a plastic or man-made leather imitation, you probably noticed that they can cause the feet to feel hot and uncomfortable. A leather jacket, when worn in either cool or warm climates, adjusts to the outside temperatures. The secret is its absorbency and insulating properties. It is significantly porous and adjusts to various climate conditions.

Lasting Moldability

When leather is forced over a form such as a shoe last, it conforms to it and retains that shape not only during the period of lasting but during all the years it is worn.

All of these combinations have made leather a unique material that far outshines imitations.

PROCESSING LEATHER

The processing of hides and skins into leather requires 20 individual stages before it may be used for apparel, accessories, and upholstery coverings. All of these operations bear a certain relationship to each other, and the tanner must exercise strict control of these stages to head off problems.

Receiving and Storage

The hides and skins arrive in a cured state that protects them from protein-destroying organisms. At the hide house, they are sorted for thickness and weighed into bundles. Each bundle is marked and identified in terms of size, weight, type of skin, and any other information that would be helpful for later processing. The hides or skins then travel through the tannery as a unit or a batch.

Soaking

As a result of the curing process, the hides and skins will have lost a lot of moisture. This must now be restored, so that the chemical processing that follows can fulfill its purpose.

The soaking is done in water to which chemical wetting agents and disinfectants are added. Proper soaking takes from eight to twenty hours, depending on the thickness of the hides, after which they are cleaner, softer, and easier to manipulate.

Unhairing

Through either mechanical or chemical means, the hides are now ready to have the hair, epidermis, and certain soluble proteins removed. In cases in which the removed hair is to be used for other commercial purposes, the hair-save process is used. This does not destroy the hair, as in the other techniques, but merely destroys the hair root, leaving the hair itself to be mechanically recovered. After the hair is removed, it is washed and dried and sold to textile manufacturers for use in making felt.

Trimming and Siding

A conveyor belt with a circular blade now removes the heads, long shanks, and other areas. Leaving them in place would interfere with the tannery equipment, and because these perimeter areas do not make good leather, they serve no purpose.

Fleshing

The hides and skins are then mechanically **fleshed** to rid them of excess flesh, fat, and muscle on their undersides or flesh sides. The machine is composed of a number of rollers, the most important of which is a cylinder with many cutting blades. Each hide is stretched to full width during this process to prevent bunching up, thus allowing the flesh to be totally removed.

Bating

After the flesh and hair have been eliminated, the residual chemicals from the prior stages of processing must be removed. **Bating** is a twofold procedure. The first step eliminates the lime and alkaline chemicals, and the second adds the bate, enzymes similar to those found in the digestive systems of animals. After the chemical agents have finished their jobs, the hides are again washed to rid them of all of the substances that this process has loosened or dissolved.

Pickling

Before the actual tannage, one last preparatory step called **pickling** remains. The hides are placed in an acid bath ready to receive the tanning materials used in chrome tanning, a procedure addressed in the next stage. Salt or brine is then added to the acid bath to attract and tie up the excess moisture that would otherwise cause the fibers to swell. This operation is a preserving technique, which allows the hides and skins to stay in this condition for long periods of time until they are needed.

Tanning

There are different ways in which hides and skins may be tanned or preserved. Any method chosen serves the same purpose, to convert the raw collagen fibers of the hides or skins into a stable product that is no longer susceptible to rotting.

Preservation may be accomplished through the application of oak bark, oils, or vegetable substances or, for the majority of the cases, with the use of chromium sulfate, referred to in the industry as chrome. Where oak and vegetable tannage takes several weeks to accomplish, chrome tannage is completed in four to six hours.

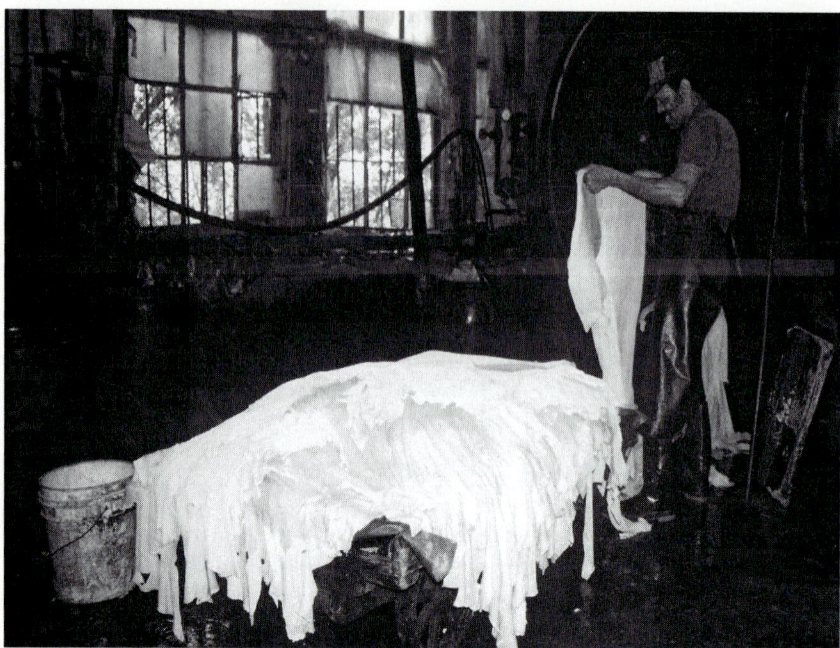

Figure 3.3 The wringing process removes excess moisture during processing. *(Courtesy of Ellen Diamond.)*

Chrome tannage produces the best-quality leather suitable for garments and accessories, and, because of the speed of operation, it certainly benefits the industries that need leather for their products.

Wringing and Sorting

At this point, the hides and skins undergo a wringing process that removes the excess moisture that has been picked up in some of the preceding stages of processing (Figure 3.3). After the moisture has been removed, the skins are sorted according to their thicknesses. The sorting is necessary because many will have to be split, as described in the next phase.

Splitting and Shaving

Hides and skins vary in degree and uniformity of their thickness. Because these variations could cause problems, any differences must be eliminated. A **splitting** machine receives the hides and skins and slices them, yielding a top or grain portion of uniform thickness and an underneath layer that is called the *split* (Figure 3.4). Sometimes, the splits in some hides are sufficiently thick to be used by themselves as leather. Because the top layers have been removed during the process, the remaining splits are void of any grain and are sometimes further processed for other uses. Suede, for example, may be a split that has been napped to raise the surface, making a valuable leather for apparel and shoe uppers.

After splitting has been accomplished, a shaving machine is used to produce a hide with overall exact thickness specifications and to open the fiber structure to enhance further processing with chemicals.

Retanning, Coloring, and Fat Liquoring

The hides are again placed in drums to perform these operations. Although each serves a different purpose in the industry, they follow one another for approximately four to six hours without interruption and are considered as a unit.

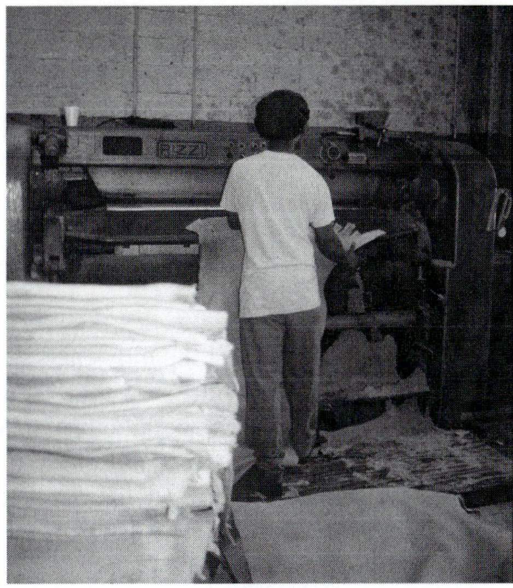

Figure 3.4 Leather hides and skins are sliced, or "split," for uniformity and to produce two layers. *(Courtesy of Ellen Diamond.)*

RETANNING

Retanning combines different tanning agents such as vegetable extracts, syntans, and mineral compounds that give the leather many valuable properties.

COLORING

The demands for leather as a fashion material requires that it be produced in many different colors. Dyeing leather is an art unto itself. Unlike the natural and man-made fibers used in fabrics that are simply colored, leather dyers must contend with several other factors not usually considered for those substances.

Being products of nature, there are built-in variabilities among hides and skins such as differences in pigmentation and grain characteristics. Although shade variations often enhance the beauty of the leather, significant coloration differences make them visibly unappealing. Another problem is the penetration of leather with dyes. One dye can rarely be used to reach the depths of the leather, requiring the combination of two or more that will work well together.

Aniline-type dyes, derived from petroleum, are used as coloring agents. They are dissolved in hot water and added to the rotating drum as the retanning step is being completed. The dyes combine with the hide fibers to form an insoluble compound that becomes part of the hide itself. How long the leather is exposed to the dye influences the resultant shade.

Literally hundreds of dyes are used today, with each offering specific benefits and properties such as resistance to fading, bleeding, and crocking (friction) and the capability to undergo dry cleaning and laundering.

The most commonly used dyes include:

- ***Acid dyes*** that easily and quickly penetrate the leather and impart a bright, lively array of colors.
- ***Metalized dyes*** that produce subdued, pastel tints.
- ***Direct dyes*** for surface use when deep shades are required.
- ***Basic dyes*** for enhancement of surfaces requiring brilliant shades.

FAT LIQUORING

To lubricate the leathers and increase their softness, **fat liquoring** is an additional wet operation makes them more pliable and increases their strength. By using oils and related fatty substances from animal, vegetable, and mineral sources, collectively known as *fat liquors*, the tanner can produce leathers that range from a firmness that is needed for shoe and boot construction and upholstery coverings to a suppleness found in today's fashion apparel.

Setting Out

Moisture must be removed again and is done so in this final stage of the wet operations. The hides are smoothed and stretched, which compresses and squeezes out the excess moisture.

Drying

Different methods are used to dry the leather. As the simplest technique, hanging requires nothing more than draping the hides and skins over a horizontal shaft and letting them dry just as you would with garments on a clothesline. To quicken the process, the pieces are moved through a large oven by means of a conveyor belt. Temperature control is imperative and usually kept at 130 degrees to minimize shrinkage.

Toggling, another drying technique, requires the use of toggles or clips, which keep the hides and skins in a stretched position. They are attached to frames that are moved along and passed through drying ovens.

Most of today's leathers are dried by means of pasting (Figure 3.5). The hides and skins are actually pasted onto 6-by-11 surface plates that are attached to a continuously moving monorail system. After the plates are scrubbed and wiped dry, a spray gun spreads a paste

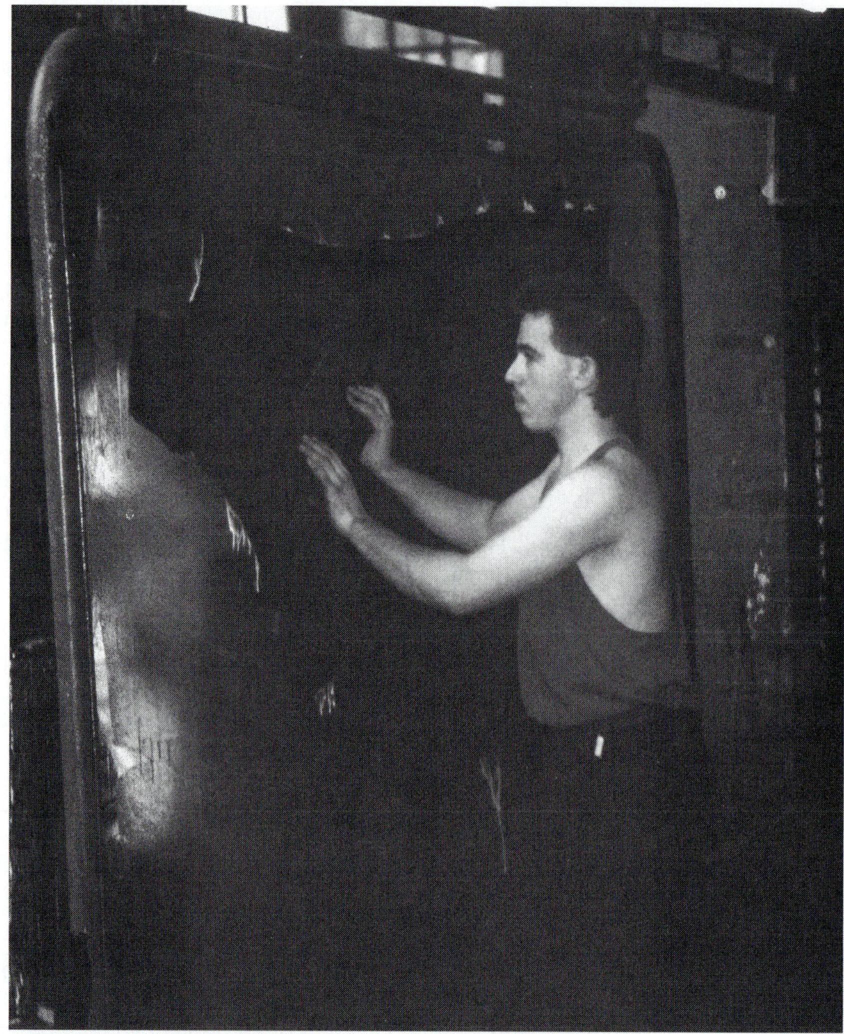

Figure 3.5 After coloring, the leather is smoothed on this frame and left to dry. *(Courtesy of Ellen Diamond.)*

over them that provides sufficient adhesion for the largest of hides. After the drying phase, the hides are stripped or peeled from the frames.

Vacuum drying is the newest of the drying techniques. This system involves the smoothing of a wet hide onto a heated stainless-steel plate covered by a perforated steel plate that, in turn, is covered by cloth. A vacuum then extracts the moisture from the leather.

Conditioning

Sometimes, the leather available at this point is too hard for use in garments and shoes. A specific degree of softness or suppleness, usually referred to in the trade as *temper*, is needed. The **conditioning** treatment requires wetting back, which involves the spraying of a fine mist of water to the leather surfaces. Several pieces of leather are then layered on each other onto a table and fitted with a watertight cover. The leather is left to dry overnight to permit uniformity of moisture.

Staking and Dry Milling

To make leather even more pliable, it is then mechanically **staked.** Through an automated procedure, the leather is carried by a conveyor belt between a large number of oscillating, overlapping fingers. Those fingers pound, hundreds of times from above and below, as the leather passes through the machines, stretching it in all directions. The sophisticated machinery today is capable of staking up to 300 large hides per hour and more than 500 smaller skins at the same time. Any excess moisture is removed through additional drying.

A different type of softening is used when soft, lightweight leathers are being produced for supple garments. The dried leather is thrown into a large dry drum and tumbled anywhere from one-half to eight hours until the dried softness and grain patterns are achieved.

Buffing

Because of the natural blemishes inherent in the leather or the scratches that might have been produced along the way, the appearances of the hides and skins usually need improvement. Although some of these markings are indicators of the authenticity of the material as leather and not a synthetic, imperfections need to be minimized. A **buffing** machine that uses a sand cylinder with an abrasive material smoothes the leather. The sanding leaves a clean, smooth surface that is now ready to receive any other finishes. Because the buffing leaves some dust on the surface, it must be removed through either rotary brushes, jets of compressed air, or vacuuming.

Finishing

To enhance the appearance of the leather and render it more serviceable, a number of finishes are used (Figure 3.6). Today's fashion leather apparel, accessories, and home furnishings indicate the use of many different procedures to give the final products their unique beauty and function. Color, initially applied during an earlier stage, may be made opaque at this point with the addition of certain pigments. Many sophisticated materials are available such as acrylate, vinyl polymers, nitrocellulose, and polyurethane that are used as coatings to render the articles resistant to abrasion and staining.

Plating

At this stage, the decision is made as to whether the leather is to have a smooth or textured appearance. **Plating** is the final step that influences these looks. The process is similar to high-pressure, hot ironing. The coating materials that have been applied are now firmly affixed to the leather. Generally, the finishing and plating procedures span four or five days, alternating each finish with another plating and repeating the operations until all have been accomplished.

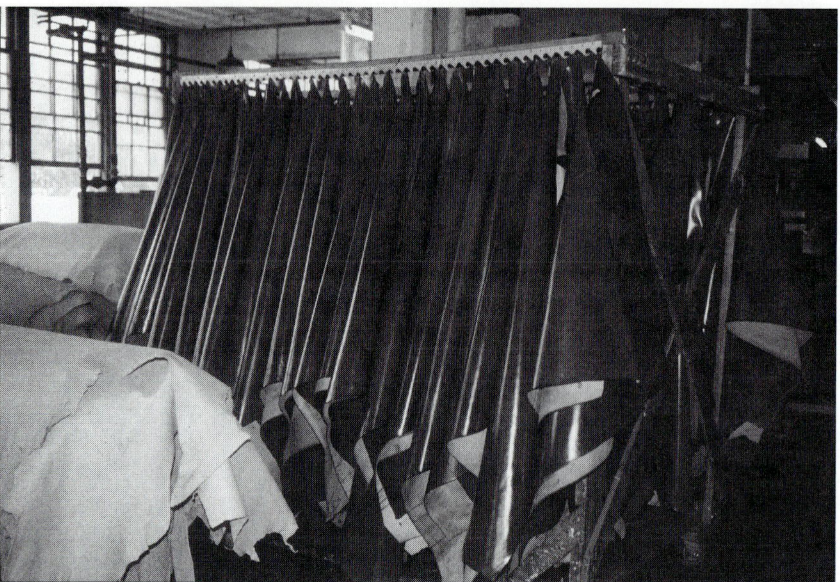

Figure 3.6 This colored, finished leather is ready for use in a variety of products. *(Courtesy of Ellen Diamond.)*

If a textured surface is desired, embossing presses capable of extremely high pressure are used. Embossing machines that are fitted with engraved plates can impregnate any desired pattern on the leather. In the case of splits, where there is no natural grain, this process significantly improves the appearance.

Grading

The leather is now graded according to thickness and color uniformity and the extent of any defects on the surface. These final **grading** measurements will dictate the price and use of the leather.

Measuring

Leather is sold to apparel, accessories, and home furnishing manufacturers on the basis of its area or size. Unlike fabric, it is irregularly shaped and requires measurement by a special machine. With the use of photoelectric cells and built-in computers, the square footage is assessed. The hides pass over a sensing device by a conveyor as a machine automatically calculates the footage. The measurements are then stamped on the flesh side of each piece.

Having gone through twenty operations for approximately four weeks, the leather is now ready to move on to the designers and manufacturers who will transform it into salable products.

FASHION LEATHER TERMINOLOGY

With the advanced technology used in the processing and finishing of leather, today's fashion consumers are the beneficiary. Through advertisements, promotions, and eager sales associates, they are alerted to a variety of new names and terms used by the industry. Some of those that are commonly heard in the purchasing market are listed for general review.

Nubuck. A leather that is lightly buffed until it takes on a fine nap that appears smoother than suede. Many of the silky suede skirts, pants, or blazers are made of nubuck.

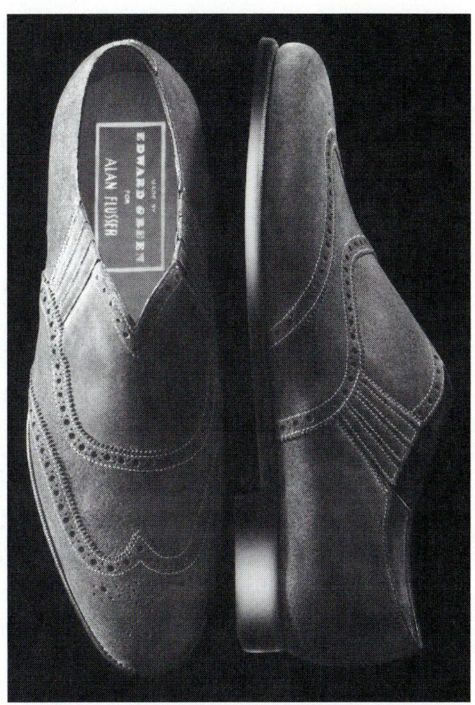

Figure 3.7 These casual shoes are made from buffed cowhide.
(Courtesy of Alan Flusser Custom Shop, James T. Murray Photography, © 2005.)

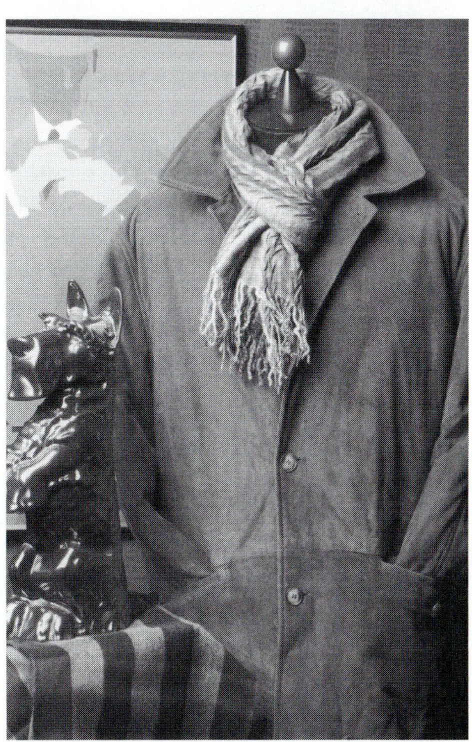

Figure 3.8 Suede jackets are made by buffing the hide's underside.
(Courtesy of Alan Flusser Custom Shop, James T. Murray Photography, © 2005.)

Buffed cowhide. Similar to nubuck except that the finish is more matte than nap; it is used often for casual shoe uppers (Figure 3.7).

Napa. A soft leather hide with a shiny, smooth, or pebbly surface.

Suede. A velvetlike surface created by buffing the underside of a hide (Figure 3.8).

Full-grain leather. When the top grain or surface is not manipulated to change it appearance; it is the best-quality leather.

Split. When new layers are created from slicing a thick hide.

Lamb leather. One of the softest and most expensive types of leather.

Shrunken lamb. A more pebbly grained leather that is achieved during the tanning process.

Distressed leather. Uneven coloration and markings achieved during tanning to give leather a fashionable, weathered appearance.

Painted leather. Opaque pigments or other materials that are applied to the leather's surface.

Aniline leather. Natural characteristics of the leather that are emphasized; transparent dyes are used in coloration.

Calfskin. Skin from a young female cow.

Cowhide. Heavy, durable leather from a mature female cow.

Embossed. Prints, commonly reptile, heat-pressed onto the surface.

Glazed finish. Surface polished to a high luster by pressurized glass or steel rollers.

Grain. Refers to the outer surface or markings or patterns on the leather's surface.

Patent. Heavily finished to give a highly lustrous, baked-enamel-type appearance.

Pearlized. Spray-on finish giving pearlized effect.

Pigskin. From pigs or hogs, commonly used for suede.

Shearling. Natural lamb pelts with the leather side often sueded and worn on the outside.

LEATHER MANUFACTURING GUIDELINES

As with any other material, natural or man-made, certain precautions must be taken when leather is made into products. The nature of the material and its relatively expensive cost to the consumer make the maintenance of specific standards important to ensure that appropriate materials are used to produce leather garments, accessories, and upholstery.

The Leather Apparel Association has developed a set of guidelines for the industry to benefit manufacturers and consumers.

The guidelines cover a wide range of areas such as the fabricating materials used in production, including glues, inner components, trims, and ornamentation.

Glues

Glues should either dissolve completely or not at all when immersed in cleaning solvents. In cases where total dissolve is important, rubber cement is suggested. When only partial dissolving is realized, unsightly markings might be permanently affixed. Testing the glue is necessary before any final decisions are made.

Tanner Identification Marks

Ink used for logos or codes stenciled on the back of unfinished skins have been known to bleed, or run, during the cleaning process. It is better to place these identification marks on scrap edges so that they can be removed during cleaning.

Inner Components

Interfacings should not be secured with glues that might dissolve during cleaning because they tend to shift and distort the garment. Polyester or other fill that increases warmth should be securely tacked at intervals to prevent shifting and distortion.

Linings

White or light pilings should be made removable when used with dark leathers because some of the garment color might run during dry cleaning and discolor the linings.

Buttons

As some types of buttons melt when placed in solvents, they should be tested first before they are attached. Although replacing buttons seems to be a simple procedure, the disintegrated buttons will often adhere to the leather, ruining the garment.

Zippers

Thin plastic zippers should be avoided because they may melt. Heavy plastic or metal is preferred.

Combining Fabrics

Many garments combine leather with other decorative fabrics. Some have different shrinking tendencies; these must be assessed to avoid damage from cleaning.

Embossed Designs

If thin, weak leather is embossed, the patterns can be altered during cleaning. Test cleaning is recommended to determine if the embossed leather can withstand the solvents.

Multicolored Garments

If more than one color is used, the garment should be test cleaned to make certain that one color will not bleed into another.

Cleaning Outfits

Because one part of an outfit may require cleaning and the other not, it is important to test and make certain that the two will match after the cleaning process.

EMBELLISHING LEATHER

Many leathers used in fashion products are embellished to add glamour. Some of the methods used include beading and fringes (Figure 3.9).

CARE OF LEATHER

With the significant expense involved in the purchase of leather garments, accessories, and upholstered furniture, it is imperative that strict attention is paid to the care of these products. Without these precautions, the life of the product might be shortened and the aesthetic quality hampered. These safeguards are not only beneficial to consumers, but also to manufacturers who can avoid problems by passing safeguards on to their retail clients.

1. Garments should be stored on broad hangars and free to breathe the air. Plastic coverings should be avoided to prevent the leather from drying out.
2. When caught in the rain, the leather should be left to dry naturally. Heat will cause damage.
3. Wrinkles will generally iron themselves out. If pressing is necessary, place a layer of heavy paper between the garment and the iron, which should be on a low setting without steam.
4. Hems may be repaired at home with a small bit of rubber cement.
5. Hair sprays and perfumes should not touch the garments, and neither pins nor badges should be attached. All of these could cause irreparable damage.

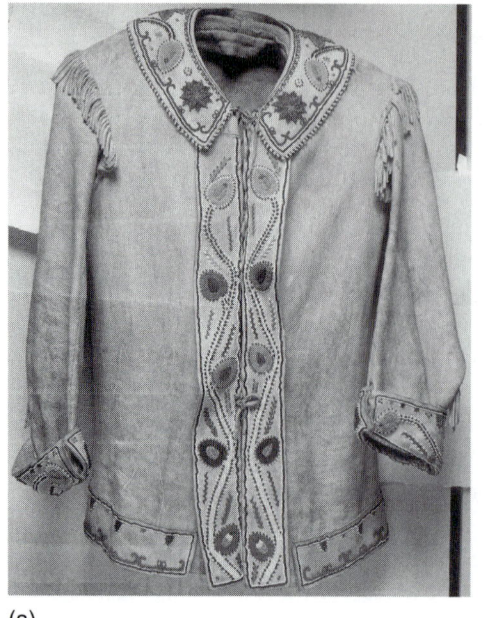

(a)

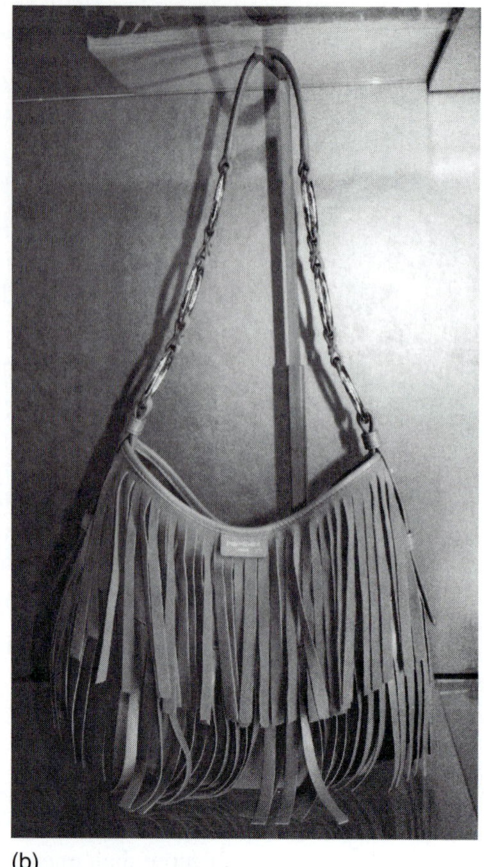

(b)

(c)

Figure 3.9 (a) Beading adds pizzazz to leather. *(Courtesy of Dorling Kindersley Media Library, Lynton Gardiner.)* (b) Fringe turns sueded leather into a fashion standout. *(Courtesy of Ellen Diamond.)* (c) Leather teamed with "torn" jeans completes this contemporary look. *(Courtesy of Donna Karan International.)*

6. Dirt may be wiped away with a soft, dry sponge or cloth. Napped surfaces may be brushed.
7. Make certain that if you use a conditioner, it is appropriate for your type of leather.
8. Professional, special dry cleaning is necessary to maintain the garment. Traditional dry cleaning techniques could cause damage.
9. Matched garments should be cleaned together because most treatments will change the color.
10. Water and stain repellent agents may be applied. They should be used immediately after purchasing of the garment and after each cleaning.

TRADE ASSOCIATIONS

As in every other industry, associations have been organized to help members address the problems associated with their businesses and to provide information to make the industry more responsive to consumer needs. One of the oldest is Leather Industries of America, which was founded in 1917, and one of the newest is the Leather Apparel Association. A brief description of their respective goals and efforts captures their missions.

Leather Industries of America

In its own words, this association seeks "to foster, develop, and promote scientifically the art of tanning and the leather industry, and the mutual welfare and improvement of those engaged therein, and to supervise, classify, and systematize the exportation, importation, and distribution of hides, skins, leather, tanning materials, and their products."

Leather Industries of America (LIA) assists its members by interfacing with the government to intercede in the problems associated with exports and trade restrictions; maintaining a research laboratory to provide technical and environmental information on leather; offering technical education through the presentation of seminars; supplying statistical services on imports and exports, trends, offshore competition, and the nation's economy; and arranging shows and meetings such as The Accessory and Garment Leather Show in New York, the USA/LIA Pavilions at the Hong Kong International Trade Fair, and the Semaine du Cuir, the world's largest international leather fair.

Leather Apparel Association

This not-for-profit organization was established in 1990 to "sponsor the industry's aggressive marketing campaign to increase the demand for leather garments and associated products and services."

Unlike the LIA, this organization is specifically associated with the manufacturers of leather outerwear, sportswear, evening wear, and active wear. It does not represent tanners.

The Leather Apparel Association develops consumer and trade publicity programs, educational materials, and extensive advertising and market research to help each company in its membership build a stronger, broader, more profitable business. Its membership network includes both large and small organizations.

Internet Resources for Additional Research

www.absoluteastronomy.com/encyclopediá/l/le/leather.htm provides information and analysis of the world of leather.

www.pawscave.dircon.co.uk/IML/leath.htm offers information on the differing costs of leather.

Merchandise Information Terminology

Hides
Skins
Kipskins (kips)
Tanning
Fleshing
Bating
Pickling
Splitting
Retanning
Acid dye
Metalized dye
Direct dye
Basic dye
Fat liquoring
Conditioning
Staking
Buffing
Plating
Grading
Nubuck
Buffed cowhide
Napa
Suede
Full-grain leather
Split
Lamb leather
Shrunken lamb
Distressed leather
Painted leather
Aniline leather
Calfskin
Cowhide
Embossed
Glazed finish
Grain
Patent leather
Pearlized leather
Pigskin
Shearling

EXERCISES

1. Secure as many different types of leather as possible and mount each on a foam board for display to the class. Along with each swatch, indicate the uses of each and any technical information on dyeing and finishes. Scraps and swatches are available from many sources. You may write to a tanner (enter the keyword *leather* on a search engine), visit retailers who specialize in leather furniture and offer a variety of swatches, or write to leather garment and shoe manufacturers (their names are also easily found by using a search engine). Prepare a five-minute talk to accompany the visual aid presentation you have created.
2. Examine a variety of fashion and home décor magazines and cut out five of each of the following leather goods:
   a. handbags
   b. gloves
   c. shoes
   d. wallets
   e. attaches and briefcases
   f. sofas and chairs

Review Questions

1. Which countries dominate in cattle production for use in leather products?
2. Define the term *leather.*
3. List five animals whose hides and skins are used for leather apparel, accessories, and home furnishings.
4. What are three properties of leather that make it so serviceable as a fashion material?
5. Why must leather be tanned before it is used commercially?
6. Why is chrome tannage favored over other methods?
7. Differentiate between *full-grain leather* and *split leather.*
8. List three major dyes used in leather coloring along with the benefits of each.
9. Why are leathers buffed after they have been staked and dry milled?
10. What is nubuck?
11. Describe aniline leather.
12. Explain why specific glues should be tested before they are used in leather construction.
13. Why should tanner identification marks be placed on scrap edges of the leather?
14. List five ways in which the consumer should care for his or her leather product.
15. How do the LIA and the Leather Apparel Association differ?

CHAPTER **4**

Furs

After reading this chapter, you should be able to:

- Discuss the state of the industry and its major characteristics.
- Explain the techniques used in fur farming and the role the industry plays in setting standards for its procedures.
- Describe the various stages of fur processing and the techniques used to construct fur garments and accessories.
- Prepare a list of different types of furs and the characteristics that distinguish each group.
- Discuss how the fur industry has expanded from one that primarily produced garments for special occasions to present the product as everyday apparel.

The arrival of elegantly dressed women at special galas often overshadows the events themselves. Although the opening of New York City's Metropolitan Opera season heralds the beginning of an artistic series, the stories and photographs that accompany the event, as seen in the pages of *W* magazine and the *New York Times*, sometimes seems more important than the reviews of the performance. Similarly, the purpose of the charitable gala is often shadowed by photojournalists' reports on the attendees' costumes. Fashion attention on these events during the fall and winter season usually focuses on their extravagant furs (Figure 4.1). Because the "paparazzi" are usually not allowed to enter the occasions' arenas and are therefore unable to capture the essence of what the patrons are wearing, they station themselves on the outside and record the fur creations for all the world to admire. Although this generates excitement for the industry, it is not the only market served.

Furs today are likely to be worn in everyday life. The woman hurrying to work may emerge from a taxicab or bus dressed in a mink coat. Shoppers similarly stroll the aisles of their favorite stores dressed in garments that were once reserved for more formal occasions. Even men, although the number pales by comparison with their female counterparts, are fur wearers (Figure 4.2). Young and old, the affluent and those with more limited disposable income, and people from all walks of life have embraced the fur garment as one that is not merely showy but also functional. With these new markets and a significant range of price points, the fur industry has branched out and successfully expanded its horizons (Figure 4.3).

The fur industry is made up of several segments, each of which performs a specific task before the garment reaches the sales floor. This chapter explores those segments, the marketing of the product, the types of furs available for use in apparel and accessories, the various techniques used in transforming them into garments, and the rules that were enacted to set standards for fur.

MAJOR SEGMENTS OF THE INDUSTRY

By the time consumers have a selection of fur garments and accessories from which they may choose, each product has passed through a variety of professional hands. The experts, who transform the "skins of the animals with the hair intact," the technical definition of fur, fit into three general classifications: the farmers and trappers, the processors, and the designers and manufacturers.

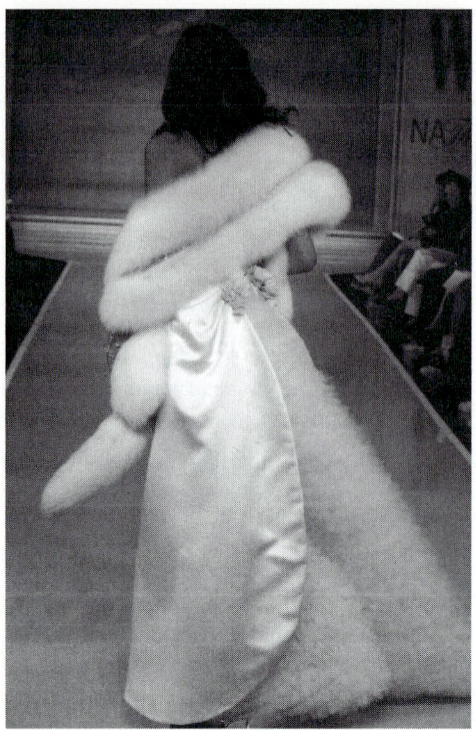

Figure 4.1 Fur stoles are used to enhance exciting ball gowns.
(Courtesy of Fur Information Council of America.)

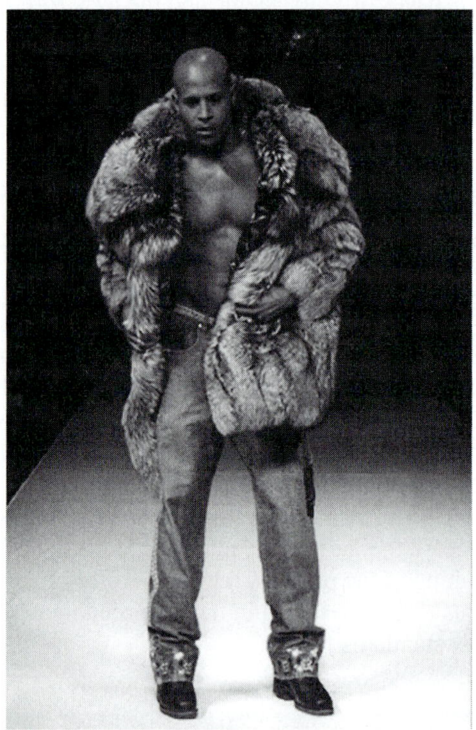

Figure 4.2 More and more men are wearing furs for every occasion.
(Courtesy of Fur Information Council of America.)

Farmers and Trappers

More than three-quarters of the fur produced in North America is raised on family farms, primarily based in Wisconsin, Minnesota, and Utah in the United States and Ontario and Quebec in Canada. Approximately 3,700 **fur farming** operations sell more than six million pelts annually at a $230 million price tag.

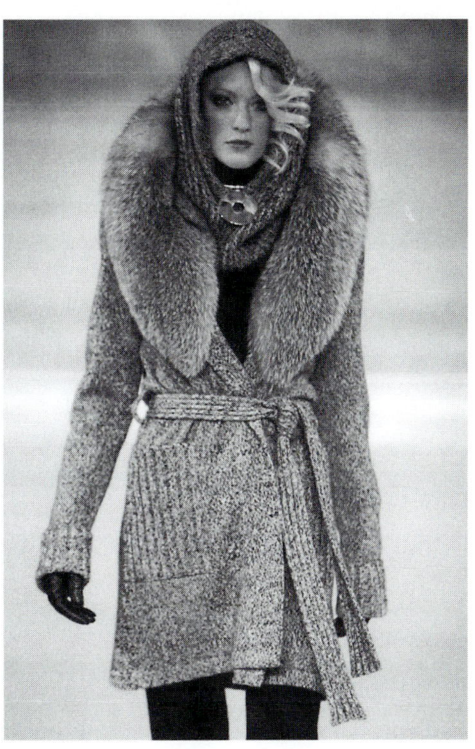

Figure 4.3 Fur trim has become a popular addition to knitted coats.
(Courtesy of Fur Information Council of America.)

Standards for the industry were developed by the farmers themselves and are administered by the Fur Farm Animal Welfare Coalition in the United States and by the Mink Breeders Association in Canada. The guidelines address such areas as farming methods, nutrition, veterinary care, and humane harvesting procedures. Coming under attack from a variety of organizations such as **People for the Ethical Treatment of Animals (PETA),** the industry has recognized the need to develop sound farming principles that cause little, if any, discomfort to the animals. The young farmer of today generally has a college degree in agriculture, biology, or business and serves at least one year of apprenticeship on a well-established farm to learn the complete annual fur production cycle.

Trappers are responsible for the procurement of furs in the wild. They no longer trap endangered species, thanks to careful control regulations at the national and international levels. Wildlife managers oversee the production, setting trapping seasons and applying quotas where necessary. Research is ongoing in the industry to make certain that the most humane methods of trapping are employed. Aside from the skills passed down from one generation to the next, today's participants learn the latest methods by taking pertinent, educational courses.

The experienced trapper knows precisely how to set the traps to make certain that only the "wanted" animals are snared.

The **pelts,** undressed skins with the hair intact, are most often sold at auction. Trappers generally sell their bounties to agents who resell them to the auction companies or, in some cases, wholesalers who keep inventories from which manufacturers may purchase. Farmers almost always sell their pelts at public auctions to wholesalers, manufacturers, or brokers. The auctions are held all over the world, with major centers located in New York City, Minneapolis, and St. Louis in the United States and London, St. Petersburg, and Montreal abroad.

Processors

Before a pelt can be turned into a salable garment or accessory, it must undergo considerable processing. This includes dressing, dyeing, bleaching, and glazing, all of which are fully discussed later in this chapter.

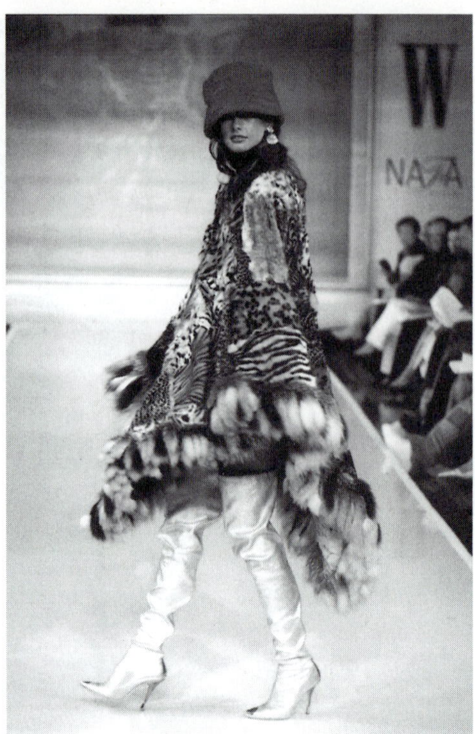

Figure 4.4 High fashion designs are now prevalent in the fur industry.
(Courtesy of Fur Information Council of America.)

Designers and Manufacturers

After the furs have been transformed into viable skins, they are ready to become part of fashion. The fur designer was once a relatively unknown individual working in the back rooms of the manufacturer's headquarters. Most companies had their own designers who primarily approached fashion design using traditional styling and silhouettes. Today, the designer is no longer an unsung hero but the individual who is often responsible for apparel and accessories.

Through the licensing route, where designers are paid to create fur collections for fur manufacturers on a contract basis and allow the companies to use their prestigious names, the industry has taken on an aura of haute couture (Figure 4.4). Names such as Oscar de la Renta, Karl Lagerfeld, and Donna Karan are found in fur salons all over the world. Of course, some unsung heroes still operate in anonymity and help deliver many of the styles to the marketplace.

After the design has been developed, the pelts are ready for production. Matching skins, cutting and sewing, and adding numerous finishing touches are all accomplished at the manufacturer's workrooms. The specifics of these stages are explored in a later section of this chapter.

PROCESSING FUR

When the shipments arrive from the auctions, they are merely undressed pelts that must be transformed into pliable, attractive skins. The feel of the dressed pelt and the beauty it offers to the wearer is a result of considerable conditioning.

Dressing the Pelts

The pelts consist of the skin or leather and two types of hair, the **guard hairs** (longer hairs) and the **fur fiber** (the soft, downlike short hairs). The initial stage oversees the removal of the substances, including flesh, that still adhere to the skin. After this removal comes a soaking and mechanical treatment known as *tanning* or *aging*, which is a process similar to that used in leather conditioning. The skins must now be rendered pliable and workable; the tanning process tends to remove some of the natural oils, which are replaced through a process known as **kicking.** This involves beating the furs against each other, which ultimately restores the lost oils. The excess lubrication necessitates removal, and this is accomplished by placing the furs in a sawdust-filled, rotating drum.

Depending on the desired final appearance of the fur, different processes may now be applied. Many fashion designers, for example, design garments that are to have velvety smooth appearances. In this case, the longer, protective guard hairs must be removed. This calls for either a shearing or plucking procedure; the choice depends on the specific pelt species. After this has been completed, the fur is again cleaned and readied for further refinement.

Dyeing and Bleaching

Many pelts are moved on to the construction area for transformation into a garment. The natural coloration may be used without any changes. Minks, for example, are produced in a variety of natural colors that make significant fashion statements without the need for enhancement. Such skins are generally of the highest quality and their natural beauty fetches better prices.

Lesser quality skins are often dull or color impaired. There might be variation in the **bundle** that requires dyeing for uniformity of color. The designer collections of today are often highlighted by colored fur garments and accessories. It is not because the skins are inferior and necessitate camouflage; the innovative use of color adds another dimension to the line and invites owners of traditional furs to purchase something extra (Figure 4.5). Bold bands of color, harlequin designs, and plaids are just a few of the end results of dyeing.

Depending on the desired effect, different dyeing techniques are used. When total color enhancement is the goal, the entire bundle of skins may be immersed in the dye bath. Not only does this dip dyeing change the fur color, it also colors the leather. If the intention is to enhance the natural color of the pelt, tip dyeing, the brushing of dye only to the hairs, is used. When the need for a particular pattern arises, stencil dyeing is the approach.

The removal of color is sometimes necessary when furs are to be lightened or blemishes need removal. In cases where pale shades are the ultimate goals, bleaching might be required before the application of dye.

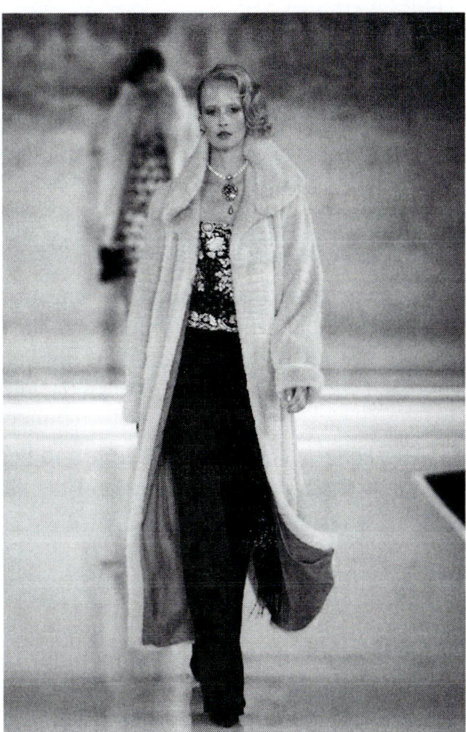

Figure 4.5 Dyeing has added another dimension of furs.
(Courtesy of Fur Information Council of America.)

Glazing

The final step in preparation for the manufacturing process is **glazing.** The fur is first sprayed with water or chemicals and then carefully pressed to add luster, evenness, and a "soft hand." Care must be exercised during this stage to avoid any damage to the skins.

CONSTRUCTING THE GARMENT

The skins are now ready for the transformation into garments by a team of skilled craftspeople. Individuals usually specialize in specific aspects of this operation, applying their expertise to the assembly-line production.

Matching the Skins

To produce a garment that is visually satisfying, the bundle of skins must be carefully arranged on the pattern. The skilled worker aligns the pelts so that they "match" or complement each other, paying attention to hair length, texture, and color, if the skins are to be used in their natural state. Distinctive markings, as in the case of lynx, must lay in close harmony so that the overall pattern will be enhanced. The patterns workers use to **match the skins** are either standard and used to produce ready-to-wear garments or specially detailed to fit a specific customer's exact measurements.

Cutting and Joining

After the skins have been satisfactorily arranged on the pattern, they must be cut and sewn. Depending on the type of fur, its quality, desired appearance, and ultimate cost considerations, a number of different techniques may be used. Furs destined to become inexpensive garments are often machine cut, with hand cutting reserved for more expensive products. One of the following methods is then chosen to join the skins.

SKIN-ON-SKIN CONSTRUCTION

Because most of the pelts are too small to be used without piecing them together, they must be sewn in some manner to produce a fur that is long enough to fill the pattern. In the production of inexpensive fur garments, **skin-on-skin construction** most likely to be used. The operator places one skin below the next and joins them until the desired length is reached. Because many skins are short haired and concealment of the seams is difficult, the end result is a telltale horizontal line around the garment.

LETTING-OUT CONSTRUCTION

To elongate the fur to the necessary length and, at the same time, eliminate the unwanted horizontal seam, the **letting-out** method is the choice. This is time-consuming and costly; thus, it is only used in the construction of quality garments.

Furs such as mink and sable are let-out. A skilled craftsperson first makes a vertical cut down the center of the pelt's dark stripe. The pelt is then cut on the diagonal into 1/8-inch strips. Each strip is then sewn above and below and repositioned into an elongated skin. The dark, center stripe is maintained and the skin is now sufficient in length without having to use horizontal seaming (Figure 4.6).

The let-out skins are then rematched and sewn together to fit the design.

SPLIT-SKIN CONSTRUCTION

Female mink skins are generally favored. They are usually silkier, lighter in weight, and narrower in appearance than their male counterparts. They are also more costly. To create a mink coat or jacket that gives the impression of the sleek, female skin, **split-skin construction** is

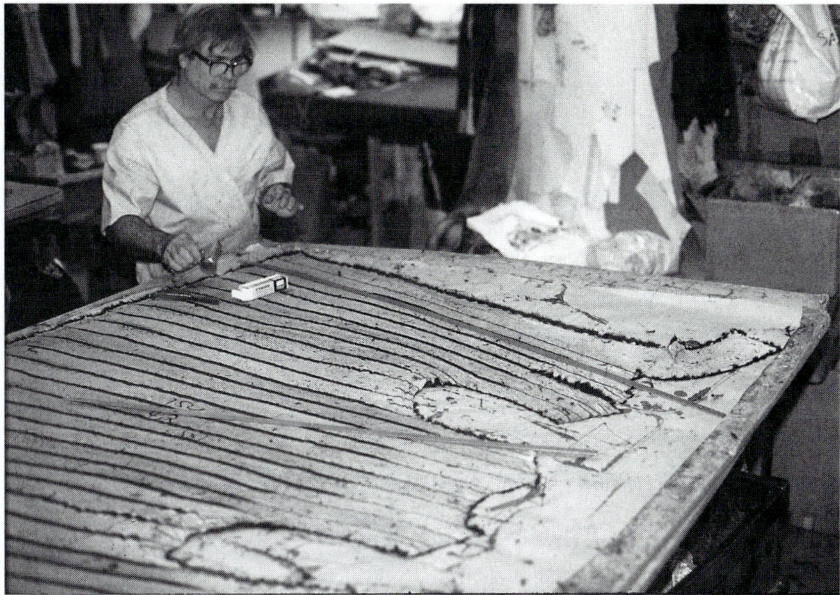

Figure 4.6 A fur technician elongates a mink pelt through the letting-out process. *(Courtesy of Ellen Diamond.)*

often chosen. The operator slices the plump, male skin down the center and now has two fur pieces with which to work. Each piece is then let out and elongated for use in the garment. The construction is still costly; however, the ultimate price is lower because fewer male skins are needed for a coat and because they are less desirable, each coat costs less than one made from the female.

WHOLE-SKIN CONSTRUCTION

When a small jacket or accessory is being produced, a full skin might be sufficient for production. In such cases, sewing or joining the skins is unnecessary. The full skin is merely cut according to the pattern in **whole-skin construction.**

LEATHERING

When bulky fur pelts are used, it is sometimes desirable to insert strips of leather or other materials between the rows of skins to eliminate bulkiness. In **leathering,** each pelt is sewn to a strip, which in turn is sewn to another until the process is competed. The strips may be carefully concealed if the guard hairs are long and bushy, rendering the garment as a full fur. The procedure also reduces the number of pelts needed and therefore makes the garment less costly.

For additional styling, sometimes leather strips are visibly displayed (Figure 4.7). In these cases, designers use a variety of materials in the leathering process.

Assembling the Garment

After the individual skins have been sewn horizontally, as in the case of skin-on-skin construction, or extended and reset through letting-out, the various pieces are assembled into either one large or several small sections. The strips or sections are carefully sewn together by machine. Those pieces are wetted down, aligned on boards to facilitate hand shaping to fit the designer's pattern, and then stapled. When the fur is dry, it will retain the curves and lines of the silhouette.

Closing the garment is the next step, which requires all of the parts to be sewn together by hand. This requires expert workmanship and calls for the most skilled people in fur manufacturing.

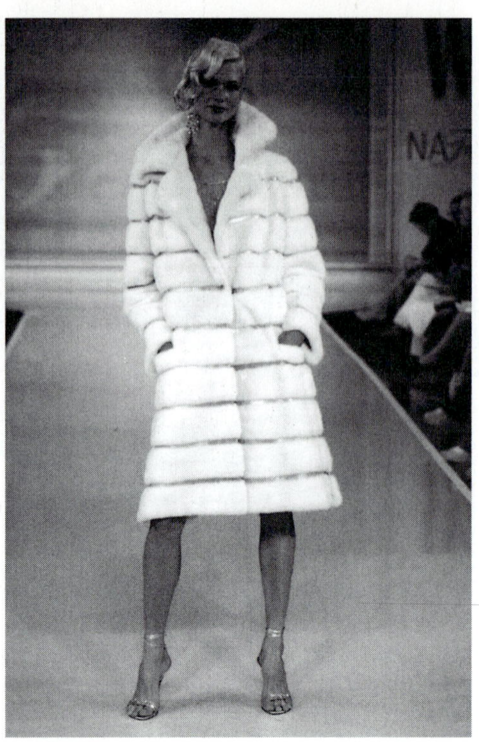

Figure 4.7 The leathering process uses different material inserts between rows of fur.
(Courtesy of Fur Information Council of America.)

Finishing the Garment

The final stage entails sewing the lining to the fur and attaching one of the several closing devices to the garment. Concealed hooks and eyes are used when invisible closure is required. Snaps are not noticeable and might also be used when no break in the line of the product is desired. Many designers are using conspicuous zippers and buttons to add a fashionable dimension to the look. Zippers are usually used for sporty or casual jackets, and buttons are used for any length garment designed to impart a less formal flare.

FURS AND THEIR FAMILIES

Before 1952, consumers were subjected to many invented fur names that added confusion to the selection process. These fur names were created by manufacturers to give credibility to less desirable furs, culminating in purchases that were not exactly what customers thought they were. Names such as "saline," to connote baby seal, and "mouton lamb" were bandied about throughout the industry.

On August 9, 1952, the federal government enacted the Fur Products Labeling Act, later amended a few times to broaden its implications, which set guidelines by which fur manufacturers, wholesalers, and retailers must abide. Advertisements, promotional materials, and garment labels must list the proper English name of the animal used in the product, its country of origin, and any color-altering techniques that were used. Dyed muskrat soon replaced the then-famous "Hudson-seal dyed muskrat." If the garment is composed of waste pieces of fur that have been assembled to give the appearance of full skins, that also must be noted.

This code has taken a great deal of the mystery out of consumer purchasing, but it still has not helped the untrained eye to discern the various subtleties of quality. These are discussed later in the chapter.

Furs are usually classified under their individual names such as mink, fox, and squirrel, each belonging to a specific family group. There are scores of furs to choose from, some more popular than others because of appearance, durability, and fashion acceptance at a particular time. The fashion designers and manufacturers strongly influence which furs are more fashionable at a given time and which furs are less desirable in terms of their fashion appropriateness. Some, such as mink, seem to be the traditional standard bearers and never lose favor through the years.

The Weasel Family

The **weasel family** collectively represents the most expensive group of furs. These include mink, the most popular of the group, as well as sable and ermine.

MINK

Every designer-fur fashion show, industry promotion, or retail salon usually features **mink** as the central point offering (Figure 4.8). The variety of natural coloration from wildlife and fur farming, its ability to be easily colored and manipulated into different appearances, and its availability at numerous price points makes it the perfect fur for many consumer markets.

Mink is extremely durable, with the best varieties originating in the northern part of the United States. It has long guard hairs and short, soft fur fibers. It provides considerable warmth, with the female species much lighter in weight than the male. Its characteristic central dark stripe adds to its natural beauty.

The industry's fashion houses and designers often ignore the typical dark-skinned Blackglama or natural, lighter-colored lunaraines that have been crossbred for color variation and opt for hot pinks, royal blues, purples, and other fashion colors that rival those that embrace woolen outerwear. To provide excitement, they sometimes pluck or shear the guard hairs to produce soft, luxurious garments that feature only the downlike fur fibers.

SABLE

Rarity and costliness are the terms that often accompany the marketing of these garments. The best quality comes from the northernmost reaches of Russia and often sells for more than $200,000 for the finest coat. **Sable** somewhat resembles mink, but its guard hairs are shorter,

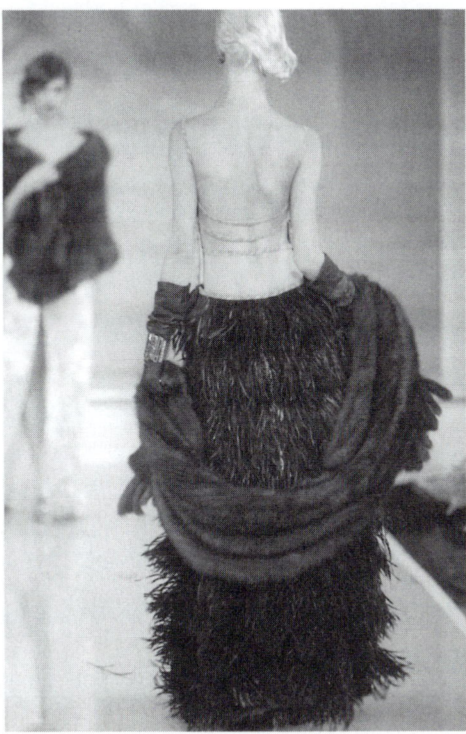

Figure 4.8 Mink adds an elegant touch to any runway show.
(Courtesy of Fur Information Council of America.)

denser, and fluffier, giving an overall bushier appearance than does mink. It is considered by the professionals in the trade to be the world's most prestigious fur.

ERMINE

Although it has not been considered a sought-after fashionable fur for many years, **ermine** still offers its own mystique. Naturally brown in color, it acquires its pure white coloration when the animal is raised in the coldest part of the United States or Siberia. The white is characteristically accentuated with dark black tails, which are used and featured in garment designs. The fur has been associated with European royalty and their pomp and circumstance, and ermine is visible in many formal or state processions.

MISCELLANEOUS WEASELS

Other members of the weasel family often make fashion statements in fur collections. Furs such as fisher, baum marten and stone martin, wolverine, skunk, kolinsky, fitch, and otter are found in a wide range of coats and jackets.

The Rodent Family

Running the gamut from the rare and costly chinchilla to the plentiful and inexpensive rabbit, the **rodent family** is a significant source of pelts. Many are used in their natural states, whereas others, because of their versatility in imitating other, more costly furs, are colored, sheared, and produced in a variety of "fun" creations.

CHINCHILLA

At the top of the scale, pricey **chinchilla** is naturally available in a variety of gray colorations (Figure 4.9). Other shades are reproduced on the ranches or farms as mutations. The fur is soft and fluffy and prone to wear poorly. It is one of the most perishable of all furs. In addition to coats and jackets, chinchilla pieces are used as collars and other adornments in fashion apparel.

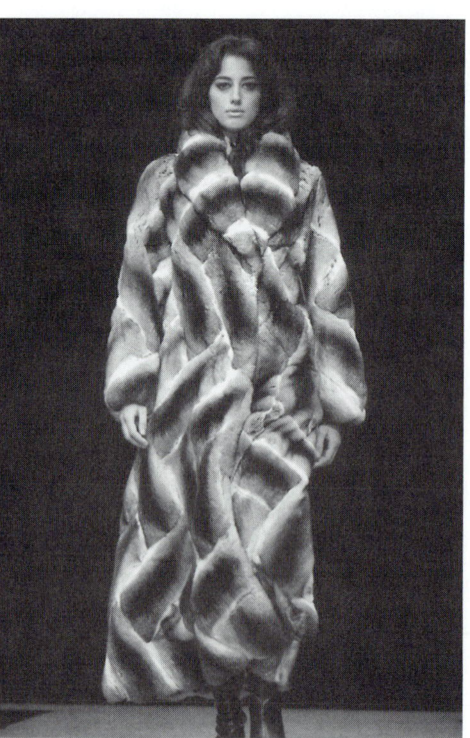

Figure 4.9 Chinchilla is a striking fur at the top of the price scale.
(Courtesy of Fur Information Council of America.)

RABBIT

Rabbit is the antithesis of chinchilla in terms of cost. It is abundant and inexpensive. It comes from many parts of the world, with the French rabbit considered the best of the species. It can imitate many furs such as beaver, seal, ermine, mink, and sable, but its problem with shedding immediately reveals it is not one of those furs. When it is newly processed, it has an appealing, fresh quality that fades quickly after repeated wear.

NUTRIA

One of the most durable furs, **nutria** is used in its natural state with both the guard hairs and fur fibers intact or is sheared or plucked to reveal only the soft, downlike fur fibers. It defies most abuse and is considered one of the most serviceable and functional furs.

MUSKRAT

Readily available in most parts of the United States and Canada, the **muskrat** has always been used as an imitator of mink, sable, and seal. With its dark stripe color-enhanced, it may pass as mink when observed by the untrained eye. Sheared and dyed, it is reminiscent of beaver. It is relatively durable and is always part of a lower-to-moderate priced collection of furs.

BEAVER

Beaver is usually plucked to remove the coarse guard hairs that protect the animal's body and then sheared to render a uniform layer of fur. Hence, the name *sheared beaver* is generally associated with this fur. It is extremely durable and is used in its natural coloring or exquisitely dyed or bleached to give it a fashion focus.

SQUIRREL

Inexpensive and plentiful, this soft fur comes in a variety of shades of gray, many with white or black markings. **Squirrel** is used in its natural state or dyed to imitate more costly species. Its one disadvantage is its lack of durability.

MARMOT

Inexpensive, **marmot** is often dyed to imitate finer, long-haired brown furs. Its guard hairs are coarse and harsh and possess a dominant lustrous appearance. It is moderately durable and serves the consumer who wants to enjoy fur ownership but hasn't the resources for something better.

The Canine Family

This group is primarily represented by fox, which comes in a variety of natural shades that have been captured in the wild or raised on farms and produced as distinctly colored mutations.

Characteristically, fox has long, lustrous guard hairs and lush fur fibers. It is showy and provides a great deal of glamour for special occasions. Its exaggerated fullness tends to make it bulky, and many coats are constructed with leather inserts between the skins to eliminate some of the bulkiness. In some cases, the leathering is concealed; in others, it is emphasized to add an extra dimension to the garment's design. Fox tends to be perishable and, therefore, not practical for daily wear.

RED FOX

Noted by their orange-reddish appearance, this variety is wild and possesses long, thick guard hairs. **Red fox** is infrequently used in coats, but does serve a market for jackets and as trim on cloth coats and suits.

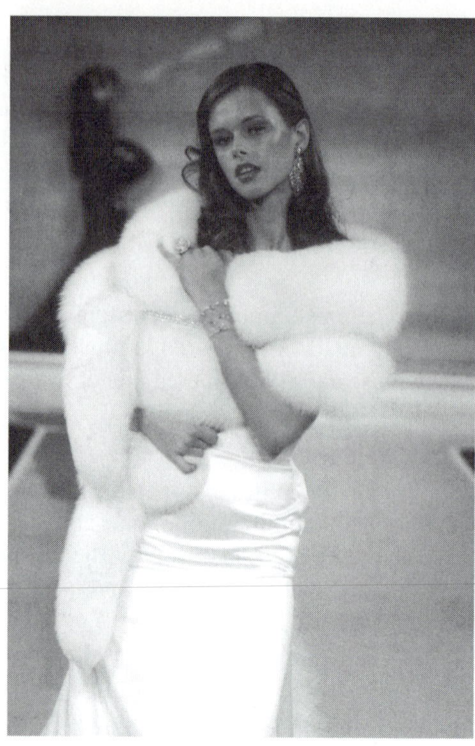

Figure 4.10 White fox is primarily used for evening wear.
(Courtesy of Fur Information Council of America.)

WHITE FOX

The whitest of the species comes from the northernmost reaches of the United States and Canada. **White fox** is extremely striking and is basically used for dramatic evening wear (Figure 4.10).

BLUE FOX

The labels indicate **blue fox;** however, the fur in the garment is decidedly brown with a blue cast or tinge. This is often misleading to the inexperienced consumer who is looking for a shade of blue. It is the **Norwegian blue fox,** developed as a mutation in fur farming, that is actually blue.

SILVER FOX

Dominated by silvery guard hairs and underscored with blue-black fur fibers, **silver fox** is generally raised on ranches. A mutation of the species is platinum fox, which has a more silvery surface than the typical silver variety.

GRAY FOX

The least desirable of the breed, **gray fox** is inexpensive and generally dyed to give the impression of silver fox.

MISCELLANEOUS CANINES

Different in appearance from fox, but nonetheless members of the same family, coyote and wolf are used for sporty or casual wear. They both have coarse guard hairs, are relatively durable, and are distinctively colored in browns and tans, speckled with white or black markings.

The Cat Family

The natural, distinctive patterns and shadings of these furs distinguish them from any other family. Although many furs from the **cat family** are favorites of fur designers and wearers, some are no longer used in garment production because they are endangered species.

LYNX

A costly fur, **lynx** is light-colored, long-haired, and fluffy. Its dark, distinctive markings on a whitish surface make these garments extremely striking. Lynx is best for jackets or three-quarter length coats; the full-length style is simply too bulky for most wearers. The fur is used extensively as trim for high-fashion apparel. Cat lynx, a cousin to the lynx, is slightly less expensive and is also used for short coats and trim.

LEOPARD

Although some species are presently unavailable for use, such as the snow leopard, its discussion is still appropriate but it is conceivable that the restriction might one day be lifted. The best quality of **leopard** fur comes from Africa, where the creamy, yellow-colored backgrounds are accentuated with black markings. The fur has moderately stiff guard hairs that lay flat. The ocelot is similar in characteristics, but it is not as costly or striking as fine leopard.

The Ungulate Family

Animals that are hoofed and feature tightly curled fur pelts are classified as **ungulates.**

PERSIAN LAMB

The best known of the group, **Persian lambs** are farm-raised animals primarily from Africa and Asia (Figure 4.11). The skins are almost always black and curly, but some are naturally colored grays and browns. The prized species are the newborn, which are called **broadtail** and are characterized by flat, water-marked patterning (Figure 4.12). Both varieties are lustrous, with broadtail costing more. When the bundles of skins are laid out for garment construction, the expert craftsperson carefully arranges each pelt next to the other to make certain that all markings are arranged in a complementary set to enhance the ultimate, overall pattern.

The fur is extremely durable and serviceable for everyday wear. Pieces that fall away during product construction are often used as decorative trim on cloth coats and suits.

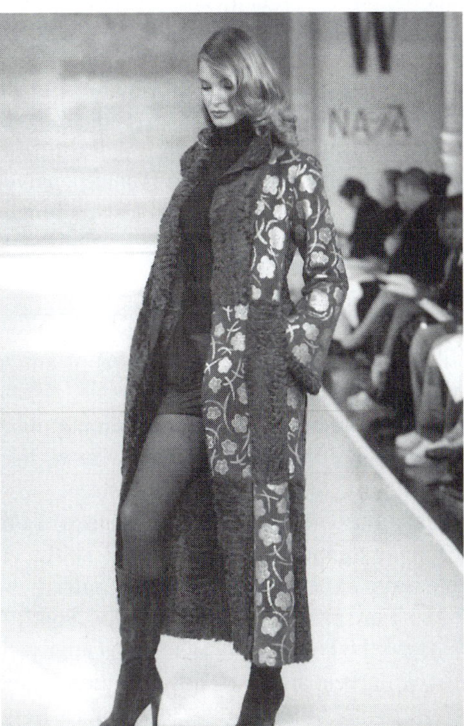

Figure 4.11 Persian lamb makes a fashion statement when it is combined with exciting fabrics.
(Courtesy of Fur Information Council of America.)

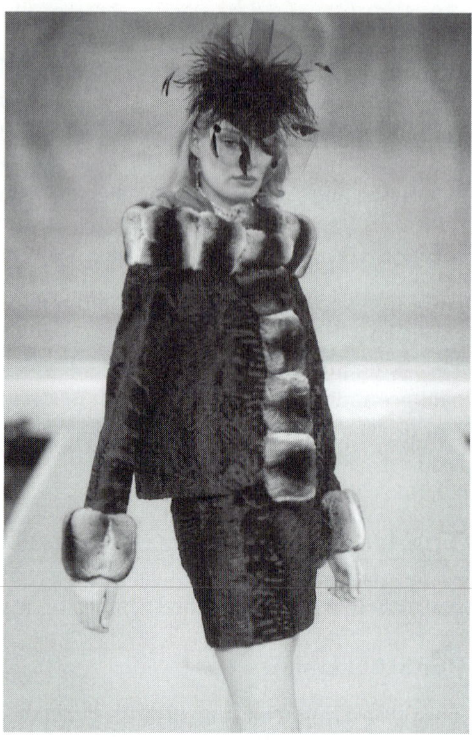

Figure 4.12 Broadtail is characterized by flat, water-marked patterning.
(Courtesy of Fur Information Council of America.)

Larger pieces are sometimes assembled and made into **fur plates,** used in making inexpensive attire.

SOUTH AMERICAN LAMB

This fur is inexpensive and durable and provides the wearer with considerable warmth. **South American lamb** is used to produce mouton-processed lamb and broadtail-processed lamb. The former is achieved through shearing the fur and electrifying the remainder to relax the pattern. It is then dyed. The latter is sheared, leaving a marked undercoat that resembles broadtail. Both are relatively inexpensive furs.

LESSER KNOWN SPECIES

Caracul lamb has short, wavy, flat fur that primarily comes in white, but is also available in black or brown. Kidskin is inexpensive and perishable; pony skin is a heavier version of kidskin. They are all used in less expensive garments and trim.

Miscellaneous Furs

In addition to the specific groups of animals, categorized as families, others do not fit any general classifications.

The raccoon has remained a popular fur for many years. It was once the darling of college football game spectators who warmed themselves in the abundantly thick, fur coats. Eventually adapted for regular street wear, the raccoon coat has transcended many periods in fashion. These furs range in shades of browns and grays and are sometimes color enhanced to make them more attractive. They are versatile and can be plucked and sheared to resemble more expensive furs such as nutria.

Fur seal comes from Alaska, South Africa, Siberia, and Japan, with Alaskan seal considered the best quality. The skins are dyed numerous colors that range from the lightest tints to the darkest shades. They are durable and give the wearer a great deal of practicality.

MARKETING FUR GARMENTS

Although most fashion products are similarly marketed to the consuming public, the fur industry uses some approaches that are almost exclusively its own. These actions are necessitated by such factors as the significant cost of the merchandise, the size of the farms that raise the animals, and the protests of animal rights activists.

Some of the following marketing strategies are used by the fur industry.

Licensing

As initially discussed, renowned apparel designers have entered the fur industry through licensing agreements with fur manufacturers. Their names, when conspicuously placed on fur labels and in advertisements, often generate additional interest in the merchandise. Rather than assessing the value of a costly fur that is produced by an unknown designer in terms of style and quality, the recognizable signature gives the garment fashion credibility. Close inspection of the collections carried by fur retailers reveals an increasing number of the designer-licensed furs.

Consignment Selling

When a buyer goes to the market for ready-to-wear, accessories, and most other fashion merchandise, he or she is ready to expend budgeted dollars for the goods. In the case of furs, however, this is not always the rule. Because of the cost of the items, with individual pieces occasionally costing upwards of $100,000, the amount needed to stock an inventory is often prohibitive. Most fur manufacturers approach the problem by offering their inventories on the basis of **consignment selling.** That is, the retailer signs an agreement that provides inventory that need not be paid for until, and if, it is sold. In that way, the producer gets customer exposure and the retail merchant has a sufficient number of garments from which customers may choose. The consignment route may be used as a means of developing a basic inventory over a full season or for a short period of time when retailer promotions take place. If you ever read about a store's three-day fur sales event, for example, that promises a large selection of garments at lower-than-usual prices, you can be certain that the regular selection has been expanded via the consignment route for the sale period. The pieces that are sold are paid for, and the remainder is returned to the manufacturer.

The Sales Arenas

Selling to the consumer is accomplished at many different types of "sales floors." They include the typical fur specialty store that feature off-the-rack as well as custom-made garments; manufacturer's salons that, in addition to serving as production points for wholesale purchasers, deal with private clientele who want the feeling of dealing with the design source; department stores that have separate departments that are usually leased and operated by independent producers who have entered into formal arrangements with the stores; catalogs that usually feature lower price point furs; Web sites that are generally owned by fur manufacturers or wholesalers; and fur expositions or "fairs" that move from arena to arena for a few days each.

The **fur exposition** has become a successful marketing tool for the industry. Typically, a promoter or major fur specialty retailer arranges with several vendors to supply large inventories on consignment for a few days. Sports arenas, convention centers, and other large facilities are stocked with items that have been advertised at lower-than-traditional prices. Unusually large crowds are drawn to these events because of the magnitude of the cooperative effort. The events usually take place at the end of the season, enabling suppliers to rid themselves of unwanted inventories and retailers to make a quick profit.

OVERCOMING ADVERSE PUBLICITY

No other segment of the fashion industry has ever had to deal with the problems generated by animal rights activists. So vocal and effective have their campaigns been that some major retailers have closed fur salons in their stores. To counteract the negative atmosphere that these groups have established and to bring sales levels to the position they once enjoyed, the fur industry participates in a variety of marketing strategies. These include advertising campaigns that underscore the humane treatment of animals on fur farms; the preparation and distribution of numerous pamphlets that attempt to make the fur fancier more knowledgeable and to dispel the myths that their opponents disseminate; appearance by industry representatives on national talk shows to do battle with their adversaries; and legal battling to control customer harassment at entrances to stores that sell furs.

CARE OF FURS

The nature of the fur garment requires specific care and attention to be paid so that it can afford customers long-lasting wear. Some simple rules follow that will help the fur retain its original beauty and serviceability.

1. Warm, dry places for daily storage should be avoided so that the leather portion of the fur will not dry and crack. Hang in a cool closet, on a fur hanger that is sufficiently large and durable for shape retention, and the garment will retain its freshness.
2. If the fur is wet, it should be left outside of the closet to dry and never left near a heater. The extreme warmth could crack the leather.
3. Sitting on most furs could cause unsightly matting and damage. Whenever possible, during long seated periods, the fur garment should be opened and loosely draped over the wearer.
4. During summer months, furs should be placed in cold storage to avoid the damage wrought by high temperatures.
5. Furs should be cleaned and glazed once a year to remove the excess oils that have built up and to restore the luster.
6. Damage should be repaired as soon as it occurs to prevent possible major problems that could shorten the life of the garment.

Internet Resources for Additional Research

www.efbanet.com/pdfs/EuroSocioEconomic.pdf provides socioeconomic information on European fur farming.

www.fur.org is the Fur Information Council of America that offers a wealth of information about furs.

www.nafa.ca/page.asp?/corporate/links.asp provides information on types of furs, classic styles, and recycling furs, with links to trade organizations, expositions, and media that specialize in furs.

Merchandise Information Terminology

Fur farming
PETA
Pelt
Guard hairs
Fur fiber
Kicking
Bundle
Glazing
Match the skins
Skin-on-skin construction
Letting-out
Split-skin construction
Whole-skin construction
Leathering
Fur Products Labeling Act
Weasel family
Mink
Sable
Ermine
Rodent family
Chinchilla
Rabbit
Nutria
Muskrat
Beaver
Squirrel
Marmot
Canine family
Red fox
White fox
Blue fox
Norwegian blue fox
Silver fox

Gray fox
Cat family
Lynx
Leopard
Ungulates
Persian lamb
Broadtail lamb
Fur plates
South American lamb
Caracul lamb
Consignment selling
Fur exposition

EXERCISES

1. Using the photographs of fur garments that have appeared in fashion magazines such as *Elle*, *Harper's Bazaar*, and *Vogue*, prepare a PowerPoint or other visual presentation on the industry at this time. Furs that fit into specific families should be grouped together.

   In addition to artwork, each piece should be accompanied by details that include whether or not the fur has been colored, obvious processing, and anything pertinent to its design. Each group should also feature a composite chart that lists its overall characteristics, price points, advantages, and disadvantages.
2. Make arrangements to visit a fur manufacturer or retailer to take a video of the company's collection or slides of individual items. Develop a narrative to accompany the products captured on tape or slides that addresses the characteristics of each. The company should be alerted that this is for educational purposes.
3. Visit a fur manufacturer, designer, or retail merchant to collect scraps of fur that may be used for a visual presentation. The pieces should be mounted on a board and accompanied by information that is important to the use of the various fur types.

Review Questions

1. What are the two methods by which furs are procured for use in garment construction?
2. How do fur trappers learn their skills and, thus, prevent unnecessary cruelty to animals?
3. Describe the method used by most fur farmers to sell their wares to the industry.
4. In what way have fur manufacturers attracted renowned apparel designers to play a role in the fur industry?
5. Why must pelts be "dressed" before they are made into garments?
6. How are furs dyed?
7. Explain the process of glazing and the advantages it affords the fur.
8. Which methods of construction are used to join skins?
9. Describe the method of letting-out and the advantages derived from its use.
10. What are the reasons for using the leathering process in the construction of some fur garments?
11. Name the piece of legislation that was enacted to protect the consumer from unscrupulous practices.
12. What rules were prescribed by this law?
13. List the three costliest furs in the weasel family.
14. Discuss two advantages and disadvantages of rabbit fur.
15. What is the difference between blue fox and Norwegian blue fox?
16. Are broadtail lamb and broadtail-processed lamb the same?
17. Why is consignment selling an approach used in the marketing of furs?
18. Discuss the use of fur expositions.
19. How is the fur industry counteracting the negativism of animal rights activists?
20. List some of the steps fur owners must take to care for this apparel.

CHAPTER **5**

Metals and Stones

After reading this chapter, you should be able to:

- Discuss the various types of precious metals used in fashion accessories, flatware, and hollowware.
- Explain how base metals are used in combination with the precious types.
- Describe the process of alloying.
- Describe the characteristics that are unique to the different types of natural stones.
- Understand the different technical terminology used in the markets of metals and stones.
- Differentiate among the various cuts used for stones.

On display at the Tower of London are the United Kingdom's crown jewels. Istanbul's Topkapi Palace is laden with such jeweled treasures as the 86-carat Spoonmaker's Diamond. The lavish Egyptian gold and silver pieces at New York City's Museum of Natural History date back more than 4,000 years. Common costume jewels of imitation stones and ordinary metallics abound in every flea market. The richness of the real and imitation are found in virtually every fashion consumer's wardrobe.

The diamond has symbolized betrothal for as long as anyone can remember (Figure 5.1), and turquoise encased in the "squash blossoms" has hung around the necks of Native American tribal chieftains. However, metals and stones need be neither rare nor precious to make a fashion statement. Barbara Bush, former first lady and a member of one of America's wealthier families, made fashion headlines with her preference for imitation pearls. Her embrace of the modestly priced, man-made imitation gave the industry a product that had fashion credibility and was within every consumer's reach.

A full complement of metals and stones is used in fashion apparel, accessories, flatware, and hollowware. The precious group, those having intrinsic or real value, is primarily for jewelry, flatware, and hollowware. The others are used for costume, or fashion, jewelry and for accessories such as belts, handbags, and other items. In the apparel market, stones and metallics are found on dresses, sportswear, sweaters, and suits. Collectively, these materials constitute a range from the rarest to the ordinary and from the priciest to the dollar variety. Designers creating for every price point regularly craft the whole spectrum of metals

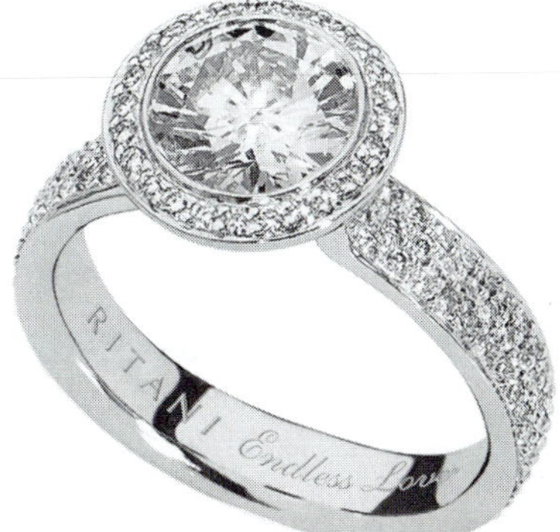

Figure 5.1 The diamond ring has long symbolized betrothal.
(Courtesy of Ritani.)

and stones. Although the master jewelers such as Harry Winston, Cartier, and Tiffany design masterpieces for a selected few, others continue to toil with every conceivable raw material so that even those with limited funds can make lasting fashion impressions.

This chapter focuses on metals and stones as materials of fashion, their characteristics, and their processing. Chapter 12, "Jewelry and Watches," deals with the various wearable accessories that use these materials, and Chapter 15 covers flatware and hollowware, the products that enhance table settings.

METALS

Characteristically, all metals have shiny surfaces that can either be enhanced to give them a brighter look or treated to alter or dull their appearance. They are **malleable,** enabling them to be twisted, bent, or pounded into a variety of shapes; they can even be elongated into wire-like threads that may be used to weave designs. After they have been extracted from the ground and separated from the natural ore, they may be used by themselves or combined with other metals. In the case of jewelry for adornment purposes, the metals are most often alloyed or plated with other materials.

An **alloy** is a combination of two or more metals. By using this technique, several advantages are achieved. Color variations are often the result of an alloy. For example, when a small bit of silver is combined with steel, the result is a silvery appearance. This increases the beauty and adds value to the new metal. Some metals in their pure form are too soft to use for most purposes. Gold, for example, is extremely soft and is usually alloyed with a base metal such as copper to add strength.

Plating is the process in which one metal is coated with another. By applying the more appealing metal on the surface and the lesser one inside, the final product takes on a better appearance. This may be accomplished either through dipping one metal into another one that has been heated, bonding the layers of metals together, or through a technique called **electroplating.** In this relatively inexpensive process, the metal used to plate another is dissolved and, through an electrical current, is attracted to the other. Often, a precious metal such as gold or silver is plated over a base such as copper, which produces an attractive metal at a low cost.

Considerations such as cost, appearance, availability, durability, workability, and color indicate the methodology that will be used to transform the raw material into one that is useful for accessories, apparel, flatware, and hollowware.

Precious Metals

Metals that are costly and relatively rare are known as *precious metals*. In the case of accessory use, precious metals are reserved for jewelry and watches; for home use, flatware and hollowware are their end products. They are simply too costly for use as garment adornments.

The most expensive of this group is platinum, followed by gold, and then silver. Their prices fluctuate every day, contributing to an increase or decrease in the prices charged for the finished products. Gold, for example, was once a "controlled" metal and sold at $35 per ounce. When the restriction was eliminated, the cost of gold skyrocketed on the open market and sold for as much as $850 an ounce. As of this writing, the price has steadily hovered around the $350 mark. Platinum costs even more, and silver costs considerably less. Silver, at this time, sells for about $6 an ounce, making it a precious metal that can be most easily marketed.

PLATINUM

Because of the extreme cost, platinum is used exclusively as settings for fine quality diamonds (Figure 5.2). However, most diamond ring settings that have the appearance of platinum are actually white gold, a less costly metal. Platinum is a soft metal, and it must be alloyed to give it strength. The finest platinum products are usually 90 percent platinum and 10 percent iridium, a metal with considerable strength. Unlike silver, which tarnishes, platinum does not.

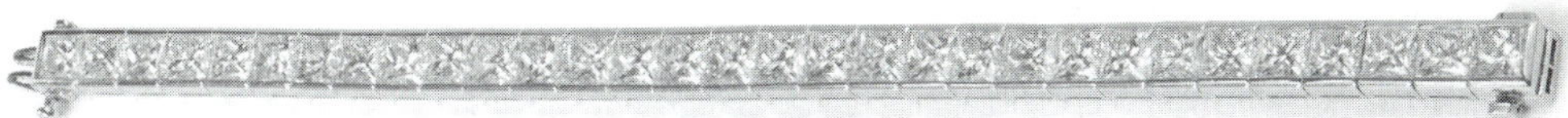

Figure 5.2 Fine diamonds are sometimes set in platinum.
(Courtesy of Julius Klein Diamonds.)

GOLD

In its natural state, gold is a bright yellow metal that is extremely soft. Thus, it must be mixed with other metals to be usable for commercial purposes.

For jewelry, the metal is either karat gold, gold-filled, rolled-gold plate, or electroplated.

Items that are labeled as **karat** gold cost the most. The designation refers to a certain part pure gold and the rest comprising other metals such as copper and nickel. For example, **14 karat,** or 14K as it is labeled, is fourteen parts gold and ten parts of another metal. The total weight must add to twenty-four, gold in its purest form. In most European countries, the predominant gold alloy is **18 karat.** To be considered karat gold, there must be a minimum of 10K gold in the alloy.

In addition to giving it strength, alloying may also alter the gold color. The base metal used will change the color.

Gold-filled items are composed of thin sheets of gold that have been rolled and adhered to a base metal. The karat gold is melted and rolled and pressed onto the base. If the term **gold-filled** is used, the amount of gold in the product must be a minimum of 1/20 of the total weight of the item.

Rolled-gold plate is similar to gold-filled, except that its gold content is less. The amount of gold used must be at least 1/40 of the total metal's weight.

When an inexpensive piece of jewelry or trim requires the shiny look of gold, electroplating is the answer. It uses the thinnest gold surface, which ultimately might wear away from the base metal.

SILVER

Its relative low cost and shiny white surface makes it an extremely valuable precious metal for use in jewelry. As with other precious metals, silver is too soft to use alone. It is alloyed with copper for more expensive jewelry pieces that bear the name **sterling silver.** For less costly designs, it is electroplated.

Sterling silver is an alloy of pure silver and copper. The silver provides the luster, the copper the strength. To be classified as such, the alloy must contain 925 parts silver and 75 parts copper.

As in the case with gold, less costly silver jewelry is achieved through electroplating. To maintain the silvery look for many years, the base metal must be heavily coated.

Base Metals

Available in large quantities at comparatively low prices, **base metals** are used as alloys with the precious varieties. Because they are either malleable, easily transformed into various shapes, or have considerable strength, they are extremely valuable in jewelry production.

COPPER

One of the most important base metals for jewelry, copper is alloyed with gold to produce karat gold and silver for sterling silver in precious jewelry. For less expensive ornamentation, in addition to mass-produced jewelry such as buttons, copper is alloyed with zinc to produce brass and tin to form bronze.

CHROMIUM

This lustrous, bluish-colored metal offers durability and tarnish resistance. It is ideal for inexpensive, shiny jewelry and flatware when plated on brass, copper, or steel.

IRON

Iron is the main ingredient in the use of steel. Its extreme strength and durability make it a perfect base metal for stainless-steel watch casings.

NICKEL

This silver metal is used to add hardness and whiteness when alloyed with other metals. When white karat gold is needed, nickel's natural color and distinct durability produce the perfect alloy.

TIN

Tin is a soft, lustrous, silver metal. It is easily shaped and, therefore, excellent for jewelry and other ornamentation that requires twisting. It is the main ingredient in pewter, a grayish metallic alloy that is primarily used in the production of pitchers and other home furnishings, and sometimes in fashion jewelry.

Metal Production and Ornamentation Techniques

A variety of techniques are used in the transformation of metals into viable materials for use in jewelry, embellishments on fashion apparel and accessories, and home products.

Annealing. The process of heating metals to make them more workable.

Rolling. Pressing metals into sheets so that they can be cut or bent to the required shape.

Drawing. A technique that produces metal wires that can be woven into designs. The metals are forced through a series of holes, each more narrower than the previous, until the desired thickness is achieved.

Forging. The heating and hammering of metal into shapes.

Welding. When two or more metals are to be joined together by heat and pressure.

Casting. Melting metals and then pouring them into a mold.

Engraving. Scratching a design into metal by hand or machine.

Florentining. Engraving the surface of the metal with a series of fine scratch marks.

Chasing. Tapping a design into a metal surface.

Etching. Through the use of acid applications, eating away certain portions of the metal to achieve the desired effect.

Antiquing. The application of chemicals to darken the metal to give it an old or antique appearance.

STONES

We all know that the fabulously emblazoned, stone-encrusted evening gowns and sweaters are not really diamonds, emeralds, and rubies, but imitations that are made to resemble the real thing. However, when a sparkling engagement ring is being shown, it is difficult to tell if the stones are diamonds or something else that bears exceptional similarity. In the case of the diamond, another natural stone, the zircon, may be used as an imitation. The eye is often fooled by a chemically produced stone such as strontium titanite, which is marketed under the trade name Fabulite. Fabulous fakes are not restricted to diamonds. They are produced to imitate emeralds, rubies, sapphires, and every other stone. Although the real and imitations offer similar visual impressions, the prices for the two groups are at extreme ends of the price spectrum.

The stones used for jewelry and other enhancements are categorized as natural, synthetic, simulant, or imitation. All of these may eventually become part of a designer's creation.

Natural Stones

Those that are classified as **natural stones** are either mined or, as in the case of pearls, found in the sea. As with any natural products, the considerable variations are influenced by the environments in which the stones are formed. Unlike the synthetics, which are laboratory created, each natural stone has a distinct appearance or personality of its own.

The stones are identified in any number of ways. Although color often indicates a particular kind of natural stone, such as green for emeralds and red for rubies, the color test is not always conclusive. Many natural stones are available in a host of colors; for instance, there are yellow diamonds and pink rubies.

Hardness measurements may be used to differentiate natural stones. Each stone has its own distinct degree of hardness and can be judged on that basis. The **Mohs Scale of Hardness,** developed by Friedrich Mohs in 1882, is still the most commonly used means of hardness measurement. Mohs chose ten well-known minerals and assigned them numbers in order of their scratch harness (Table 5.1).

Under the Mohs scale, diamonds with a hardness of 10 can scratch any mineral (Figure 5.3), while topaz, with an 8 rating, can scratch anything from quartz down to talc.

An even more precise measurement of scratch hardness can be made with a sclerometer. The stone is mounted and a sharp diamond point is drawn across it. The pressure on the point is regulated with the addition of weight, until the stone is scratched. The weight is then often compared with predetermined values. The values in Table 5.2 were determined with the sclerometer. It should be noted that scratching can damage a stone and should not be used on a stone that has been fashioned.

Other methods of identification consider gravity and light refraction. Each stone has a specific gravity that may be tested by dropping it into water and comparing it with the preestablished numbers of each type. When light enters a stone, the light is slowed and bent away from its normal course. Each stone has its own angle of light bending and may therefore be classified as a result of this test.

Natural stones are subdivided into two categories: precious and semiprecious.

Precious Stones

Diamonds, rubies, sapphires, emeralds, and natural pearls are classified by jewelers as - **precious stones.** Although some might argue that the pearl isn't really a stone, it is generally acknowledged as such by those in the trade.

Diamond

The only precious stone that is made entirely of one chemical composition, carbon, is without question the one that receives the greatest amount of attention from the consuming

TABLE 5.1 The Mohs Scale of Hardness

*Mineral**	*Hardness*
Diamond	10
Corundum	9
Topaz	8
Quartz	7
Feldspar	6
Apatite	5
Fluorite	4
Calcite	3
Gypsum	2
Talc	1

*Different stones fall within each mineral category. Ruby and sapphire, for example, are in the corundum classification, and emerald and aquamarine (known technically as beryl) have the same hardness as topaz.

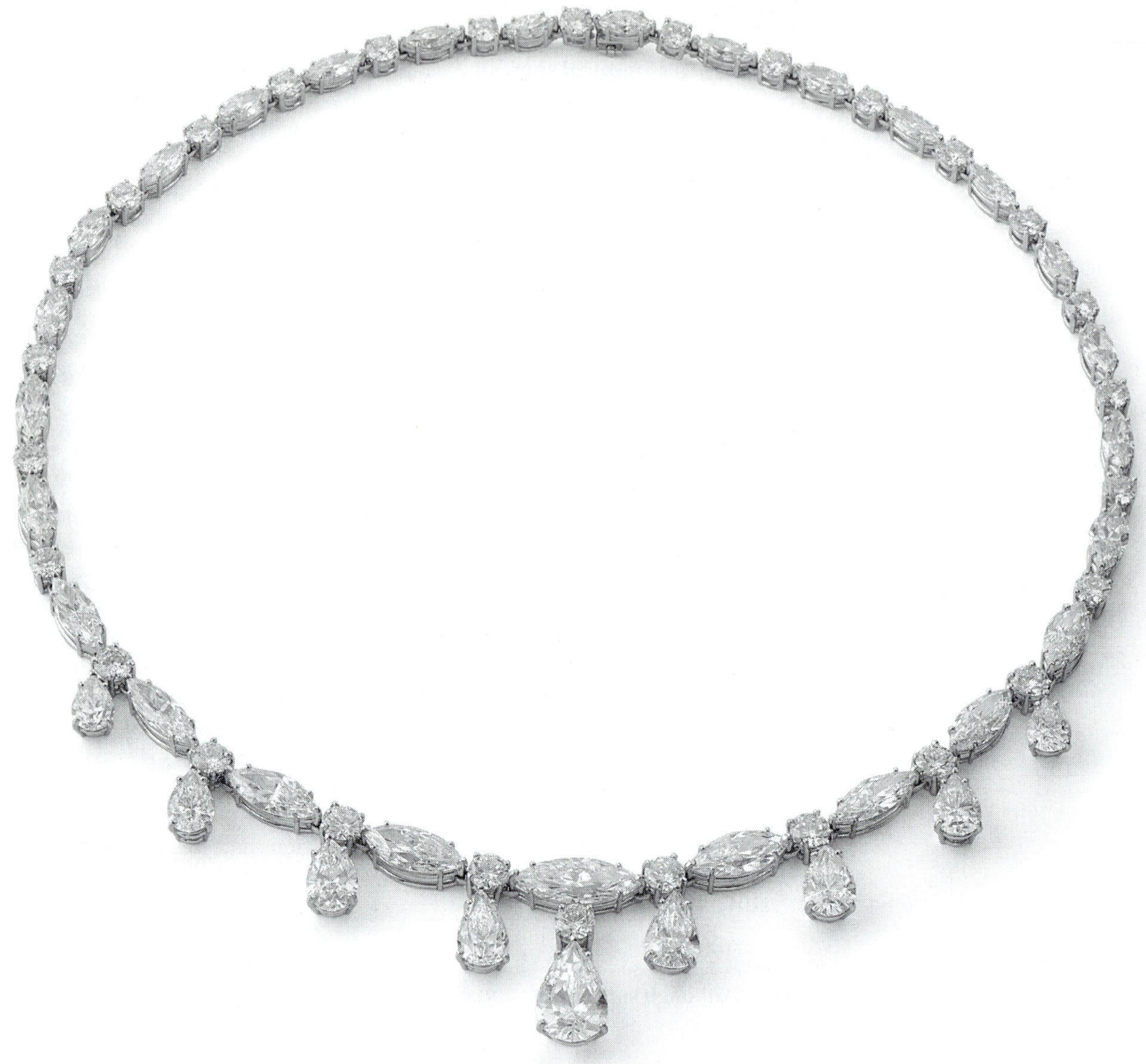

Figure 5.3 Diamond is the hardest stone.
(Courtesy of Julius Klein Diamonds.)

TABLE 5.2 Hardness Measurements Determined with Sclerometer

Mineral	*Hardness*
Diamond	140,000
Corundum	1,000
Topaz	459
Quartz	245
Feldspar	191
Apatite	53.5
Fluorite	37.3
Calcite	15.3
Gypsum	12.03
Talc	1.13

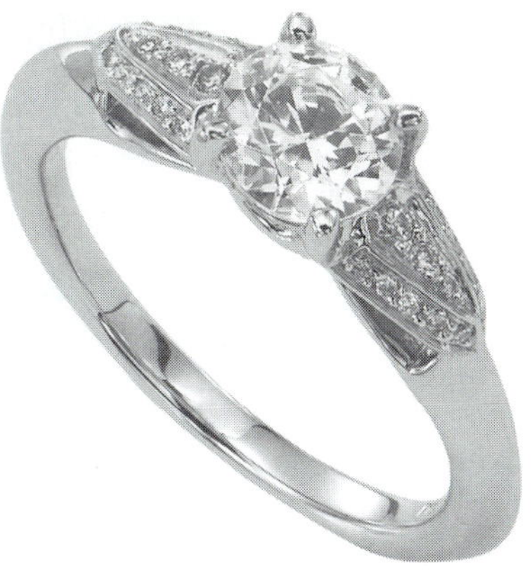

Figure 5.4 Diamonds are assessed in terms of carat weight, color, clarity, and cut.
(Courtesy of Ritani.)

public. Long the symbol of betrothal, it also signifies success and achievement and is treasured by a large segment of the population. Not all diamonds are created equal, however.

Diamonds are formed anywhere between 75 and 120 miles below the earth's surface, where the necessary conditions of temperature and pressure exist, and then are forced to the surface by volcanic action. First discovered in India about 500 B.C., the stone's deposits are in many different parts of the globe. A large proportion of the world's diamonds come from Australia, South Africa, and Russia; many professionals consider the Russian diamonds as the best in quality.

Diamonds and other stones are measured in carats. One carat equals 0.2 grams. It would take 142 carats to equal one ounce! Because fractions of a carat can significantly alter the price, it is necessary to be precise in measuring. The carat is broken down into points, with each representing $1/100^{th}$ of a carat. In other words, there are 100 points to a carat.

To evaluate the worth of a particular diamond, the jeweler makes an assessment based on the **four Cs:** carat weight, color, clarity, and cut (Figure 5.4).

The beginning point is usually the carat weight. This does not mean that an s-carat stone is more costly than one that is half the size. The final value will be determined when all other factors have been considered.

Although most consumers think of diamonds as colorless stones, they come in a variety of colors. There are yellow, gray, brown, and even black diamonds. Some of the colored stones are so rare that they cost more than the conventional types. They are classified as fancies.

The degree to which a diamond is free of blemishes and **inclusions** (a term to describe internal imperfections) is known as its *clarity*. It is virtually impossible to find a stone that is free of imperfections. However, when neither a blemish nor an inclusion is observed under ten-power magnification of the **jeweler's loupe** (Figure 5.5), the stone is considered to be flawless. Such specimens are rare and highly prized. Of course, many stones contain imperfections that are visible to the naked eye and have inclusions that could affect durability. These stones are significantly less valuable than those with limited imperfections.

Next, the cut of the stone contributes to its value and cost. A talented diamond cutter can cut the natural stone in such a manner as to minimize flaws. When observing the rough stone, skilled craftspeople must determine which style of cut will best serve the stone in terms of retaining as much weight as possible while producing an eye-appealing diamond. The various cuts are discussed later in this chapter as they apply to different types of stones.

Finally, the stones are graded according to the four Cs. The industry standard for grading, established by the **Gemological Institute of America (GIA),** is adhered to by the world's jewelry professionals.

Some of the more renowned diamonds that have become historically significant are: the Empress Eugenie, a fifty-one-carat perfect diamond; the Eureka, a yellow diamond with a weight of 21.25 carats rough that was cut to 10.73; the Cullinan I and II, the former weighing 530.20 carats and the latter 317.40, both fashioned from the Cullinan with a rough weight of 3,106.75 carats; and the Great Table, a pink stone measured at 250 carats!

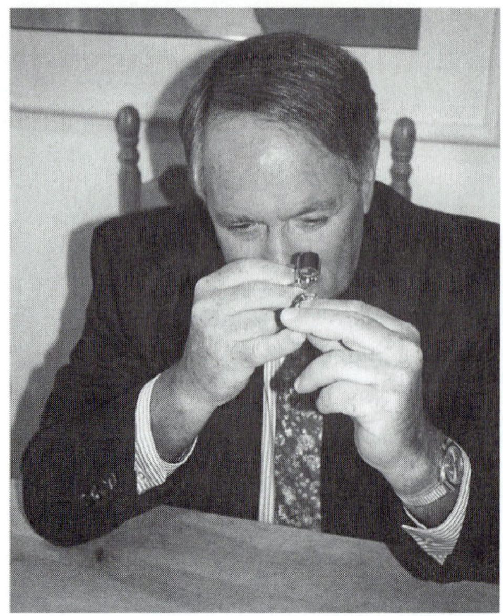

Figure 5.5 The jeweler appraises a diamond with a jeweler's loupe.
(Courtesy of Ellen Diamond.)

RUBY

The most valued of all gemstones, the ruby is a variety of the corundum family. Its rare, red characteristic makes it more costly than another member of the same family, the sapphire. This hard stone is sometimes referred to as *oriental ruby* to distinguish it from its close relative, the spinel ruby. The latter cannot match the hardness, density, and value of the ruby. Colors range from deep red to rose red. The most valued are those that are tinged with a bit of purple, which professionals sometimes call *pigeon's red.*

SAPPHIRE

Also a member of the corundum family, the sapphire is a transparent, highly valued precious stone. It is basically made of the same substance as ruby, but its coloration ranges from pale blue to deep indigo, the rarest. Sapphires are also occasionally found colorless or in shades of yellow, green, pink, and purple, sometimes confusing them with other stones. In such cases, their true identity may be determined only by the hardness tests.

EMERALD

The emerald is generally recognized by its deep green color. It is a member of the beryl family, as is the less expensive aquamarine. The emerald is the only precious stone of that family, the others being classified as semiprecious. The emerald is softer than the other precious gemstones, with a hardness rating of 7.5. In ancient times, the emerald was considered to have many virtues, including the prevention of epilepsy and an ability to drive away evil spirits.

PEARLS

Natural pearls are formed when a tiny irritant such as a speck of sand invades the oyster. As a means of alleviating the irritation, the oyster coats the tiny matter with a nacreous solution, the same element that coats the oyster's shell, thus eventually forming a pearl. The most valuable of the pearls are those that are perfectly round and formed next to the oyster's body. The translucent quality and iridescent color make it a desirable gem. Those that are found as formations attached to the oyster's shell are labeled **baroque pearls** and are irregularly shaped.

Unlike the other precious stones, which are measured in carat weight, pearls are measured in millimeters. The larger the millimeter, the greater the cost. When made into necklaces or bracelets, the matching of size and color determines the cost.

Although most pearls range in color from a creamy beige to a faint pink tint, they are also formed in colors that include yellow, brown, green, blue, and black.

Semiprecious Stones

In addition to the rare, precious natural stones, many **semiprecious stones** are significantly beautiful. They are, of course, less expensive than their precious counterparts, but nonetheless they are important to the jewelry industry. We explore those that are especially popular.

ZIRCON

This transparent stone comes in a variety of colors, including yellow, orange, and red. In its colorless form, it is often used to imitate the diamond. Although it has significant sparkle, it does not have the fiery brilliance of the diamond and, because of its softness, tends to scratch easily.

TURQUOISE

This stone ranges from deep blue to a light shade of green. It is opaque and has a soft, smooth surface that scratches easily. It is used in a wide range of jewelry products and is especially prized when teamed with sterling silver in Native American–designed pieces such as the "squash blossom."

ALEXANDRITE

This transparent stone features a greenish tinge under normal daylight and dramatically changes to red under artificial light. The **alexandrite** is common in small sizes, but when it weighs more than two carats, it is relatively scarce and costly, compared with other semiprecious stones. A weight of three carats easily commands a $20,000 price tag.

CAT'S-EYE

This translucent stone ranges in color from yellow to emerald green. It feels velvety to the touch. When properly cut, the **Cat's-eye** produces a bright, white light down its center. It symbolizes long life, and some owners value the protection it offers from the "evil eye."

CORAL

Coral ranges from semitransparent to opaque. Its coloration runs from white to deep red. The latter is the costliest of coral. The majority of stones found in jewelry are red-orange in color. Although much of the coral used for jewelry is cut and fashioned by craftspeople, a significant amount of this stone is used in its uncut stage.

AMBER

Amber is somewhat different from the other semiprecious products. It is not a stone; it is petrified tree sap. In its natural formation, colors generally range from yellow to dark brown. The lightest of the gems, amber can be distinguished by its ability to float. As a test to determine its authenticity, it may be immersed in a slat-water solution. Only amber will float.

AMETHYST

One of the most popular of the semiprecious stones, **amethyst** ranges in color from light to dark purple. It is the birthstone of February. Available in large weights at a modest price, this durable stone will provide the wearer indefinite years of use.

ONYX

A member of the quartz family, **onyx** ranges from semitranslucent to opaque. Its coloration includes the spectrum of colors from red to apricot, with white evident in some stones. It is usually the stone used in carved cameos. Although many people think black onyx is a variation of the natural stone, this is not the case. It is a dyed version of **chalcedony,** a variety of quartz.

AQUAMARINE

This is a member of the beryl family, as is emerald, but **aquamarine** costs considerably less than the precious emerald. It ranges in color from light blue to dark blue, with the latter the more valuable. Spectacular rings that bear as much as a fifteen-carat stone are available at relatively modest prices; however, they are becoming increasingly scarce.

GARNET

A hard, durable stone, the **garnet** comes in a variety of shades of greens, reds, yellows, and oranges. When a brilliant green is desired, but emeralds are too costly, a fine garnet is a much more affordable alternative.

JADE

Jade comes in two varieties, jadite and nephrite. The former is the more expensive and is naturally available in green, a white and green combination, light gray, pink, brown, yellow, orange, and lavender. The most desired is the emerald-green color, often referred to as *imperial jade*. Nephrite colors are more limited, with dark green its mainstay, and nephrite costs much less than jadite.

OPAL

Each **opal** features a brilliant array of colors, somewhat like a rainbow. Color is the major characteristic for judging its value. The costliest of the variety is the black opal, which is extremely rare. A gem that is about the size of a lima bean can cost as much as $50,000. To "extend" the black opal, it is often produced as a doublet, a combination stone that uses both an opal and a less expensive variety in its presentation. Combination stones are explored later in the chapter.

LAPIS-LAZULI

Lapis-lazuli is a natural, opaque blue stone. The most prized variety is deep blue, with no traces of gold or silver specks in the piece.

TOPAZ

This versatile stone comes in yellow, a range of browns, red, and shades of green; sometimes it is colorless. Many stones are sold as **topaz,** but they are generally imitations of the real variety. Most are quartz topaz, which costs considerably less.

CULTURED PEARL

A **cultured pearl** is cultivated with the assistance of people. It is produced by the insertion of an irritant such as a bead of mother-of-pearl into the oyster (Figure 5.6). The oyster is then

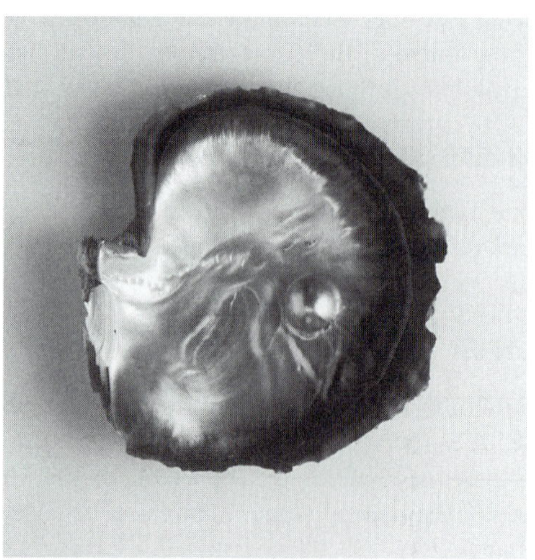

Figure 5.6 The cultured pearl is formed by the insertion of an irritant into the oyster.
(Courtesy of MIKIMOTO.)

returned to the water and over a period of several years, it secretes a substance around the bead to form a pearl. Fine cultured pearls are extremely expensive, with the costliest possessing the same qualities as its precious, natural counterpart. The BIWA cultured pearls are grown in fresh water rather than sea water and are cultivated much faster. Pearls of any type are either smooth and round or are the irregularly shaped baroque type.

Other semiprecious stones that are used by jewelers, but to a lesser extent than those discussed, include: andalusite, a hard, durable stone in a wide color range; bloodstone, a dark variety of quartz; labradorite, a grayish, opaque stone; moonstone, a milky-white, transparent member of the feldspar family; obsidian, a dark-brown, inexpensive stone used for Mexican jewelry; peridot, the birthstone for August that comes in shades of green; rhodochrosite, a soft stone that ranges from white to deep rose; serpentine, a green stone that is sometimes used as a jade substitute; and spinel, which is available in reds, oranges, blues, greens, purple, and black. The various types of spinel are often confused with ruby, sapphire, amethyst, and garnet.

Synthetic Stones

Is it a natural stone that has been mined and fashioned by the jeweler or has it been manufactured to look like the "real thing"? Some **synthetic stones** are so perfectly produced that they easily fool the untrained or unsuspecting. In many cases, only the eye of a professional jeweler can distinguish the imitation from the natural gemstone.

These man-made reproductions of mined stones have essentially the same chemical compositions, structures, and visual and physical properties of the stones they mimic. Some of the more popular synthetics are those that simulate precious emeralds, rubies, diamonds, and sapphires and many of the costly semiprecious varieties such as opal and turquoise.

The new technologies for making the synthetics are so advanced that, on occasion, even the professional jeweler can make a mistake. These costly mistakes can be verified only when actual testing is undertaken.

Simulants

Anything that is marketed as look-alikes for natural stones are called **simulants,** or imitations. Unlike the synthetic group, these have none of the properties inherent in the real stones that they imitate. Glass, for example, has been carefully cut and backed with a foil surface to imitate diamonds. Not all simulants, however, are produced to fool the public. When used as a trim on apparel and accessories or as elements in elaborate, inexpensive jewelry, only the less informed would believe the rhinestone was actually a diamond.

Ceramics have often been manipulated to resemble turquoise or coral. When the prices are comparatively low, it is most certainly true that the final product is not the real thing.

With today's shortage of real ivory, plastics are being manufactured as imitations for use in jewelry and apparel ornamentation.

Some of the more popular simulants or imitations are successfully marketed today as diamonds are YAG (yttrium aluminum garnet) and GGG (gadolinium gallium garnet).

Birthstones

For hundreds of years, specific gemstones have been associated with particular months of the year. The **birthstones,** a name given to the stones that fall within each month, have not always been the same throughout history. Today, the jewelry industry follows the birthstone list established by the Jewelry Council of America in 1952.

Some months have a single stone earmarked for them, whereas others have two or more (Table 5.3).

TABLE 5.3 Birthstones

Month	*Stones*
January	Garnet
February	Amethyst
March	Aquamarine or bloodstone
April	Diamond
May	Emerald
June	Pearl, moonstone, or alexandrite
July	Ruby
August	Peridot or sardonyx
September	Sapphire
October	Opal or pink tourmaline
November	Topaz or citrine quartz
December	Turquoise or zircon

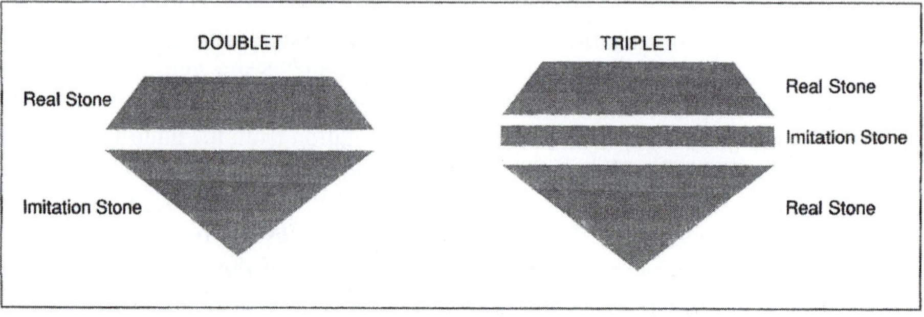

Composite stones.

Figure 5.7 Composite stones are made of two or three parts.

Composite Stones

A stone with more than one part is called a **composite.** The combination of different stones is used to enlarge the size of the stone or enhance its color.

The most popular composites are called doublets and triplets. **Doublets** use two parts, and **triplets** use three. The different stones are held together with cement.

In the case of the doublet, the natural stone is on top, which is seen, with the bottom a glass imitation. Triplets use the real stone at the top, a glass insertion in the middle, and a real stone at the base. Figure 5.7 shows how the parts are engineered to make up the composites.

Today, combination stones are less frequently manufactured because of the excellent quality of synthetics now available. Some combinations that have been created in the past, however, are still available today.

Most doublets use the garnet as the top portion of the creation. Its excellent luster and durability account for its popularity. The garnet-topped doublet, for example, uses a blue-glass bottom for a sapphire look-alike piece and a green-glass bottom when an emerald appearance is the choice. Sometimes, a colored cement is used to fuse two colorless stones, resulting in a colored stone.

Cutting Stones

Most of the rough stones must be cut to enhance beauty and sometimes to hide imperfections or inclusions. For fashion purposes, the occasional use of an uncut stone may be in order. Coral, for example, may be cut or left in the rough. In the case of pearls, of course, no cutting is necessary; the natural beauty lies within the shapes as they come from the oyster.

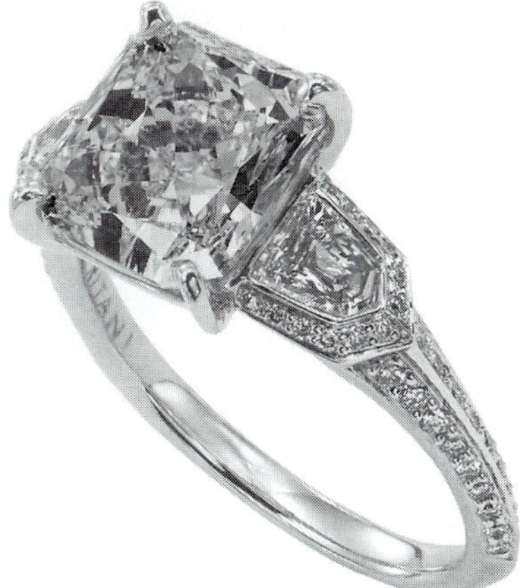

Figure 5.8 This square cut diamond is an example of a faceted cut.
(Courtesy of Ritani.)

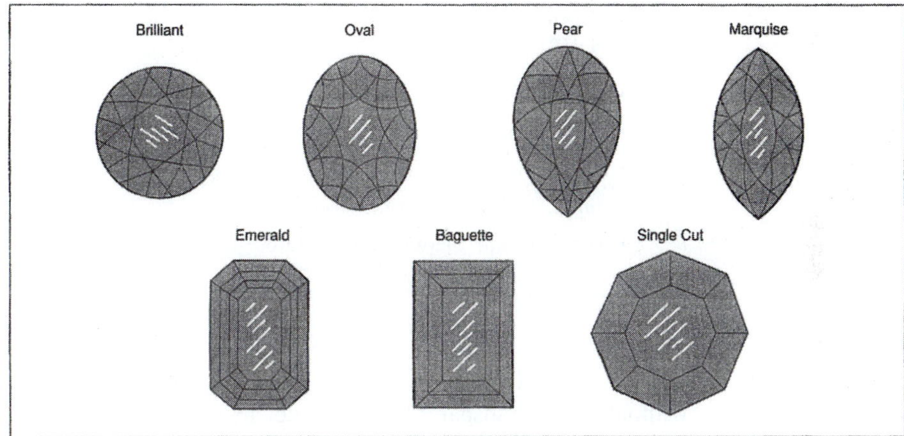

Figure 5.9 Faceted cuts are designed to make the stone more desirable.

Stones are either faceted or cabochon cut. **Facet** refers to the series of faces or planes that make up the cut (Figure 5.8). **Cabochon,** on the other hand, is a facetless cut that produces a smooth, rounded surface.

FACETED CUTS

The **lapidary,** or stonecutter, examines each stone to determine which type of faceting would make it most desirable when finished. There are many different types of faceted cuts from which to choose (Figure 5.9).

- *Brilliant.* Sometimes referred to as a full or round cut, it imparts the greatest amount of "fire." It is usually the traditional choice for engagement rings.
- *Emerald.* This name is used because it is the most popular method used for cutting emeralds. Diamonds and other stones, however, are often emerald cut. Its facets are similar to miniature steps, which is why it is sometimes referred to as the *step cut.*
- *Pear.* It is rounded at the top and tapers down to a point, resembling a teardrop. It tends to make the stone seem larger than the round or emerald cut varieties of the same weight.
- *Marquise.* If visual size is important, this cut gives the impression that it is larger than round stones of the same weight.
- *Oval.* The newest cut, the oval is actually a variation on the round cut.
- *Baguette.* Small rectangular stones may be baguette cut to flank a larger stone.
- *Single cut.* A variation of the round or brilliant cut, it features fewer facets and is used for small stones.

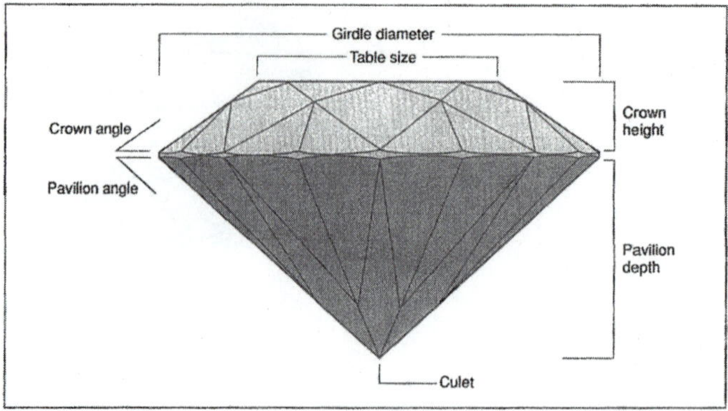

Technically labeled faceted stone.

Figure 5.10 Faceted stones are evaluated based on these attributes.

Faceted stones are discussed in the trade and evaluated in terms of the following attributes (Figure 5.10):

- *Crown.* the top of the stone
- *Girdle.* the widest part of the stone
- *Culet.* the lowest part of the stone
- *Table.* the flat, top of the stone
- *Table spread.* the width of the table

CABOCHON CUT

When a smooth, rounded surface is desired, this type of cut is used. It is less complicated than the faceted types. Stones that feature this cut are translucent, letting the light through without being transparent, or opaque, in which light cannot come through. Coral, jade, labradorite, moonstone, opal, turquoise, and some alexandrites are cabochon cut.

Internet Resources for Additional Research

www.jewelrysupplier.com is a resource that features a variety of information about precious metals, gemstones, crystals, and minerals.

www.host33.com/casting offers step-by-step instructions on molding, melting, pouring, and casting metals.

http://minerals.VSGS.Gov/minerals/pubs/commodity/gold/ is designed to help consumers make informed decisions about a precious metal purchase.

www.indygem.com/productinfo_diamonds.htm features a comprehensive analysis of diamonds, colored stones, and precious metals.

Merchandise Information Terminology

Malleable	Rolling	Precious stones
Alloy	Drawing	Zircon
Plating	Forging	Turquoise
Electroplating	Welding	Ruby
Karat	Casting	Sapphire
14 karat	Engraving	Emerald
18 karat	Florentining	Pearls
Gold-filled	Chasing	Four Cs
Rolled-gold plate	Etching	Inclusion
Sterling silver	Antiquing	Jeweler's loupe
Base metals	Natural stones	Gemological Institute of America (GIA)
Annealing	Mohs Scale of Hardness	Baroque pearl

Semiprecious stones
Alexandrite
Cat's-eye
Coral
Amber
Amethyst
Onyx
Chalcedony
Aquamarine
Garnet
Jade
Opal
Lapis-lazuli
Topaz
Cultured pearl
Synthetic stones
Simulants
Birthstones
Composite stones
Doublet
Triplet
Faceted cuts
Cabochon
Lapidary
Brilliant cut
Emerald cut
Pear shape
Marquise cut
Oval cut
Baguette
Single cut
Crown
Girdle
Culet
Table
Table spread

EXERCISES

1. Using the listing of birthstones in the chapter, select the one for your birthday. Prepare an oral or written report on your birthstone. The information can be obtained from entering the word *birthstone* on any search engine, or directly contacting any of the following:

   The Gemological Institute of America
   Jewelry Council of America
   American Gem Society
   Local jewelers
   Jewelry manufacturers

   The report should feature drawings, advertisements, photographs, and any other illustrations that feature your birthstone.
2. Select one of the many alloys discussed in the text. For the one chosen, prepare a report that discloses:

   The alloy's composition
   The benefits of the alloy
   The jewelry or tableware for which the alloy was formed

Review Questions

1. Define the term *malleable* and how this characteristic of metal enables the jewelry designer to create different designs.
2. What is an *alloy* and why is it used in jewelry production?
3. Describe the method of electroplating.
4. Differentiate between items that are labeled *karat gold* and *gold-filled.*
5. For what major reason is silver not used in its pure form in jewelry?
6. What is sterling silver?
7. Name some of the base metals used in alloying and discuss the advantage it brings to the final product.
8. How do jewelers identify stones?
9. What is the Mohs Scale of Hardness?
10. List the five stones that are considered to be precious.
11. Differentiate between *carat* and *karat.*
12. How do jewelers use the four Cs to assess the value of diamonds?
13. Discuss the difference between the natural and cultured pearl.
14. Does color definitively disclose the name of the stone?
15. Are synthetic stones and simulants the same?
16. What is a doublet and why is it produced?
17. Describe the job of a lapidary.
18. List and briefly describe three faceted cuts.
19. Name the various parts of a faceted stone.
20. How do cabochon cuts differ from the faceted varieties?

CHAPTER 6

Glass, Ceramics, and Wood

After reading this chapter, you should be able to:

- Discuss the different materials used in the manufacture of glass and the benefits they provide.
- Distinguish between soda-lime glass and lead glass and the major differences between the two types.
- Describe glass blowing and the products produced as a result of this process.
- Explain the reason why hard-surface plastics are used in place of glass.
- Discuss the manufacture of chinaware.
- Differentiate between earthenware, ironstone, and stoneware.
- List the major types of wood that fall into the hardwood and softwood categories.
- Explain the purpose of veneering.

Wherever the world-renowned Dale Chihuly exhibits his glass masterpieces, crowds are likely to gather. The unique, masterful handling of glass into pieces that range from the monumental to the traditional, in a multitude of shapes, indicates that the material can be manipulated into forms that were once rarely considered feasible. Of course, glass is also seen in other products such as jewelry, apparel enhancements, and an ever-increasing number of products for the home, including drinking vessels and decorative accessories.

What has become popular and exciting material for both the home and personal wear are ceramics. Once reserved for dinnerware ranging from fine china to more utilitarian dishes, ceramic pieces now are featured in art galleries and museums and adorn the homes of discriminating consumers. In addition to the home furnishings arena, adornments such as broaches and necklaces and apparel enhancements are also catching the attention of designers and consumers.

Whether it is exquisite wood parquet floors installed by master craftspeople, decorative urns and candlesticks produced on the lathe by brilliant woodworkers, jewelry, or trim that transforms simple apparel into eye-appealing costumes, wood has become a material that continues to make exciting fashion statements.

These materials, once taking a back seat to the likes of textiles, leather, furs, metals, and stones, have become fashion staples. Through the ingenuity of the designers who use them and the many new techniques now available in their manufacture, glass, ceramics, and wood have become important elements in the fashion arena.

GLASS

While many of us still consider glass merely for its function in numerous products, the wealth of home furnishing designs and wearable accessories indicate that the world of fashion is being treated to the decorative aspects of this material. Colors from the subtle to the bold are used in fashion as never before. In home furnishings, for example, glass fixtures, stained glass windows, vases, and other decorative items created by Louis Comfort Tiffany feature the most magnificent iridescent colors.

Several types of glass are formulated to produce to different effects and properties, and many techniques provide the purchaser many options.

Materials Used in Glass Manufacture

Several components may be used in the production of glass:

Sand. The main ingredient in the manufacture of glass. Technically known as silicon dioxide, about half of the earth's surface is composed of it.

Sodium carbonate. Also known as soda ash, a white powder that is mixed with sand.

Limestone. Added to the batch to improve hardness and chemical resistance.

Potash. A grainy white powder that decomposes into potassium oxide and becomes part of the glass. It yields pure, colorless glass.

Stabilizers. Different substances added to the glass mixture to give any physical and chemical properties important to its ultimate use.

Lime. Also known as calcium carbonate, used to improve hardness and chemical resistance to the glass.

Aluminium oxide. Added to the batch to improve chemical resistance and increase viscosity.

Lead oxide. Yellow and red lead used to make glass more brilliant.

Barium oxide. Used as an alternative to lead to produce lighter-weight lead crystal and brilliance in the products.

Coloring agents. Generally metallic oxides used to produce browns, grays, reds, oranges, and yellows.

Opacifiers. Fluorine materials added to make the glass opaque.

Sodium oxide. A fluxing agent to lower the melting temperature of sand.

Major Glass Groups

Three main types of glass are used for commercial production: soda-lime glass, lead glass, and borosilicate glass.

Soda-lime glass is the most common and widely produced type of glass. Primarily used for bottles, everyday drinking glasses, and flat glass windows in storefronts and glass doors on case furniture, its nonporous surface can easily be cleaned.

Lead glass is commonly known as *lead crystal.* Its relatively soft surface is excellent for decorating purposes such as grinding, cutting, and engraving. Fine-quality drinking glasses, vases, and other decorative items are usually lead crystal.

Borosilicate glass is primarily used for home products such as high-power lamp bulbs and cooking dishes safe for oven use.

Glass-Making Techniques

Numerous techniques are used in the production of glass and glass products. Some are used in the formation of different products, and others in their decoration and enhancement.

- **Glass blowing** is the technique of using air pressure to expand a hot bubble of glass. It is used more than any other process in glass production (Figures 6.1 through 6.8). With the use of a blowpipe, molten glass is inflated like a bubble and either freely formed or blown into a mold, to produce the desired shape. Small pieces are generally made by one blower, while large-scale "art" productions are the efforts of teams (Figure 6.9). Contemporary glass sculpture of enormous proportions is best appreciated by the intricate and colorful works of Dale Chihuly and his team of artists.
- **Casting** is the process by which the glass batch is poured into prepared metal, wood, or sand molds.

- **Slumping** is a molding method that places glass in the mold, lets it melt down in the kiln, and continues to refill the mold until it is completely filled. Once it has cooled, the mold is opened and the object is removed.
- **Stained glass** uses many pieces of glass assembled with the use of metal strips between them. It was popularized by the work of Louis Comfort Tiffany.
- **Laminating** is the process of gluing layers of glass on a flat surface.
- **Sandblasting** is used to achieve an engraved or etched pattern on decorative glass. It is accomplished by blasting a stream of sand with compressed air pressure.
- **Engraving** is a technique that cuts designs and patterns into glass objects by holding them against a rotating copper wheel.
- **Pressing** is when molten glass is pressed into predesigned molds.
- **Annealing** is the process that gradually cools the glass to decrease the potential for breakage.

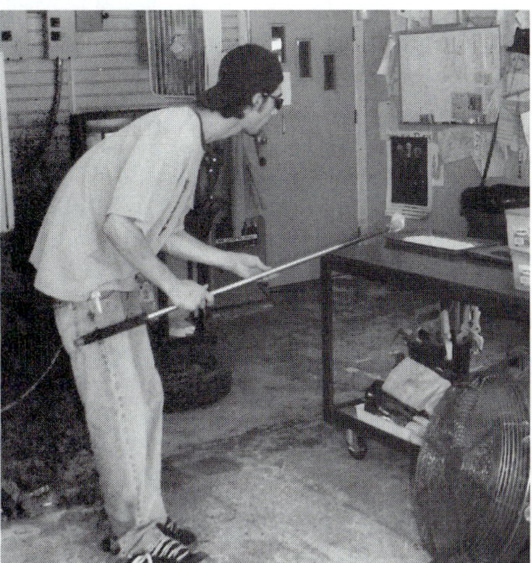

Figure 6.1 A glassblower's assistant adds glass particles to a glass ball that has been heated.
(Courtesy of Ellen Diamond.)

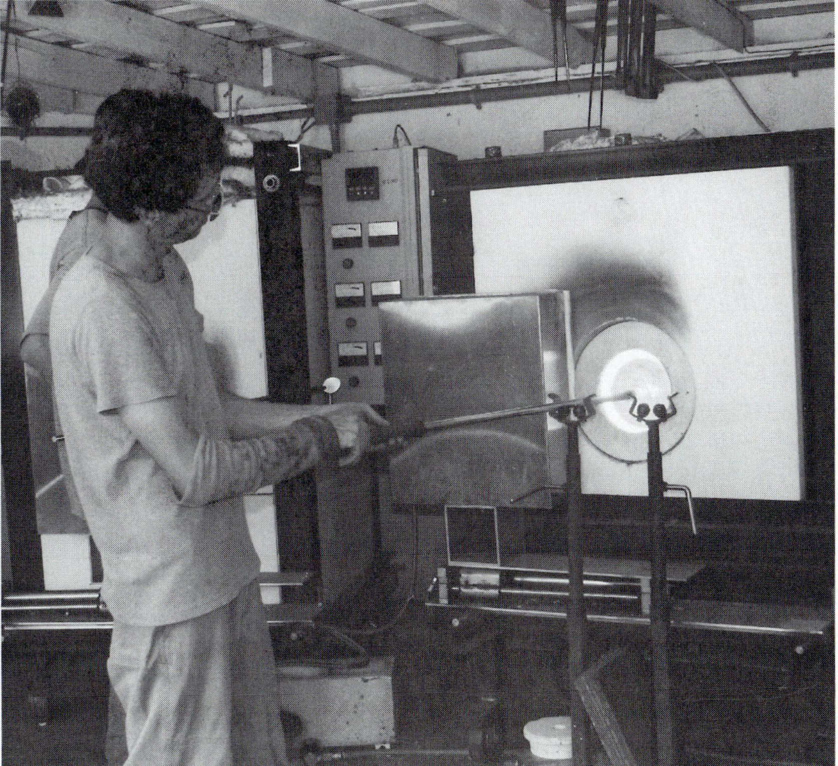

Figure 6.2 Glass is heated in a kiln.
(Courtesy of Ellen Diamond.)

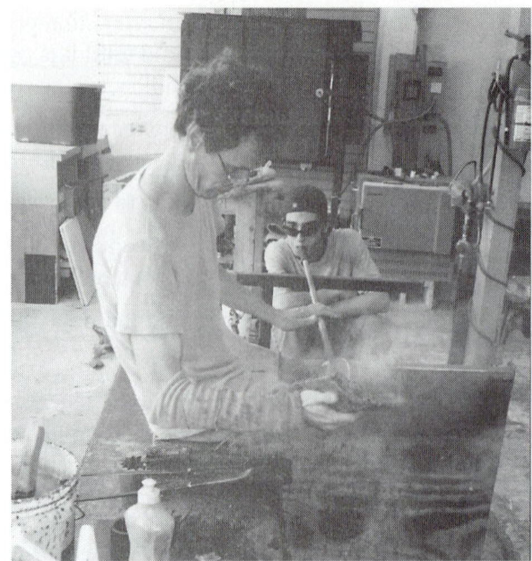

Figure 6.3 Glass is being blown and shaped.
(Courtesy of Ellen Diamond.)

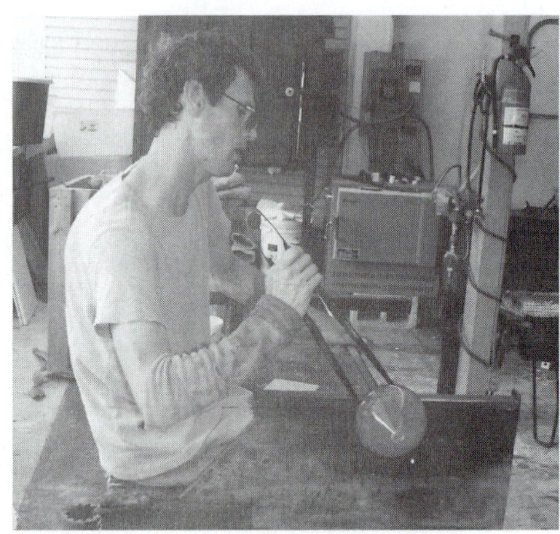

Figure 6.4 Glass is continuously shaped and made ready to be spun.
(Courtesy of Ellen Diamond.)

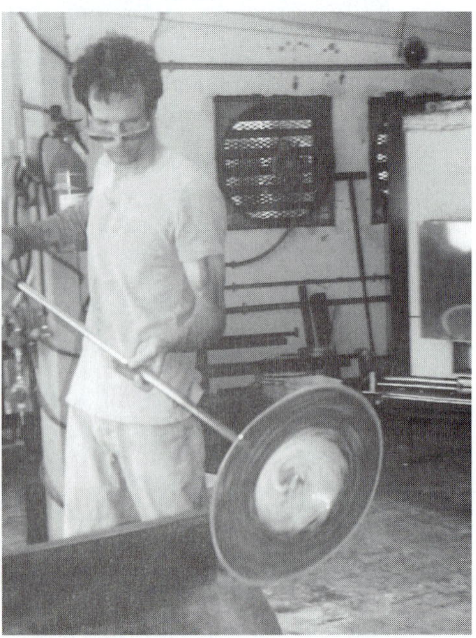

Figure 6.5 Initial spinning gives preliminary shape to the glass bowl.
(Courtesy of Ellen Diamond.)

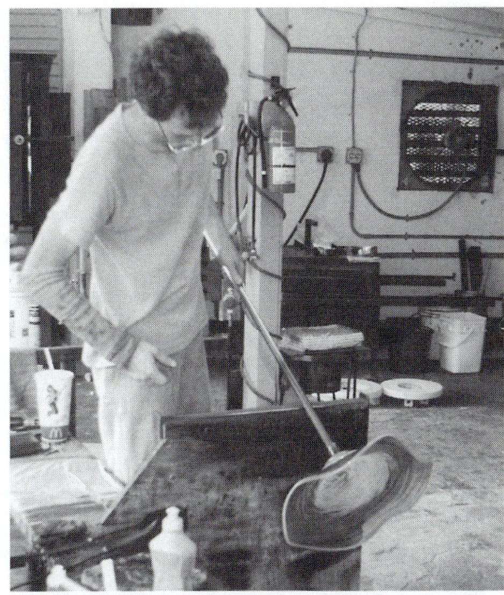

Figure 6.6 Continuous spinning, along with gravity, gives the bowl its rippled effect.
(Courtesy of Ellen Diamond.)

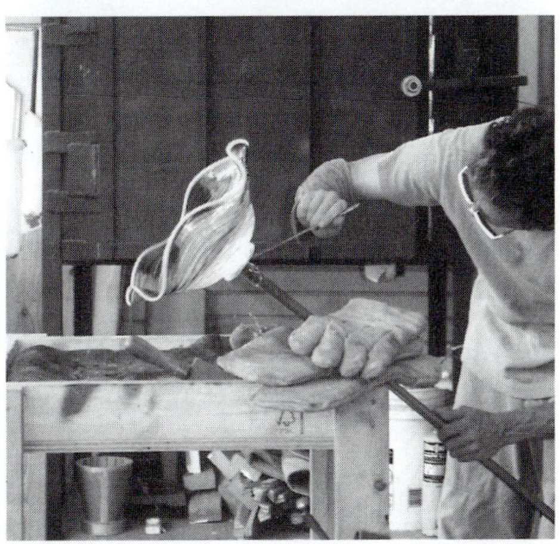

Figure 6.7 The finished bowl is removed.
(Courtesy of Ellen Diamond.)

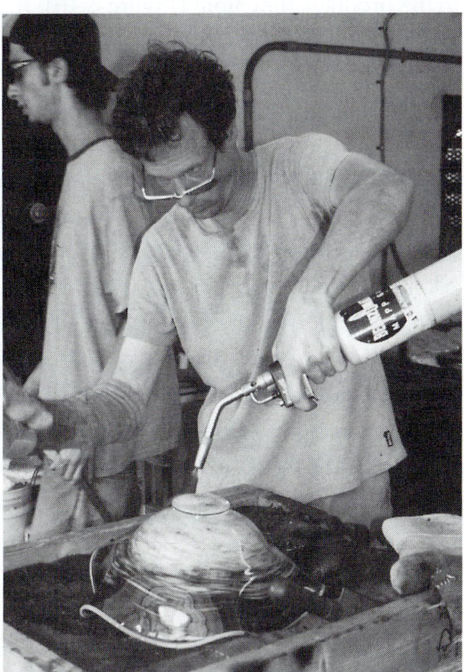

Figure 6.8 The base of the bowl is heated to make it perfectly flat.
(Courtesy of Ellen Diamond.)

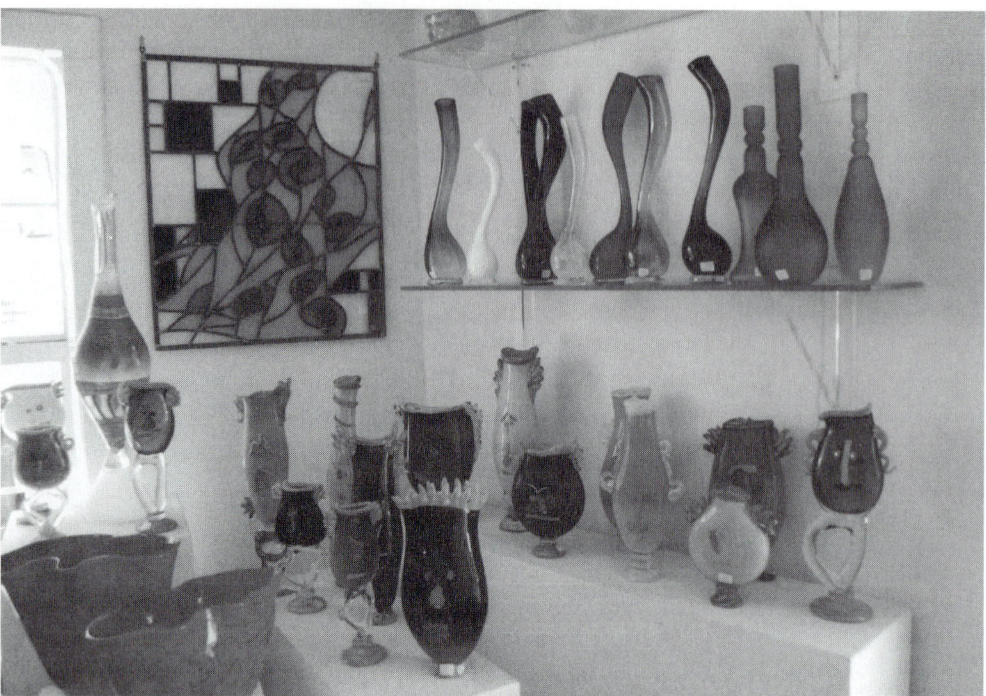

Figure 6.9 These vessels were produced by a glassblower. *(Courtesy of Ellen Diamond.)*

Glass Types for Home Décor and Accessories

Industry professionals, ranging from those in the creative aspects to salespeople, use a common vocabulary of glass in their everyday endeavors. Some of the more common types of glass include:

Flat glass. While it is chiefly for windows, flat glass is also extensively used for decorative mirrors and tabletops. It comes in a variety of thicknesses depending upon its use.

Glass containers. While they are primarily utilitarian in nature, they also add pizzazz to the products they hold (Figure 6.10). In the perfume industry, for example, the bottle that houses the product is often as carefully designed as the product itself. Similarly, wine bottles are second only to the vintage as an important selling tool.

Colored structural glass. More and more glass is used in decorative building facings and tabletops. This heavy plate glass can withstand a great deal of pressure.

Opal glass. When a milky appearance is required, as is sometimes the case with lighting fixtures and tableware, **opal glass** is the material of choice.

Heat-resistant glass. With ability to expand without cracking when heated at high temperatures, heat-resistant glass is the choice. It is extensively used in cookware.

Depression glass. Either in color or clear patterns, this is machine-pressed glass. **Depression glass** was initially made during the 1930s and sold in the old five-and-dime stores. It was inexpensive, but its brittleness caused it to wear poorly.

Stained glass. Popularized by Louis Tiffany and often referred to as *Tiffany glass* even if it is created by a different artist, it is comprised of sheets of colored glass attached with metal strips (Figure 6.11).

Glass Alternatives

Fashion designers and manufacturers have embraced glass alternatives such as Lucite, melamine, and others for use in their products. These engineered materials are either translucent or opaque and provide the producer and ultimate user with many benefits. They may be

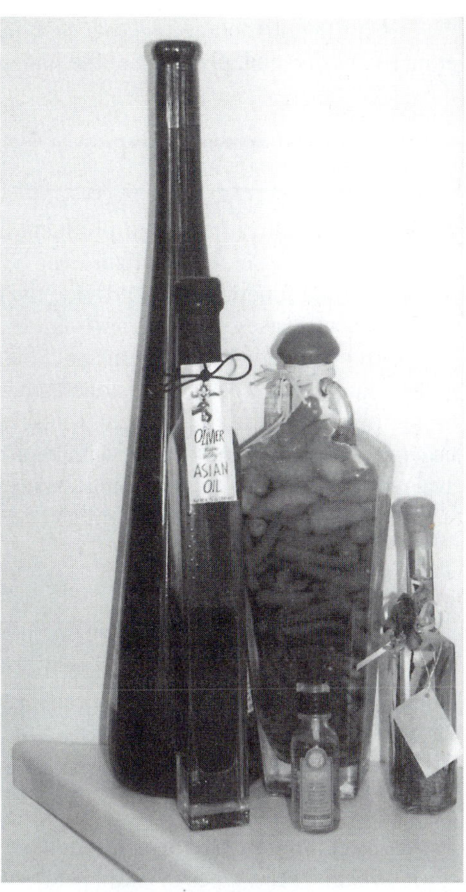

Figure 6.10 Glass containers add pizzazz to products.
(Courtesy of Ellen Diamond.)

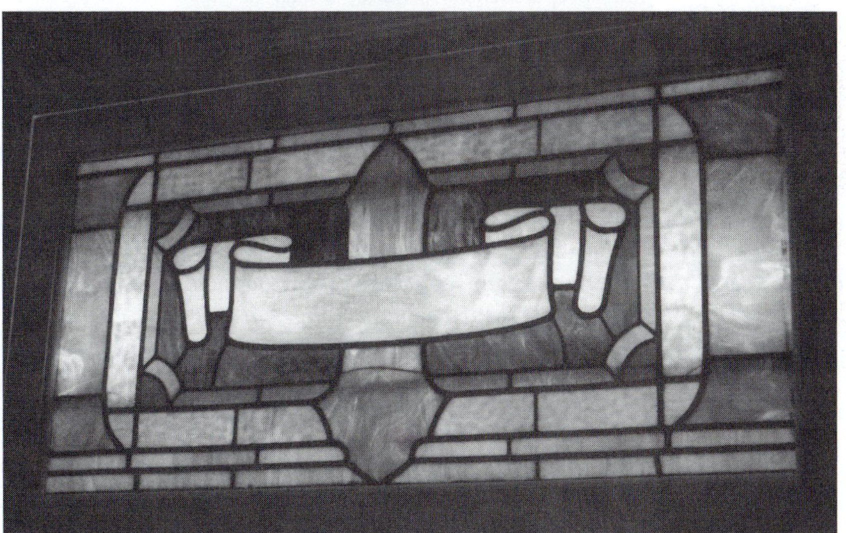

Figure 6.11 Stained glass panels are being used as decorative enhancements.
(Courtesy of Ellen Diamond.)

colored to meet the demands of the fashion industry and enhanced with different finishes such as embossing and etching.

Many jewelry designers are choosing hard-surface plastics for the production of cost-saving, fashion-forward creations. Home furnishings manufacturers often choose Lucite for tabletops, accent furniture, and drawer pulls. Producers of dinnerware often choose melamine because of its natural resistance to absorption and other plastics for outdoor dining because of their resistance to breakage. Moderately priced plastic buttons that are both functional and fashionable are increasingly chosen in place of such natural materials as ivory.

With the advantage of cost, ease in manufacturing, durability, and the ability to be attractively finished, plastics are the natural alternatives to glass.

CERAMICS

Although a wealth of ceramic products has been used in the home for centuries, today's varieties are more extensive than ever before. These objects made of baked clay are both decorative and functional and provide the consumer with what seems to be limitless choices of dinnerware, vases, flooring and wall tiles, and artistic sculpture of museum quality.

From the traditional patterns of china that have graced households for hundreds of years to the contemporary designs of stoneware artisans continue to create, table settings have never been more exciting. Tiles, once merely considered products for utilitarian flooring, have become more and more artistic with replicas of ancient patterns and newly designed motifs available at a variety of price points. Many art galleries and museums have embraced ceramic sculpture as an an exciting art form and continue to elevate its presence in their collections.

Ceramic Classifications

While all ceramic objects are made from baked clay, different ingredients and production techniques result in a wide variety of finished products, ranging from the modestly priced to the costly.

CHINAWARE

Basically, **chinaware** or *china*, a term that is commonly used to describe the product, is primarily a mixture of two types of earth, petunse and kaolin. When they are mixed together and carefully prepared, they produce a clay or paste that is either molded into the desired shapes or thrown on the potter's wheel and gradually shaped by hand. A variation on traditional, or oriental, china is **bone china,** a material that was first introduced by Josiah Spode around 1800. It also has the ever-important kaolin as its base, but includes bone ash in the paste mixture. Its advantages are increased chip resistance and a whiter appearance than the oriental type.

When handles, knobs, and other embellishments are added to the china pieces, they are attached with *slip*. This thick, creamy substance is shaped by hand and set in place on the items. They are stored away until they dry and the time is set for firing. Firing the pieces over high heat is the next step. They are either fired with or without a glaze. Sometimes, one firing is initially used, with subsequent firings to achieve the required state. Oftentimes, if the item is glazed along with the initial firing, subsequent glazes are generally applied. These extra glazes are baked into the china. It is up to the potter to determine the number of times the glazes must be applied to the product. Most glazes are colorless, which enables the pattern to show through.

To give china a distinctive appearance, it is decorated in any number of ways. Decoration may be accomplished before glazing by means of engraving or embossing or with any imaginative applications. If the white china is to be colored, it may be achieved either by using a colored underglaze before glazing and firing or applying gold and enamel colors and then firing a second time. This second, or overglaze, gives permanence to the piece and makes it suitable, in the case of dinnerware, for dining without fear of discoloration or absorption.

An overview of china styles and merchandising is presented, along with the other ceramic classifications, in Chapter 15.

EARTHENWARE

Technically, pottery that has been "lightly" fired is called **earthenware.** Left unglazed, it absorbs water and is problematic for dining purposes. To alleviate the problems of porosity, the fired object is covered with fine, ground glass powder, suspended in water, and then fired for a second time. During this second firing the fine particles fuse with the earthenware, giving it a glasslike surface, and making it suitable for dining.

There are two distinct types of earthenware: (1) creamware and (2) majolica, faience, or delft. **Creamware** is the result of covering the earthenware body with a transparent lead glaze, cream in color, thus giving it its name. **Delft** is tin-glazed earthenware, first produced in Delft, Holland, in the seventeenth century and later produced in England. It is notable for its fine decoration and thinness. It is often embellished with manganese purple before it is fired with a blue underglaze. One of the more popular delft patterns are imitations of the Chinese blue and white products.

IRONSTONE

A variation of earthenware is known as **ironstone.** This hard, white product is extremely strong. It was introduced in England in the early nineteenth century as a substitute for porcelain or china. It was mass produced and marketed to the more cost-conscious consumer. Ultimately it was manufactured in the United States where rich deposits of clay were available in New Jersey and Ohio. Although it never replaced fine china as the dinnerware of choice for elegant dining, it was abundantly used for everyday meals.

STONEWARE

Pottery that is fired at higher temperatures than traditional earthenware is called **stoneware.** Even when left in an unglazed form, it is relatively free from absorbing liquids. It is extremely strong, making it a popular choice for everyday dining (Figure 6.12). Since it is nonporous, it need not be glazed; when a glaze is used, it is merely for decorative purposes.

COOKWARE

Often referred to as flameware, this type of ceramic can withstand the shock of being exposed to open flames or preheated ovens. It is not unusual for **cookware** to remain intact at temperatures of several hundred degrees. It can be taken from the freezer to the oven for the purpose of cooking. It is similar to ovenware, but ovenware cannot be exposed to open flames.

The Language of Ceramics

When consumers and fashion professionals engage in discussing ceramics, a common understanding of some of the terms used in their manufacture and sales is essential.

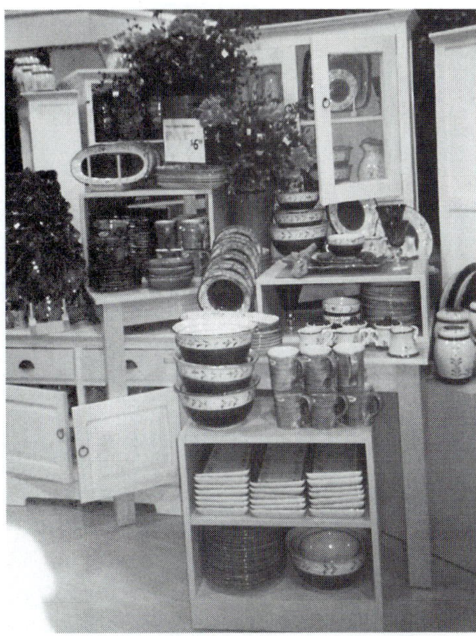

Figure 6.12 Stoneware is an excellent choice for casual dining.
(Courtesy of Ellen Diamond.)

Some of the often-used terms to describe ceramics production are defined in the following list.

- *Bone china.* translucent pottery that uses bone ash as a primary ingredient.
- *Coiling.* a hand-building technique of coiling a long rops of clay into a cylindrical shape (Figure 6.13).
- *Firing.* heating the clay pieces to temperatures that will make them into durable ceramics.
- *Glazing.* mixture of various materials and coloring agents to give the piece a glasslike surface and make it more durable and nonporous. Different degrees of glazing result in different functional and decorative finishes.
- *Kiln.* the oven in which ceramic pieces are fired. The many different types of **kilns** range from the basic to the sophisticated (Figure 6.14).

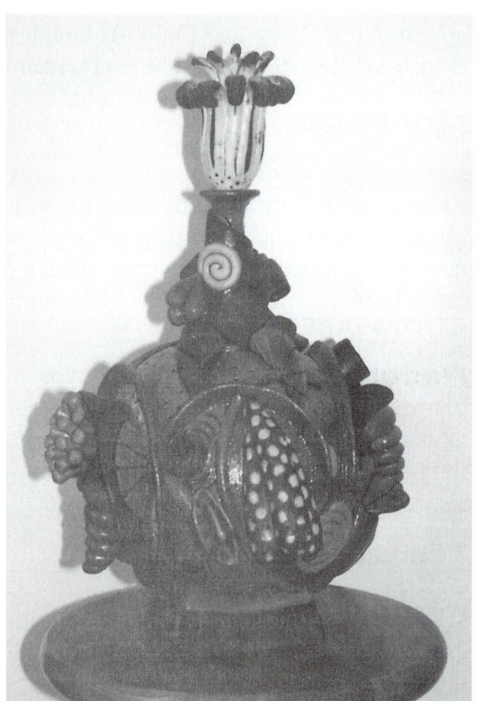

Figure 6.13 Coiling was used to create this unique artwork.
(Courtesy of Ellen Diamond.)

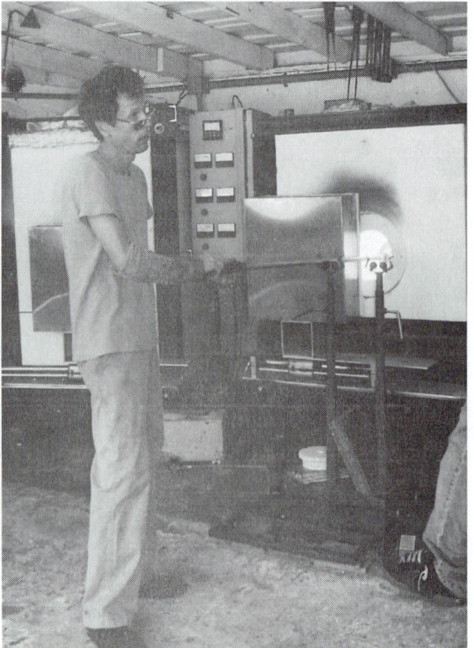

Figure 6.14 Kilns are used to heat glass.
(Courtesy of Ellen Diamond.)

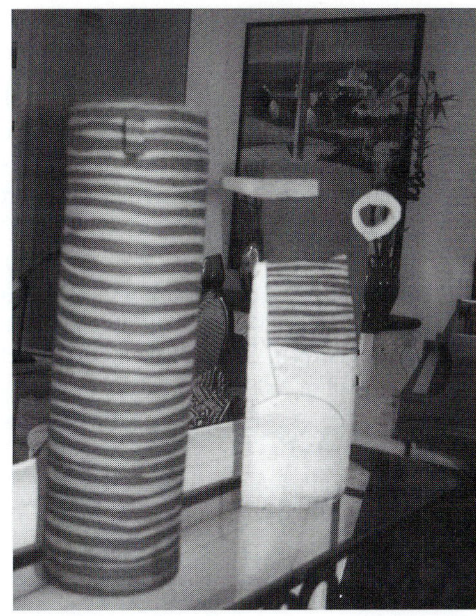

Figure 6.15 The raku technique was used to create this piece.
(Courtesy of Ellen Diamond.)

- *Porosity.* the ability to absorb water and other liquids.
- *Potter's wheel.* a rotating platform skilled potters use to produce a perfectly cylindrical shape.
- *Raku.* a technique originally developed in Japan and used primarily to create decorative pieces. In **raku,** the piece is taken from the kiln and placed in a raku pit while very hot. The pit is filled with combustible pieces that immediately ignite. The fire and smoke create an atmosphere that gives a wide variety of finishes to the pieces. The result is a uniqueness that produces a one-of-a-kind item (Figure 6.15).
- *Leaching.* unintended interaction of lead glazes that are not carefully formulated and fired with the foods stored in ceramic ware.

Potential Hazards of Ceramics

Although the use of ceramic products continues to increase, several risks are involved in their use. Specifically, the problem involves the use of lead glazes, and corroded glazes.

- *Lead glazes.* While lead glazes remain the most commonly used glazes on earthenware and older bone china and porcelain, they may cause problems if not properly formulated and fired at a high temperature. If this is the case, the lead may *leach,* or move away from the glaze, into the food stored in or on ceramic ware. When properly fired, the lead is sealed and not apt to cause harm. Today, raw or free lead is rarely used. Instead, the lead is compounded with silicate, making it less dangerous. One way to determine the ceramic ware's safety is to look for such words as *lead-free, nontoxic,* and *dinnerware safe* to identify lead-free glazes.
- *Corroded glazes.* If the ceramic ware has a corroded glaze, it is extremely dangerous, and should never be used to serve food or drink. The telltale sign of the corrosion is a chalky-gray residue after the item has been washed. Old tableware and highly decorated ceramic ware are often the culprit and should be tested. This can be accomplished by bringing it to a professional chemist.

Reducing the Risks of Questionable Ceramic Ware

Some of the ways in which the risks may be minimized or eliminated include:

- Not using questionable products to store food or drink.
- Not using highly acidic foods such as citrus juices, cola, salad dressings, vinegar, coffee, and tea.
- Not using questionable china on a daily basis.
- Not heating or microwaving old china.
- Not reheating coffee in a microwave.

WOOD

While wood has long been used as both decorative and functional materials in the home, recent years have seen an enormous gain as a favorite of interior designers and consumers. Parquet, hardwood floors have become artistic additions to what were once considered modest homes, and those that are found in more stately environments have taken on the excitement that was once reserved for palatial villas. The ingenuity and creativity of interior designers, and those who follow their plans in meticulous installations, have often created patterns that bring as much interest to a room setting as the furnishings and artwork. Of course, wooden furniture, from the handcrafted to the commercially produced varieties, has been a standard for case products such as chests and tables for hundreds of years.

The use of wood does not stop there. Artists are hand-carving wood for use in decorative home accessories, frames for paintings and mirrors, statuary that has made its way into elegant art galleries and museums, and tableware that includes dinnerware, service trays, drinking vessels, and handles for flatware. More commercially focused, "hand-turned" items produced on the lathe are less costly but oftentimes equally striking.

The significant number of varieties, finishes, and uses as both decorative and functional products make wood an extremely desirable raw material.

Types of Wood

Hundreds of types of woods are used for decorative purposes. The one that is best suited for a particular project such as a parquet floor might be inappropriate for use in a hand-carved product. Those who work with wood and those who sell it must be familiar with the various types and the purposes for which they are suited.

Basically, wood falls into two main classifications. Traditionally, they are either in the **hardwood** or **softwood** category. Those of the former group come from leaf-bearing trees; the latter, from cone-bearing trees. Despite these terms, the reality is that hardwoods can be very soft, and those in the coniferous group may actually be quite hard.

Let's examine some of the more popularly used woods, along with their characteristics.

Hardwoods

MAHOGANY

Although there are many grades of mahogany (a topic to be discussed later in the chapter) and considerable price differences among them, collectively they have the same characteristics. They are fine-grained with a reddish-brown color and feature various "designs" such as stripes, ribbons, ripples, and other effects. The best quality comes from the Caribbean, where the wood is strongest and hardest. Philippine mahogany is really not mahogany, but uses the name nonetheless; it is poor quality because of its lesser durability and beauty and inability to take finishes. One of the prized types, called "crotch" mahogany, is primarily used for figurines because of the beautiful markings and is greatly valued by interior designers.

A great deal of period furniture such as Empire and Federal is constructed with this wood, as are the reproductions of early American designs.

CHERRY

Sometimes referred to as **fruitwood,** cherry is a close-grained wood that is warp resistant and doesn't generally shrink when finished. Colorations range from light to reddish brown, with a deeper reddening when exposed to sunlight. It was used for original American colonial furniture and also for French provincial furniture. Furniture made with this wood is either solid or veneered.

WALNUT

One of the more versatile woods used today, walnut is a popular choice for furniture makers. Characteristically, it is fine-textured, strong, and easy to work with. In its natural state, the color range is light to dark brown, and the wood takes finishes very well. Used in both the solid state and veneers, it is a favorite for eighteenth-century reproductions.

OAK

With more than sixty species, oak is the most widely used hardwood. The stock comes from two basic varieties: red and white. It is a heavy, strong wood, making it ideal for flooring (Figure 6.16). It resists moisture and stains well when different colorations are attempted. In addition to its use as decorative flooring, oak is a favorite for desks and other solid-wood furniture.

MAPLE

With more than 100 species available, maple is widely used for fine flooring and furniture. Commercially, its hardness makes it appropriate for bowling alleys and other surfaces where a great deal of abuse is common. In furniture construction, maple is especially used for less-expensive and medium-priced pieces. Since it resembles cherry wood and can be finished to simulate it, it is a substitute for that wood when price is a factor.

TEAK

Resistant to moisture and rot and extremely durable, it is an excellent choice for outdoor furniture. For interior use, it is often the choice for contemporary Scandinavian designs. Characteristically, it is often strong-grained. It is used both in its solid state and as a veneer. With costs generally high, veneer use is popular.

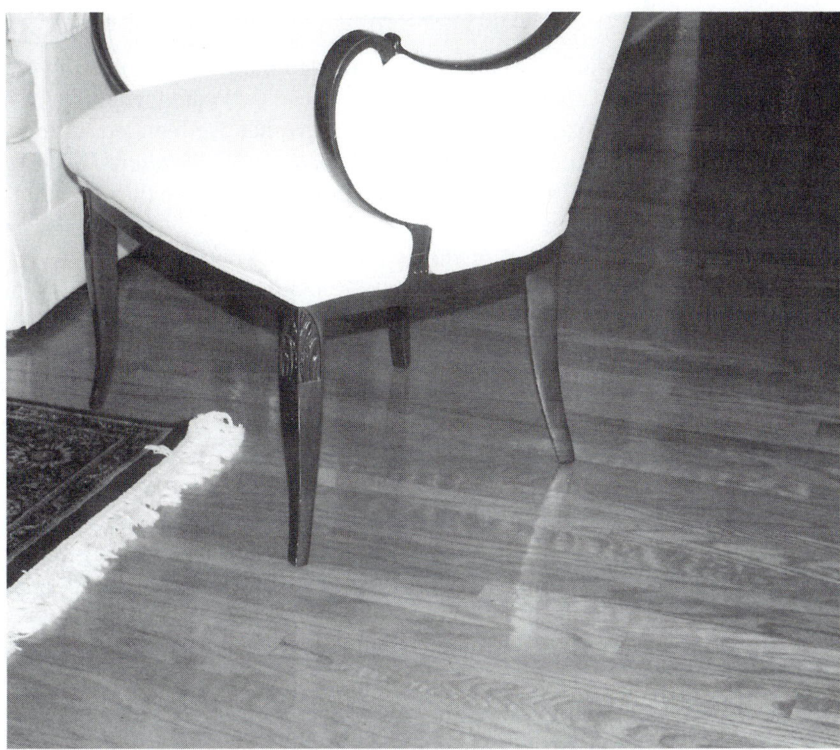

Figure 6.16 Oak is a popular choice for hardwood flooring.
(Courtesy of Ellen Diamond.)

Softwoods

PINE

With more than 100 species, most of which come from the Northern Hemisphere, pine is the most widely used of the softwoods. In its natural state, its coloration ranges from white to pale yellow. For a host of decorative purposes, such as wood paneling, "knotty" pine is often the choice. Country furniture makes significant use of pine either with "pickled" or white-painted finishes. Occasionally, it is used in its natural state with an oil finish.

FIR

Because of its uniformity in texture, fir is used where evenness is desired. It is easily finished either in its natural state or dyed to numerous shades. Often millwork, the decorative trim used in interior design, is made of fir. It is usable as a solid piece of wood or as a veneer.

REDWOOD

Redwood comes mainly from trees that grow as tall as 300 feet in the Pacific areas of the United States. It is an excellent choice for outdoor furniture since it is resistant to sunlight, moisture, and a host of insects. It is easily finished with a natural coat of varnish or other protective materials, or it may be color-enhanced with a light reddish stain.

CEDAR

One of the characteristics of cedar is the fresh odor that it imparts, making it a perfect lining for clothes closets. It also has moth-repellent qualities that prevent moths from damaging the garments in closets lined with it. For decorative purposes, builders often choose cedar on the homes they design. For interior spaces, it is often the choice for Venetian blinds.

Engineered Wood

In addition to the aforementioned hardwoods and softwoods, the industry has **engineered wood** that does not fall into these two categories. There are two types: *particle board* is composed of refined wood chips that are blended with adhesives and pressurized to produce wood panels, and *medium density fiberboard* (MDF) uses wood pieces that have been cooked in steam and made into fibers that are then blended with adhesives and pressed into wood panels.

With all of the available hardwoods and softwoods, the layman might wonder why these engineered products are manufactured. First and foremost is cost. These products are considerably less costly than the "real thing." In their favor, however, the engineered varieties are extremely warp resistant and are unlikely to split. Environmentalists also offer the fact that these procedures ensure that the use of harvested trees is maximized.

Carving Wood

Many homes and offices feature a number of different hand-carved pieces to augment their functional furnishings. Wood carvers have many different types of wood from which to choose, some for the ease in which they may be carved, others for the natural grains they impart, and still others for their ability to be easily finished.

Before selecting the individual piece of lumber, the carver must consider many factors such as the freshness of the wood (which may have a great deal of moisture in it, making it difficult to carve), or the quickness in which it was dried (often causing cracking). The right drying time is essential for carving and the creation of an attractive piece.

Basswood, butternut, and pine are all easy to carve, making them excellent woods for the carver. Mahogany is considered to have medium carving difficulty. More difficult carving is attributed to cherry and walnut, and the most difficult are maple and oak.

Veneering

Many finished products make use of veneers instead of solid wood. **Veneering** is the process of applying one sheet of wood to another. The top layer is the more expensive type and gives the user the desired appearance. The bottom layer, to which the top layer is adhered, is less expensive, making the end product less expensive. Thus, a considerably more attractive piece is available at considerably less expense to the buyer. The bottom layer may even be plastic rather than wood.

In the wood industry, several types of veneers are used in furniture construction. The most commonly produced are *curl veneer,* in which the finished product resembles a curl; *burl veneer,* a design that resembles a tortoise shell; *oyster veneer,* a pattern accomplished through the use of many small pieces that, when completed, resembles an oyster shell; and *inlaid veneer,* a process that involves large sheets of wood to be cut into strips and then rearranged geometrically.

Finishes

The applications or finishes used on wood are either functional or decorative. Enhancement of the natural wood makes it more pleasing to the eye and also renders it more practical for commercial use.

A variety of finishes may be applied.

- *Fillers.* When a smooth surface is required on open-grain woods such as oak, fillers are the answer to solve the problem.
- *Sealers.* Before a final finishing coat is applied, base coats of sealers are sprayed on the wood.
- *Glazes.* If a sheen is desired, slow-drying pigments are sprayed to achieve the effect.
- *Synthetic coatings.* A wide range of synthetics and polyesters are often sprayed on the wood to increase durability along with a high gloss. Using this process eliminates the necessity for hand rubbing.
- *Oil finishes.* Certain hardwoods, such as walnut, can be color-enhanced by means of applying coats of linseed oils. The individual coats are repeated after a couple of days of drying.
- *Polyester finishes.* Where durability and high gloss are the objectives, polyester is the solution. Polyester is available in many colors and can produce surfaces that are scratch-resistant.
- *Color washing.* If a slight tinge of color is desired, thinned paints are applied over the dried surface of the wood and wiped off with a rag or brush.
- *Gilding.* This is the application of applying thin sheets of gold leaf to the wood to give it an antiqued look.
- *Lacquering.* If the objective is extremely high gloss, a resin varnish is used. After each application, sanding is used, until sufficient coating effect is achieved.
- *Spattering.* With the use of "trained hands," spattered effects can be accomplished by "flecking" a wet brush that has been imbedded with paint.

Turning

When specific desired shapes are needed on such furniture parts as legs or arms, or for use in the production of artistic, decorative accent pieces, craftspeople use lathes to create them.

The more skilled the craftsperson, the more likely the end result will be more fully realized. The piece of wood that is to be **turned** is attached to the lathe that continuously spins as the craftsperson carves the wood (Figure 6.17). There are numerous variations of turning, with each resulting in a particular style. The most commonly used include *ball turning,* a process that produces a "string" of balls that resemble a string of pearls; *bamboo turning,* the result of which is similar to the shape of natural bamboo; *rope turning,* a process that produces a finished product that resembles rope; and *reed turning*, in which the end result is much like rope.

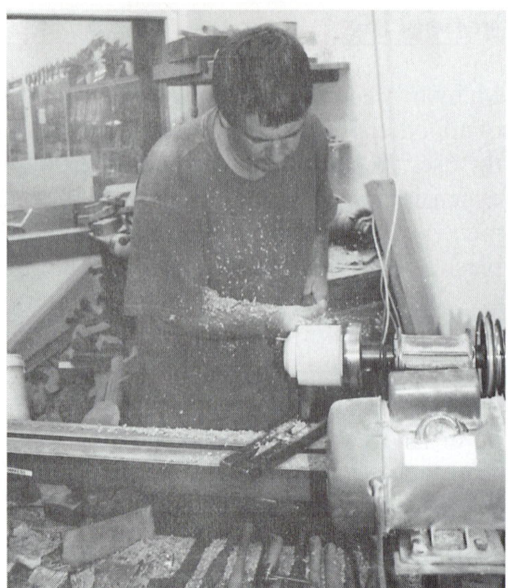

Figure 6.17 A craftsperson uses a lathe to carve wood.
(Courtesy of Ellen Diamond.)

Internet Resources for Additional Research

www.o-i.com/about/corporate/glassmfg.asp is an excellent site that features the complete glass manufacturing process.

www.beyond.fr/themes/glassworks.html features pictures and descriptions of the stages of glass blowing.

www.answers.com/topic/ceramics provides a wealth of information on ceramics.

Merchandise Information Terminology

Soda-lime glass	Annealing	Firing
Lead glass	Opal glass	Kiln
Borosilicate glass	Depression glass	Potter's wheel
Glass blowing	Chinaware	Raku
Casting	Bone china	Hardwood
Slumping	Earthenware	Softwood
Stained glass	Creamware	Fruitwood
Laminating	Delft	Engineered wood
Sandblasting	Ironstone	Veneering
Engraving	Stoneware	Turning
Pressing	Cookware	

EXERCISES

1. Using the Internet, research two of the famous glass designers, such as Louis Comfort Tiffany and Dale Chihuly, or any other. The names may be obtained by using such search engines as **www.google.com** or **www.askjeeves.com,** and entering specific names or *glass artists*. Once you have decided upon the individuals to write about, make certain that you elicit the following information:
   - The type of glass-making techniques they use
   - The colorations and how they achieve them
   - Whether they work(ed) alone or as part of a team
   - The types of creations in which they specialize(d)
   - Typical prices for their designs

2. Visit a retail outlet that offers a selection of ceramic ware in their merchandise assortment. By questioning a sales associate or through the use of pamphlets and brochures that are usually available in these stores, determine the differences between chinaware, earthenware, and ironstone. Make certain that for each you include price ranges, methods of decoration, advantages and disadvantages, and manufacturer brands.
3. Closely inspect two types of wood flooring for use in any room in your home. Comparisons should be made between natural hardwood such as oak, and the variety that has been prefinished. Using the following chart, fill in the spaces to provide comparisons for individuals wishing to install a wooden floor.

COMPARISON CHART		
	Natural Hardwood	*Prefinished Flooring*
Installation techniques		
Wood types		
Prices		
Advantages		
Disadvantages		
Comments		

Review Questions

1. What is the main ingredient in glass production, and what is its technical name?
2. In what way does soda-lime glass differ from lead glass?
3. How does a glass blower accomplish his or her designs?
4. Which types of materials are used for glass molds?
5. Why are many glass products annealed before they are used in everyday situations?
6. How would one describe *depression glass*?
7. Instead of using glass for some projects, what substitutes could be used that give a similar appearance?
8. What is *bone china,* and how does it differ from oriental china?
9. In what way does traditional earthenware differ from ironstone?
10. Discuss the advantages of ceramic cookware.
11. How is the potter's wheel used to create ceramic pieces?
12. What is *raku*?
13. Are hardwoods always harder than softwoods? Explain.
14. By what other name is cherry wood known? What are some of its characteristics?
15. Why is teak often used for outdoor furniture?
16. What is engineered wood, and what are the two categories that make up the designation?
17. Why are veneers sometimes used in place of solid wood?
18. What is veneering?
19. Why are polyester finishes applied to wood?
20. What is turning?

SECTION THREE

Apparel Classifications

CHAPTER 7

Designing and Producing Apparel Collections

After reading this chapter, you should be able to:

- Discuss the design elements used in the creation of men's, women's, and children's wear collections.
- Identify the various principles on which design is based.
- Briefly outline the steps in the execution of a sample garment.
- Explain how the cost of the product is determined.
- Discuss the stages that make up the manufacturing process.

With their creative juices flowing, apparel designers are ready to take the challenge of creating collections that will capture the hearts and minds of professional buyers and, ultimately, those who purchase them for their wardrobes, the consumer (Figure 7.1). Creating unique designs is a formidable task that comparatively few can accomplish. Today, the most successful of these talents are greeted with both fame and fortune in some cases, they achieve the stardom that was once reserved for the entertainment industry.

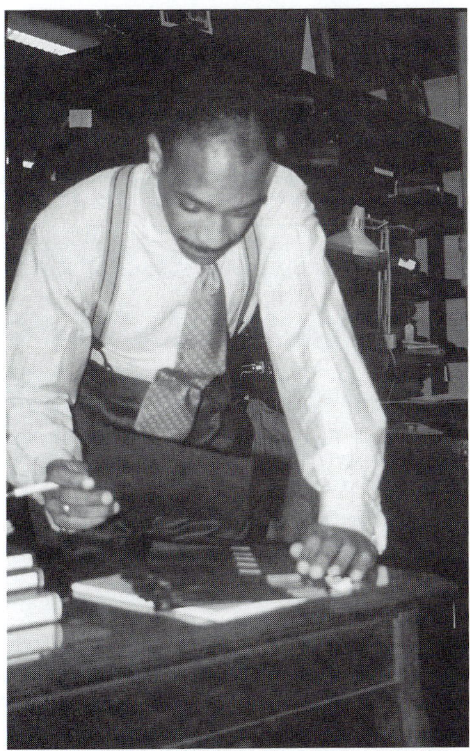

Figure 7.1 The designer develops a line using all of his creative talents.
(Courtesy of Ellen Diamond.)

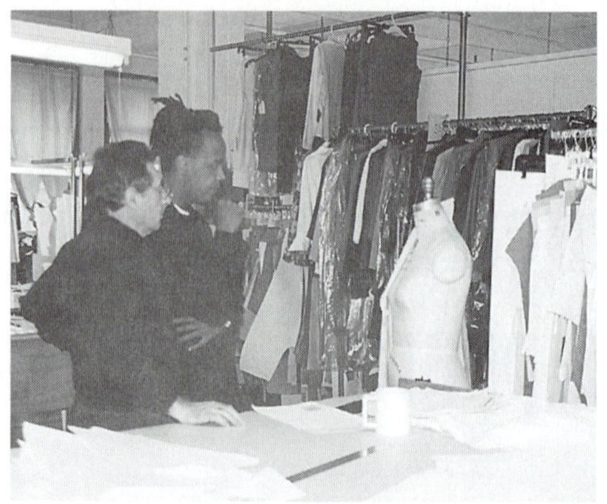

Figure 7.2 The designer often calls on the pattern maker to discuss the new design.
(Courtesy of Ellen Diamond.)

Bringing their designs to fruition is an accomplishment that requires intense dedication, design acumen, and a complete knowledge of the materials that will eventually comprise the items they create. As we have seen in previous chapters, an abundance of textiles, leather, furs, and ornamental enhancements are there for the taking. It is how these elements are selected, manipulated, and used in original ways that make the ultimate design a potential winner.

The design phase is just one aspect in the development of an apparel collection. While the ability to adapt different styles and silhouettes requires design competency, the magic of bringing it to the consumer lies in the hands of the manufacturer. He or she must be able to properly cost the items and apply the appropriate production processes to manufacture collections that will be enthusiastically received. The techniques employed must be carefully addressed and carried out by professionals who have mastered their individual skills to deliver the finished product on time and in accordance with preestablished standards (Figure 7.2).

The design and manufacture of apparel are virtually the same for each of the apparel classifications. Whether it is men's, women's, or children's clothing, the "rules" are the same, thus warranting one general discussion. In the remaining chapters of this section, each of the classifications will be separately explored in terms of their individual categories, size ranges, silhouettes, styles, and details.

DESIGN ELEMENTS

Inherent in every good design is a complement of ingredients that work together. The designer selects these **design elements**, with the company's overall concept in mind, and blends them into a garment that will be fashionable as well as functional. In fashion design, the basic elements are color, fabrication, silhouette, details, and trim. While one may serve as the dominant force, each plays a vital role in the creation of the garment.

It should be understood that these same design elements are part and parcel of all fashion products. As we will learn later in the text, designers of wearable accessories and furnishings for the home must also address the basic elements that make up their products.

Color

Rarely does one of the other elements rival the initial impact made by color on the potential customers (Figure 7.3). It is often the first thing that we see when we take an overview of a particular department in a store, catalog, or Web site. To take advantage of this reaction, many designers and manufacturers often present groups of clothing within a collection in a specific color. Just as the ultimate consumer is inspired by color, so are the professional buyers who purchase them for their model stocks.

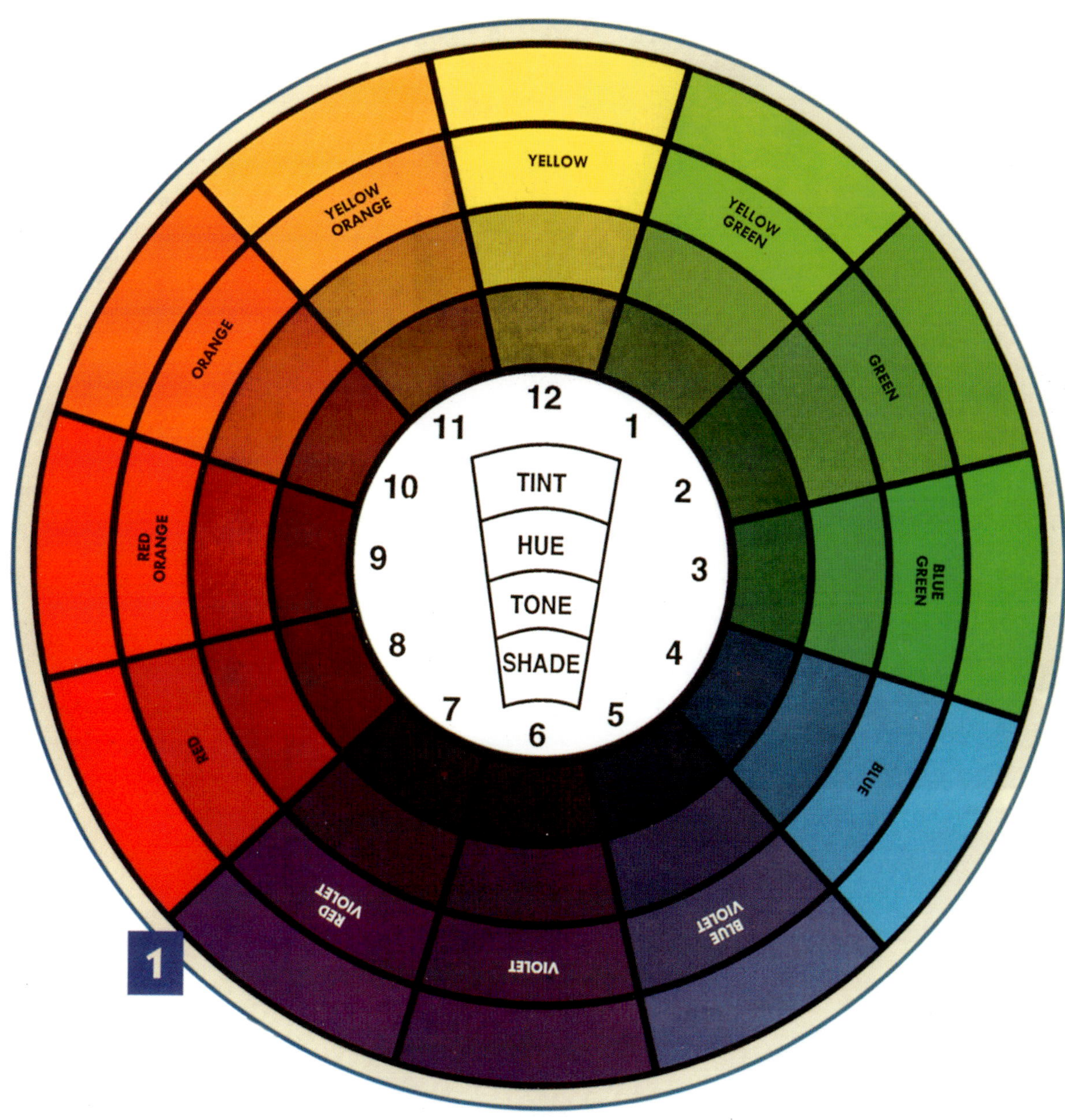

Color plays a dominant role in fashion. *(Courtesy of Ellen Diamond.)*

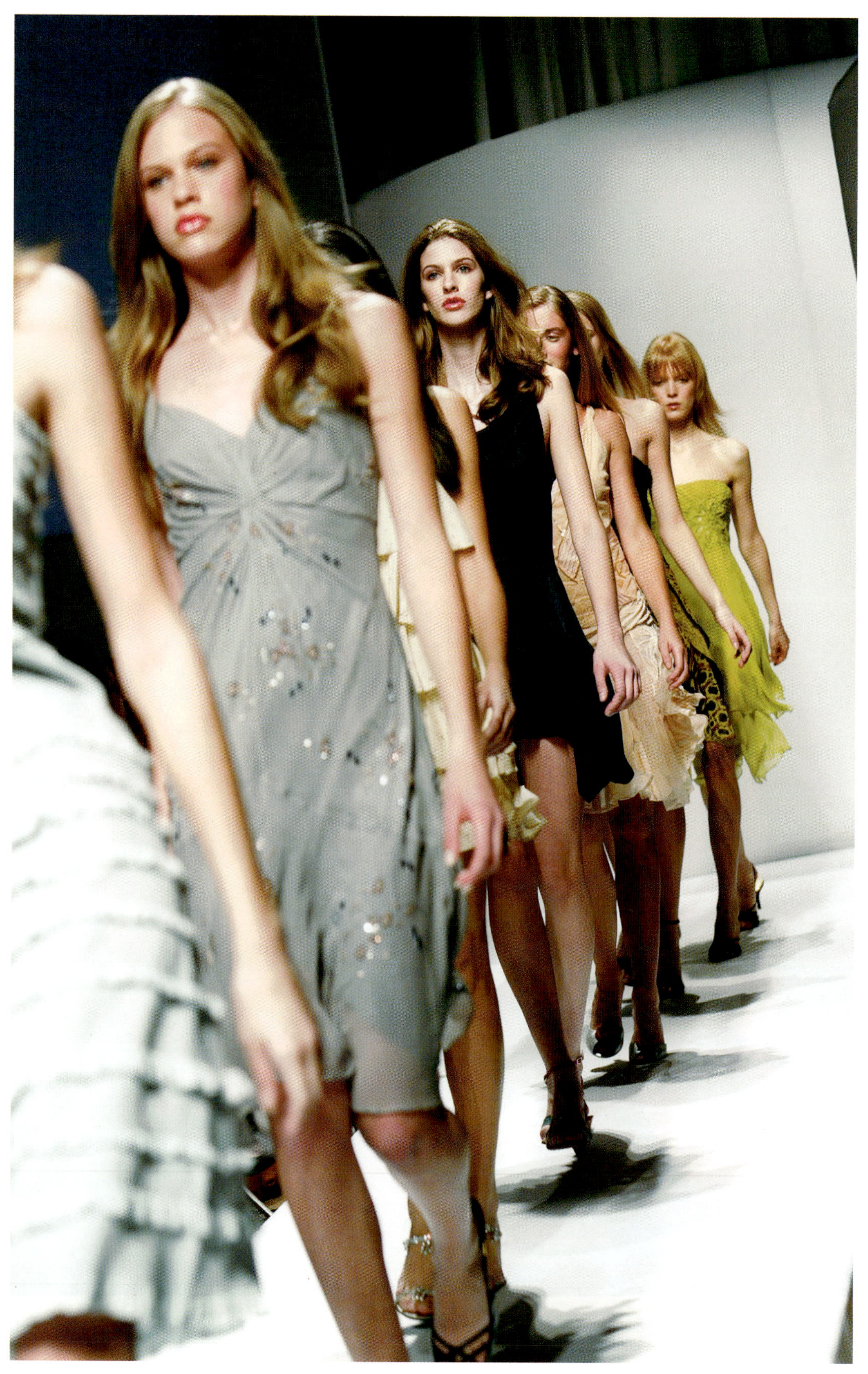

The fashion parade features the latest designer collections.
(Courtesy of Getty Images, Evan Agostini.)

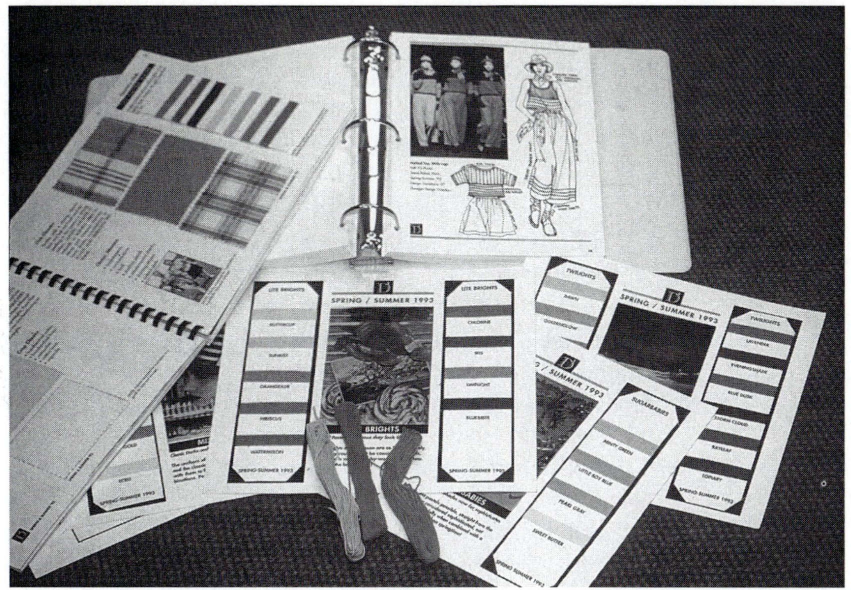

Figure 7.3 Color is a critical design element and must be selected with care. *(Courtesy of Ellen Diamond.)*

COLOR THEORY AND SELECTION

There are color rules to address and color rules to ignore, the decision coming from those who chart the company's design philosophy. Some designers are traditionally oriented in terms of color use, while others are sufficiently gifted to rely on their instincts to come up with color combinations that defy the rules of the game.

When safety is the approach to be followed, the use of the **color wheel** is generally the primary tool that designers use. This simple tool, which is shown in a color section of the text, displays three primary colors and three secondary colors from which a multitude of combinations may be achieved. The primaries are yellow, blue, and red; the secondary colors are orange, purple, and green. Their placement on the wheel enables the user to develop color harmonies that are both technically correct and pleasing to the eye.

In any discussion of color, designers regularly use the terms *hue*, *value*, and *intensity*. **Hue** is the technical name of the color; **value** refers to the lightness and darkness of the hue; and **intensity** signifies the hue's brightness or dullness. When the colors are augmented or enhanced with the neutrals, black and white, any array is possible.

Table 7.1 features some of the many color combinations that can be pulled from the color wheel.

TABLE 7.1 Combinations from the Color Wheel

Color Combinations	*Characteristics*
Monochromatic	The simplest of the schemes; one basic color is used; variations are achieved by using different values intensities, and neutrals.
Analogous	The use of two adjacent colors on the wheel; the addition of neutrals gives more freedom to color harmony.
Complementary	The use of two colors that are opposites on the wheel; allows for the designer to achieve color intensity.
Split Complementary	The use of one color on the wheel in combination with two colors that flank the initial color; allows for greater freedom of color choice.
Double Complementary	The use of two sets of complements on the wheel; produces a great deal of color intensity.
Triads	The use of three colors on the wheel that are equidistant from the other two.

In addition to deciding on the appropriate scheme for their projects, designers must also be aware of the psychological impact of colors. Red is associated with romance; yellow offers a "friendly" image; orange imparts warmth; blue, a favorite among people, provides restfulness and quiet; green is refreshing and peaceful; and purple lends itself to the dramatic in fashion.

Materials

The term *materials* refers to any products such as fabrics, leather, furs, metals, stones, and anything else the designer chooses to use in the creation of the finished product. He or she must assess each item and select the materials that are best suited for it. The feel or "hand" of the fiber, its visual effect, or function plays an important part in the selection process. Leather choices range from the softest to the stiffest and must be considered in terms of the product's ultimate use. If it is a fur offering, then luster, markings, durability, and uniqueness must be addressed before the design is created.

Designers spend many hours scouring the material's markets and the products available to them before embarking on their plans. Their travels take them to domestic markets and global marketplaces to obtain the best raw materials (Figure 7.4).

As we learned in the previous section, designers choose from a wealth of materials. Only those with a complete understanding of the technical and aesthetic merits of each product will have a greater chance to design finished products that will attract both the professional purchasers and ultimate consumers.

Silhouettes and Details

The garment's outline or shape is known as its *silhouette*. The silhouette is enhanced with the use of details such as pockets, pleating, and buttonholes to make it unique. The silhouette's importance is paramount to the success of each garment and must be carefully considered.

In the following three chapters on women's, men's, and children's clothing, an overview is presented to show how silhouettes influence particular designs.

Trimmings

Although the basic elements such as color, materials, silhouettes, and details comprise the product's basic design, the trim often distinguishes one model from another. Decorative adornments to any design are known as *trimmings*, whereas those that are functionally oriented such as zippers are called *findings*.

Trimmings may be produced in a variety of forms. Some of the more typical types include **braid,** achieved through the interlacing of three or more strips of fabric or leather, until a narrow trim is produced; **appliqués,** small individual pieces of fabric that are either manufactured to a particular size or shape or are cut into from larger pieces of fabric, as in the case of lace; **embroidery,** motifs produced by hand or machine that use a variety of threads sewn into the fabric; *beading*, *sequins*, and *piping*, narrow strips of fabric that are used to outline and accentuate details; and *artificial flowers*, *bows*, *ribbons*, and *belts* that are part of a garment (Figure 7.5).

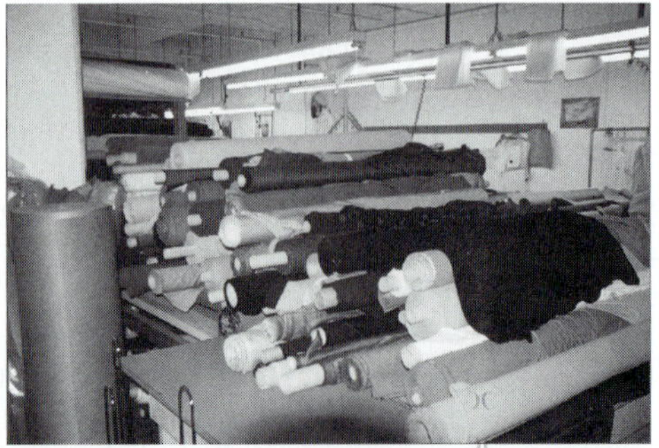

Figure 7.4 Fabric must be chosen carefully to enhance the design.
(Courtesy of Ellen Diamond.)

DESIGN PRINCIPLES

Having selected all of the elements that constitute the final product, attention focuses on the manner in which they are assembled. A relationship of all of the parts must be considered and placed in a manner that is based on the principles of design: balance, proportion, emphasis, rhythm, and harmony.

Balance

To understand **balance,** it is best to think of a scale that has two equal objects on either side. The sameness of the two pieces allows the scale on which they sit to be balanced. When designers speak of balance it is more as a visual distribution. The concept of balance is twofold: symmetrical and asymmetrical. **Symmetrical balance** approaches the design by placing two elements on either side of a central point. Using buttons down the front of a dress as a central point, with patch pockets on each side, for example, would make the garment one that uses symmetrical or formal balance. Although this approach is certainly correct and appropriate for many styles, it does not leave room for more inventive design. With the use of one oversized pocket on one side, and another, differently shaped object such as a decorative pin or flower on the other, the construction uses **asymmetrical balance** to capture attention. It should be noted that both approaches stay within the rules of balance, except that the former is formal and the latter informal.

Proportion

When the various parts are properly scaled to complement each other in the design, they are said to be in **proportion.** An example of poor proportion would be if an enormous bow were to be placed on a delicate, sleeveless, snug-fitting blouse. The body of the garment would be lost to the proportion of the trim.

A design must have a sufficient amount of unadulterated and unadorned space so that the details and trim can proportionally enhance it. The term *fashion*, however, denotes experimentation, and strict reliance on the rules tends to produce a boring garment. Designers continuously experiment with proportion and try to make their creations more exciting. The elongated jacket teamed with a short skirt, for example, might seem disproportional. When the fabrics for both parts are the same and provide the overall impression as one piece, the proportion is not only correct but more exciting.

Rhythm

When a sense of motion moves the eye from one of the design's elements to the next, **rhythm** has been achieved. It may be accomplished by one or more of many means. **Repetition,** for example, provides rhythm by placing a number of the same shapes or details in the design. A row of pleats, for example, would be indicative of repetition. **Continuous line** is exemplified by the use of a linear connection. A "path" of vertically placed tucks on a blouse moves the eye throughout the entire garment. **Progression** involves the gradual increase or decrease of one of the design elements. When a color pattern uses a hue in its purest form and then features a variety of lighter tints of that color in bands, the feeling of rhythm has been accomplished. In **rhythmic radiation,** the movement generates from a central point. A sunburst pattern may achieve this type of rhythm. **Alternation** is simply accomplished when two different elements, usually color, are used. In a yellow and orange striped motif, the two colors serve as the alternating forces that create rhythm.

Emphasis

Every good design has a central or **focal point** on which attention is focused. It is the place in the design to which the eye is initially drawn. If this place of emphasis has been carefully considered, the rest of the garment will then become the beneficiary of this featured aspect of the design. It may be achieved in a number of ways, such as through the imaginative use of trim or detail, the introduction of a striking color to an overall subtle color scheme, or the use of an unexpected material as in the case of leather ornamentation on a denim jacket.

Harmony

When all of the elements of the design work together and the eye witnesses a unified effect, **harmony** has been accomplished. The end product should underscore the intention of the design. Where the goal is subtlety, the principles used should quietly blend together, producing a low-key effect. If, however, drama is the desired effect, the principles should be handled in a manner that accentuates those elements, such as color or trim that impart excitement.

EXECUTION OF THE SAMPLE GARMENT

The complexity of the task turning out samples varies from situation to situation. The most rigorous occasions are those when a totally new collection is being readied. With the final number of pieces having been determined by the staff's merchandisers, the company's design component must now provide the various styles.

The sketches, patterns, and sample constructions are now ready to be produced.

The Sketch

The chore begins with a preliminary **sketch** by the designer. The first sketch may be nothing more than a rendering that addresses the silhouette and perhaps some detailing. It must, however, be sufficiently drawn to be understood by those who are going to develop the patterns. The design may be either be hand-sketched or created with the use of a CAD system. Many computer programs feature a wealth of shapes and details that can assist the designer by adding clarity to his or her own design. Most CAD programs translate the sketch into the pattern that will be used to cut the pieces of the proposed design.

The Pattern

The **pattern** is composed of the various parts of the design such as the body of the garment, the sleeves, collar, and pockets (Figure 7.6). It is used in the transition from the designer's rendering to the creation of the sample-size garment. The sizes used are generally those that best show off the products. In men's wear, a size 38 suit is typical and in women's wear, juniors usually are sampled in size 7 and missy in size 8.

The pattern may be achieved either through a means of draping in which a "muslin" is created by cutting the various pieces of the design on a form; through the use of the flat pattern technique, accomplished on a table, where draping is less desirable; or by means of a CAD system.

After the pattern is made, it is placed on the fabric to be cut by the individual who is responsible for making the sample. Some designers use their assistants for this purpose, whereas others use cutters (Figure 7.7).

Sample Construction

The sample maker assembles all of the pieces that complete the garment (Figure 7.8). The stitches and methods used must be appropriate for those that will be used in regular production.

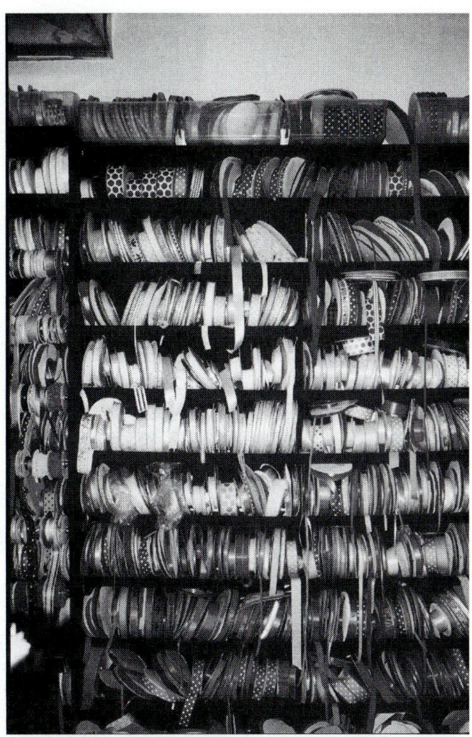

Figure 7.5 Ribbons are often used to add visual interest to a design.
(Courtesy of Ellen Diamond.)

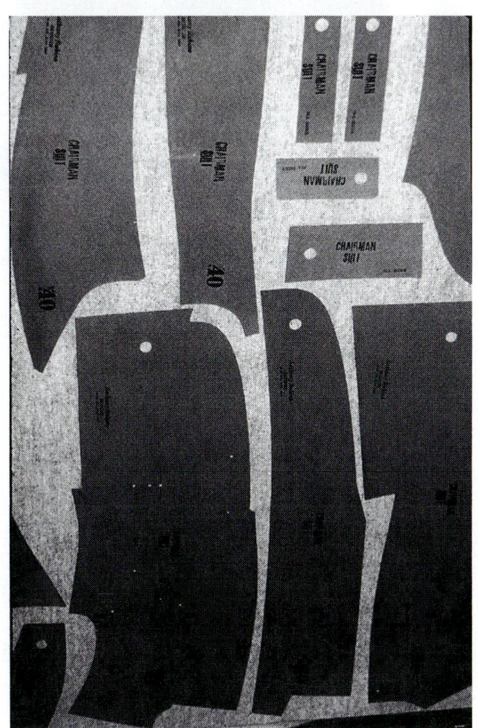

Figure 7.6 The pattern for each piece of the design must be carefully created to ensure a perfect result.
(Courtesy of Ellen Diamond.)

Often, the sample is so carefully sewn that the finished products that reach the retailers pale by comparison. If this is the case, the goods that reach the client's premises might be returned to the vendor. Care must be exercised to make certain that both the sample and the production pieces are of similar quality. Most companies employ quality controllers to make sure that this goal is achieved.

Although the garment's appearance is of significant importance to its sale, its fit is equally critical. To ensure proper fit, the garment should be tried on a live model, called the

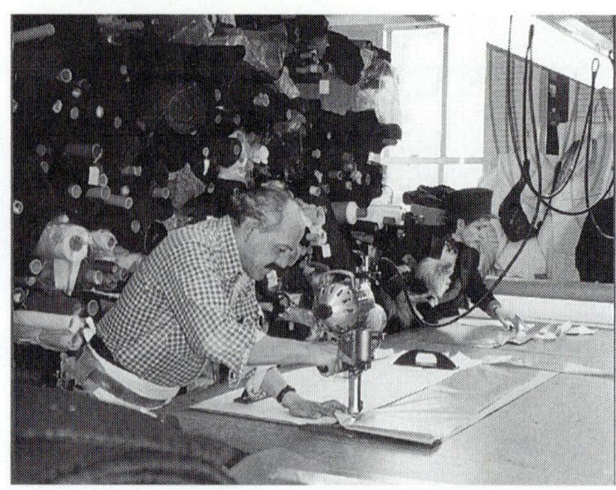

Figure 7.7 The designer and her assistant make certain that the fabric is cut perfectly for the sample. *(Courtesy of Ellen Diamond.)*

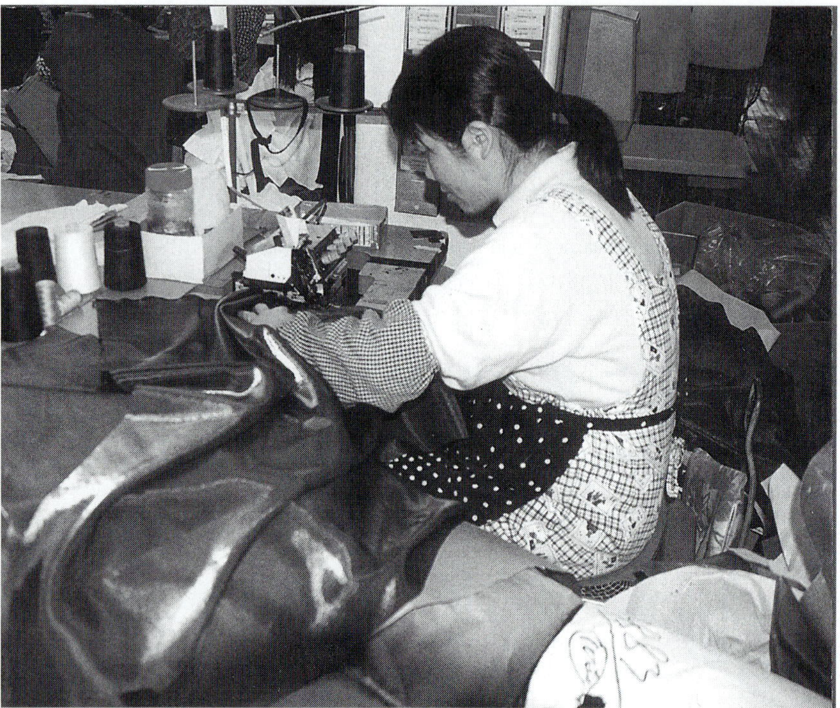

Figure 7.8 The sample maker assembles the parts to complete the garment. *(Courtesy of Ellen Diamond.)*

fit model, after the kinks have been corrected on the stationary form. As the model walks and sits, the garment's ability to satisfy the figure's formation can be assessed.

Too often, when this stage of development is lightly passed over, the products are sent back to the manufacturer.

When the tasks of the design phase are completed, the line is readied for selling, and production is about to begin.

ESTABLISHING THE COST OF THE GARMENT

Long before materials and trimmings are purchased and production schedules set, the costs of every component of the finished product must be determined. If not carefully approached, a best-selling garment might not produce a profit. Up until this time, an approximate set of costs has been established based on the designer's original model or sample. After the signal has been given to go ahead with production, these estimates must be transformed into actual costs.

Materials

The exact amount of materials must be determined and costed. If more than one material is required, then each cost must be assessed. Once this is completed, the trimmings are the next element to be considered.

Trimmings

These enhancements may include anything from buttons and bows to ornamental pins and flowers. They, along with the main materials of the garment, must be figured before production labor is determined.

Production Labor

Production labor costs include making the patterns, grading, marking, and assembling. Some of the costs are borne by the manufacturer of the garment, while others traditionally follow the **outside route** and are performed by contractors. Those that are accomplished through an in-house staff, the production is said to take place in an **inside shop. Contractors** who work for the manufacturers are said to be operators of outside shops. The expenses of both, as they pertain to the production of the product, must be carefully determined so that the appropriate whole price may be established. It should be noted, that in addition to the hourly or weekly wages of those involved in apparel production, **piece-work** costs are sometimes used in which each finished product is costed at a particular price.

Transportation

The cost of freight must also be figured for each unit. In-house production eliminates the need for shipment from one production point to another. However, today, in-house production is the exception rather than the rule. With the enormous amount of production accomplished offshore, transportation costs have steadily risen. With the ever-increasing costs of shipping, these expenses must be carefully considered so that the end result will be a profit.

THE MANUFACTURING PROCESS

The process of transforming the designer's work into merchandise that will reach retailers involves several steps, beginning with making the production pattern for each style and concluding with the finished product.

Each apparel classification has its own stages of development. Some are general procedures that cut across most merchandise products, whereas others are specific to a particular product type. The classifications addressed are appropriate to men's, women's, and children's apparel. Those that are concerned with fashion accessories and enhancements will be discussed in the appropriate chapters in Section IV.

Knowledge of the manufacturing process often enables those who sell the products to make a more meaningful sales presentation to their customers.

The Production Pattern

The original pattern is created by the designer or designer's assistant and is accomplished either by draping, flat pattern making, or the use of a CAD system. In some companies, the patterns that will be used to produce the actual garments are mere adjustments or corrections to the designer's creation.

The professional who makes the **production pattern,** who might serve a dual role by also making designer patterns, uses the same methods discussed previously. Strict adherence to the company's size standardization is perhaps the most important detail to which attention must be paid. Any consumer who tries on a variety of styles of different vendors quickly recognizes that size-standard sizing is not part of the fashion industry. The dimensions of a size 12 dress, for example, from one manufacturer may be totally different than from another. Often, a retail sales associate will say, "try a smaller size because this manufacturer makes a fuller cut." The specifications must be established by the company and carried out by the pattern maker.

Grading and Marking

After the pattern is completed, it must be graded to fit the different sizes in the range that will be produced. Designer samples and patterns in men's clothing generally are made in a size 40 regular, but the complement of sizes might range from 38 to 46 with shorts and longs needed in additional to the regulars.

The **grading** may be achieved by manual or computerized means, with the latter typically used in today's factories that mass-produce clothing. In the former, traditional procedure, the operator uses the sample pattern as a guide and creates the other sizes by increasing or decreasing the other patterns, using amounts that have been predetermined. In these manual preparations, the grader must possess specific skills because the hand, not the machine, that does the actual calculation necessary for each size. The computerized systems, which are by far more in use than the hand-crafted technique, requires the operator to take the initial pattern and mark the key points with a "digitizer" that automatically upgrades or downgrades the pattern. Once the key points of each pattern are set into the computer's memory, a pattern for each size is automatically printed. Not only does the computerized method allow for greater accuracy, but it takes a fraction of the time an operator would need to perform the functions.

After the grading is accomplished, **markers,** or pattern layouts, are constructed that measure the same width as the material to be used for the product. The markers are made of paper and traced from the pattern boards for each of the garment's components. Each part is then set out to fit as closely as possible to the next to eliminate fabric waste. As with grading, markers can be accomplished by computer.

Cutting

After the patterns and markers are generated, the fabric is spread on the cutting table in layers over which the markers are placed. The number of layers depends on the density of the fabric, with as many as 500 for sheer materials. Of course, in couture construction, cutting is typically accomplished one piece at a time.

In the mass-production situation, the cutter expertly follows the markers and guides a vibrating blade around their edges. The vertical blade is better than the circular type because it is more accurate when following the curves of some designs. The fineness or coarseness of the blade depends on the thickness and density of the material. For the one-of-a-kind products, scissors are used to make the cuts.

In many of today's production facilities, the laser beam is used in conjunction with the computer to perform the cutting function.

In cases in which a style is repeated over and over again, making it a staple in the line, **die cutting** is often used. The process resembles that of a cookie cutter. A die with sharp edges is developed when it is pressed against the layers of the material, which it easily cuts through.

Assembling

The number of different sewing steps can range from upward of 200 for fine-quality men's wear. The work may be accomplished by hand, as in the case of custom-tailored suits, or for the most part, by machine (Figure 7.9).

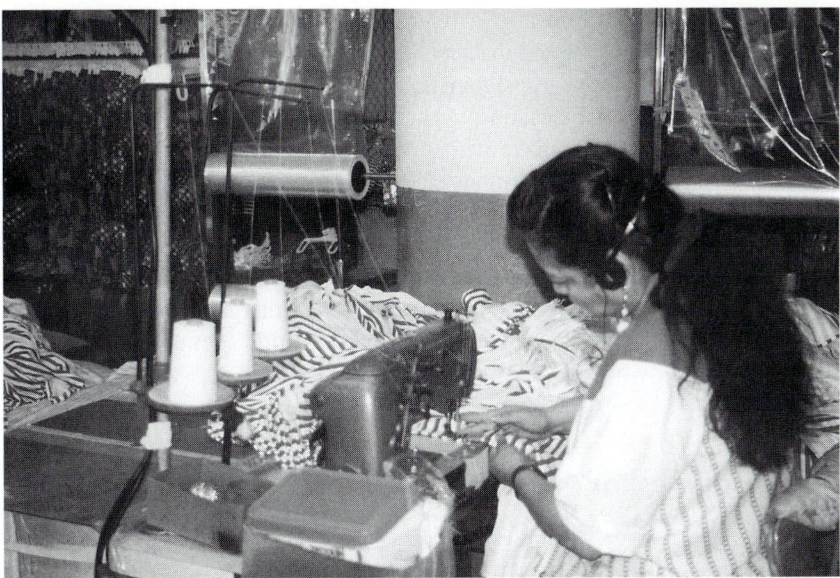

Figure 7.9 Individual workers on an assembly line produce the garments.
(Courtesy of Ellen Diamond.)

Sometimes, an individual worker may assemble the entire garment, but in the majority of cases, the final product is a team effort of assembly-line production. In the latter, individuals are trained to perform one function, passing their work to the next in the line who furnishes the next sewing effort, and so on to the last in the line. Factories using this approach place individuals performing the same operation in one section. After they complete their particular task, the batch of work is moved on to the next section for the next production step.

Although hand sewing is sometimes used, only the most expensive garments are totally hand sewn. The majority of the assembling is done by a number of power machines, with handwork, if used, left for decoration or trim.

There are several types of machines, including the **lock-stitch,** which sews a straight seam; the **chain-stitch,** which produces a looped effect; an **overlock** that sews one seam over another and enhances the appearance of some designs; the **blind-stitcher,** used for hemming; and the **buttonholer,** which effortlessly and automatically sews the buttonholes.

Some assembling involves fusing, where two pieces are **bonded** together. In the menswear industry, lesser-quality garments fuse together the facing and visible fabric of a lapel, thus eliminating the need for costly sewing.

The price and quality of the garments to be finished dictate the type of assembling techniques that will be used.

Finishing

After the garment is assembled, it moves on to the finishers who sew the buttons or provide some decorative touch. Beads may be sewn on at this stage, as might ornamentation such as appliqués and fringe. Decorative hand stitching may also be added at this point. Although some of the finishing is done by hand, much of it is accomplished by special machines.

Some of the finishes are functional rather than decorative. Pressing, for example, is important because it usually straightens a poorly sewn garment and renders it appropriate for selling. The special finishes used in the production of fashion apparel are discussed in their respective chapters.

Labeling

Any number of labels is affixed to each product. One identifies the manufacturer or designer. These are extremely important to a large segment of the consumer market because of the messages they deliver. A consumer might be aware of a particular brand's quality, and the visibility of the label helps make the sale. Another might be motivated by the status of a particular designer, and his or her name on the garment could spell a quicker sale. Throughout the decades, in fact, many designer and manufacturer labels sewn on the outside of the garment have helped to increase sales. Calvin Klein's name on the outside of the pocket brought enormous sales to the company during the designer-jean era.

Instructions for care are also found on labels, which enable the consumer not only to learn how to clean the garment but also cuts down on returns due to improper laundering. Foreign-made merchandise, by law, must list the country of origin, and this accounts for a third label that must be affixed to the garment.

The remaining chapters of this section offer a closer look at the specifics of men's, women's, and children's clothing.

Internet Resources for Additional Research

www.apparelsearch.com/computer_assisted_design.htm offers a comprehensive compilation of CAD systems for the fashion industry.

www.apparelsearch.com/techniques/color_harmony.htm features examples of color combinations.

Merchandise Information Terminology

Design elements
Color wheel
Hue
Value
Intensity
Monochromatic color scheme
Analogous color scheme
Complementary colors
Split complementary colors
Double complementary colors
Triadic color scheme
Braid
Appliqué
Embroidery
Balance
Symmetrical balance
Asymmetrical balance
Proportion
Rhythm
Rhythmic repetition
Continuous line
Rhythmic progression
Rhythmic radiation
Alternation
Focal point
Design harmony
Sketch
Pattern
Outside route
Inside shop
Contractors
Piece-work
Production pattern
Grading
Markers
Die cutting
Lock-stitch
Chain-stitch
Overlock
Blind-stitcher
Buttonholer
Bonding

EXERCISES

1. Choose an apparel classification for the purpose of evaluating its designs. After scanning a number of fashion periodicals such as *Elle*, *Gentlemen's Quarterly*, *Vogue*, *Harper's Bazaar*, and *Esquire*, select five items that attract your attention. Mount each on a piece of foam or construction board and, next to them, indicate the following:
   - The specific elements used
   - The garment's silhouette
   - The details used in each design
   - The trim used to enhance the product
   - The principles of design followed

   Each item should then be carefully critiqued in terms of how you believe it will fare in the marketplace.
2. Bring to class tubes of acrylic paint of the three primary colors and black and white. Mix the appropriate primary colors to achieve the secondary colors. When this is complete, with the addition of black and white, create tints and shades of each color.

3. Select a shirt, dress, pair of trousers, or some other garment from your wardrobe that you are ready to discard. Carefully disassemble the various parts of the design and staple them onto a foam board. Any functional or ornamental trim should also be affixed to the board.

   To estimate the approximate materials costs of the garment, measure the total yardage used and the number and types of different trim elements. After this preliminary work has been completed, visit a fabric and trimmings store to determine the costs of the same or similar types of materials found in your garment.

   Tally those costs to find out exactly how much it would cost for the materials needed to produce a copy of your garment.

Review Questions

1. What five design elements constitute a garment?
2. Define the terms *hue*, *value*, and *intensity*.
3. Which of the color combinations is the simplest?
4. How can a monochromatic color scheme be given variations?
5. How does the complementary scheme differ from the split complementary?
6. What is the nature of a triadic color combination?
7. What is the difference between details and trimmings?
8. How does symmetrical balance differ from asymmetrical balance?
9. In what way does continuous line rhythm differ from progression?
10. Why is proportion so vital to the success of a garment?
11. What is meant by the term *focal point?*
12. How is harmony in a design achieved?
13. In addition to hand sketching, how are designers producing their original designs?
14. What is a *pattern* as it refers to apparel?
15. Why is a *fit model* used before a garment can be mass-produced?
16. Define the term *inside shop*.
17. What is an *outside shop*?
18. How are patterns graded?
19. When is die-cutting appropriate for garment production?
20. What purposes do labels serve?

CHAPTER **8**

Women's Clothing

After reading this chapter, you should be able to:

- Discuss the various classifications that comprise the women's clothing industry.
- Explain the pricing structure that is used to segment women's apparel.
- List the types of size ranges used in women's wear and discuss their characteristic differences.
- Differentiate between the numerous styles and silhouettes that dominate apparel designs.
- Describe the concepts used in the marketing of women's merchandise collections.

Ever since Eve covered herself with the biblical, functional fig leaf, women through the ages have covered themselves in ways that have made fashion history. Although function has always played a significant role in the apparel world, it is the outrageous and exciting costuming that makes an indelible mark on our imaginations.

Women dressed in the fabulous ball gowns at the Metropolitan Opera's opening night and the stars who make their grand entrances on Oscar night clothed in ingenious designer creations have stolen the spotlight from the events themselves. The print and broadcast media often spend more time and space critiquing the clothing than reviewing the performances and guest appearances. The discussion of who wore what seems to remain the subject of the viewing audience longer than anything else about the eventful evenings.

Although these glamorous nights certainly generate fashion excitement, other segments of the industry play significant roles in the business of women's clothing. The appropriate business suit for the successful executive, the swimsuit that combines both fashion and function, and casual, everyday attire are all components of women's fashion apparel.

Before the 1800s, any suggestion of fashion in women's clothing was restricted to the domain of the affluent. Only royalty, the wives and daughters of heads of state, and affluent, socially prominent women could have seamstresses to create garments to suit their needs. Not until 1858, when Isaac Singer developed his sewing machine, did ready-to-wear, or prêt-a-porter, become available to the masses.

Since the beginning of the twentieth century, women's clothing has gone through many phases and stages of design. The pinched-in waistline of the early 1900s was followed by Poiret's abandonment of the full, bouffant petticoat styles and introduction of the narrow silhouette. The beaded and fringed dresses of the "flappers" in the 1920s gave way to the elegance of the strapless gowns highlighted by Vionnet in the 1930s. Padded-shoulder suits and dresses were the rage in the '40s, and the following decade saw the expansion of the sportswear market that Claire McCardell and Bonnie Cashin introduced in the years following World War II. "Mod" fashions were popularized by Mary Quant, and the minis and boots with which they were worn were featured in the collections of Courreges in the 1960s. Americans embraced unisex designs in the '70s and elegance returned in the '80s with the Christian LaCroix pouf skirt. Freedom of choice in terms of skirt length and silhouette opened the 1990s and has continued into the twenty-first century. These are just a few of the styles that have had successful runs in women's fashion apparel.

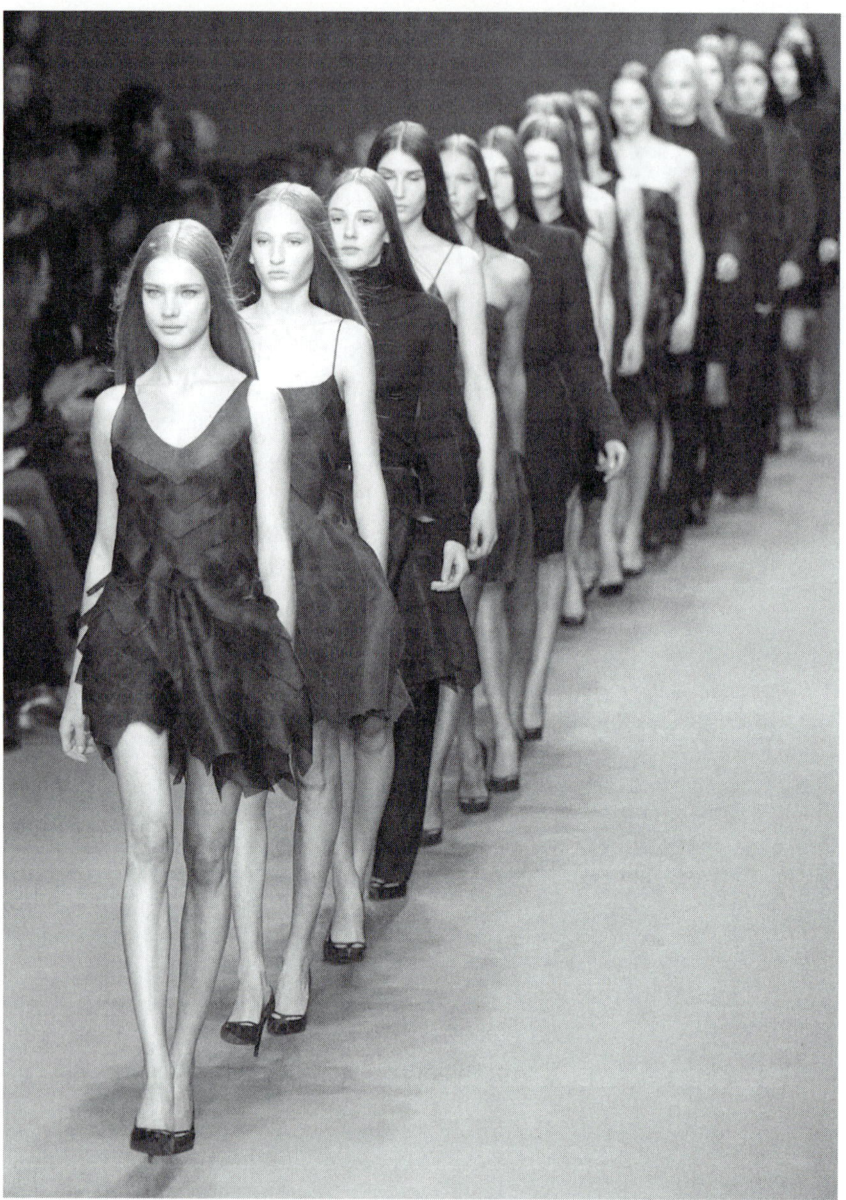

Figure 8.1 *The runway show is used to feature the latest collections.*
(Courtesy of Corbis/Bettmann, Reuters.)

In an ever-expanding global fashion market, more than 4,000 companies regularly produce clothing at every price point to fit every need and occasion. Some restrict their offerings to narrow product lines, whereas others feature collections that cut across several product classifications (Figure 8.1).

In exploring the field of women's clothing, attention focuses on the various classifications that constitute the industry, its price points, the size ranges that are produced to fit specific needs, the styles and silhouettes that are typical of women's wear and regularly find their way into fashion cycles, and the manner in which the industry markets its wares.

CLOTHING CLASSIFICATIONS

Most apparel manufacturers specialize in one specific merchandise category such as dresses or sportswear. A few of the giant companies cut across product lines and feature a wide range of merchandise. The DKNY label, for example, may be found on business attire,

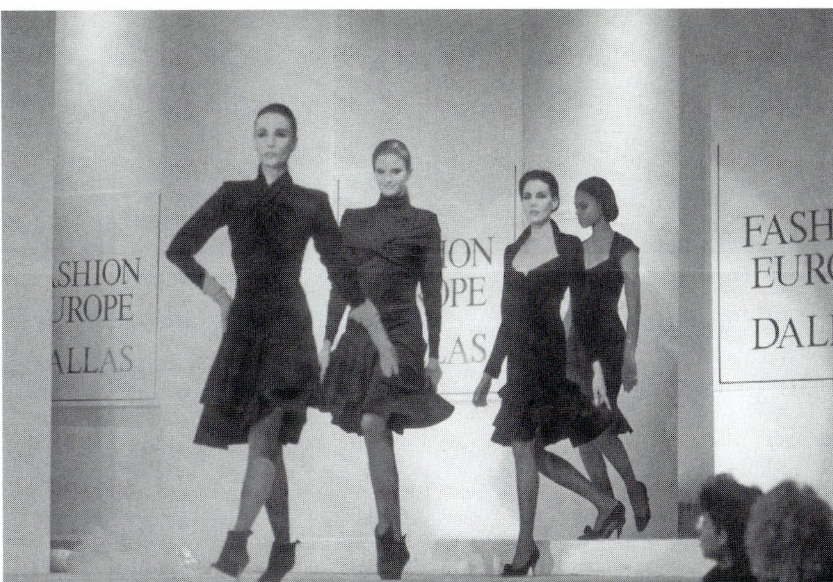

Figure 8.2 Dresses are often the mainstays of many women's wardrobes.
(Courtesy of Dallas Market Center.)

sweaters, cocktail wear, active sportswear, and other items. Some that take this diversified route often do so by manufacturing some of the merchandise themselves and by using licensees for the rest, as is the case with Ralph Lauren. Some even produce lines under different labels, as does Liz Claiborne who features Dana Buchman, a **bridge collection** under that label.

The following product classifications encompass women's clothing:

Dresses

The dress has long been the mainstay of many women's wardrobes, with styles that range from the simple to the fancy (Figure 8.2). Most manufacturers identify the particular market they wish to serve and concentrate on a specific type of dress. By specializing in a narrow segment of the classification, a company may be better able to make a name for itself in the industry and more easily able to market its line.

At times, however, even companies that regularly produce a particular "look" enter into other product variations. At holiday time, for example, even those that specialize in casual or career dressing often produce fancier collections for Christmas and New Year's celebrations.

Sportswear

Until the 1940s, the sportswear market was practically a nonentity in the apparel field. Properly attired women wore dresses for every occasion. During World War II, a more relaxed attitude toward dress emerged, and designers like Claire McCardell and Bonnie Cashin revolutionized the field with their casual clothing styles. Women who once relied entirely on dresses for every social and business engagement began to opt for the newer approach to dressing. They chose a variety of separate pieces for their wardrobes such as skirts, pants, sweaters, blouses, and jackets. These **separates** could be interchanged, or "mixed and matched" to create different outfits (Figure 8.3). Enormous enthusiasm was generated by this merchandise craze, and manufacturers that once limited their lines to dresses soon joined the bandwagon and began to produce sportswear.

Some manufacturers such as Liz Claiborne produce a variety of sportswear collections under different labels that include all of the elements of the classification, whereas others restrict their offerings to only one, such as sweaters.

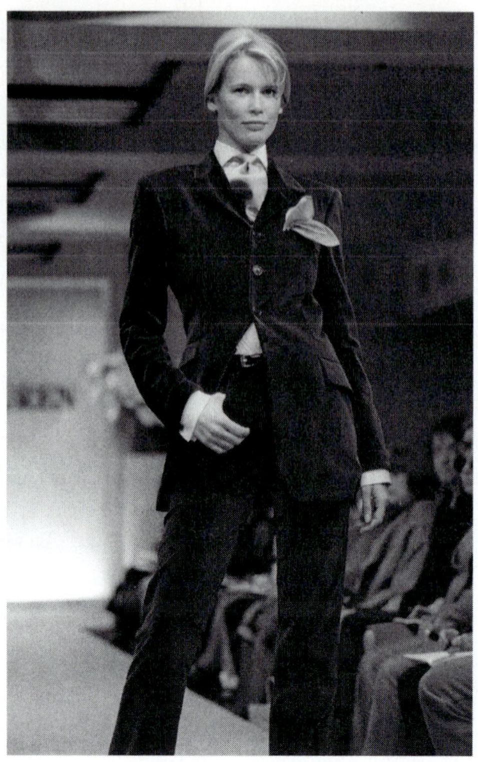

Figure 8.3 This man-tailored suit has become a popular alternative to the dress.
(Courtesy of AP Wide World Photos, Richard Drew.)

Active Sportswear

Participation in sports such as golf and tennis usually call for players to wear special attire. The manufacturers Head and Fila specialized in apparel that was expressly made for these events. Starting in the 1980s, the physical fitness craze grabbed hold in America and continues to reign today. Beyond the continued participation in the aforementioned sports, the offerings of these and other companies were expanded to include jogging suits, bicycle pants, and other items to suit participants' needs (Figure 8.4).

Although the number of people involved in these and other sports increased, making the need for these products greater than ever, another segment of the population brought the active sportswear classification into greater prominence. Significant numbers of people who had never sought the challenges of physical fitness or sports activities began to embrace the mode

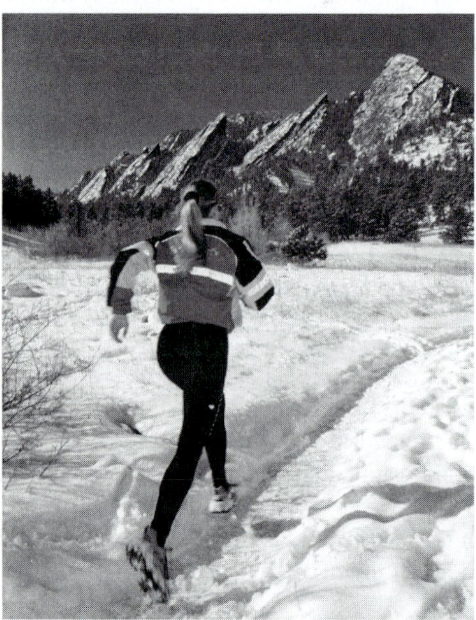

Figure 8.4 Active sportswear is a continuously growing field.
(Courtesy of Omni-Photo Communication, Inc., Phil Mislinski.)

of dress worn by those who participated in the games. It has become common to see warm-up suits, tennis outfits, and golfwear, worn with a host of different tennis and athletic shoes, at restaurants and gathering places where regular sportswear was once the order of the day.

It should be noted that the "rules" of such dress on the field have also changed. In the tennis world, once a bastion for "tennis whites," more contemporary styling and color are now commonplace. Solid color, stripes, and prints now dominate the courts and have carried over into regular daily activities. This is just one example of how fashions change and contribute to greater sales for manufacturers.

From the late 1980s on, there has been an invasion of this market by many manufacturers whose product lines have little to do with an active sportswear orientation, and many new companies have begun to capitalize on this trend in casual dress.

Suits and Coats

Although there has always been a substantial market for coats and suits, the industry significantly expanded its offerings as more and more women entered professional careers. Not only was the right dinner or occasion suit needed by women, but appropriate suits were needed to satisfy the requirements of appropriate business dress (Figure 8.5).

At the same time, the coat manufacturers also began to feature a wider and more diverse merchandise assortment to satisfy both casual wearers and women whose work assignments demand proper coats.

Many producers in this area generally restrict their lines to either coats or suits, some manufacture both, and others are makers of sportswear collections that feature a number of suits and coats in their collections. Some men's coat and suit makers expanded their businesses by offering lines for women. At Brooks Brothers, for example, the labels once primarily featured men's clothing, but today have expanded into women's coat, suits, and other apparel.

Knitwear

Although sweaters have played an important role in casual dress since the 1940s, the knitwear industry has never been as important as it is today. In addition to the more tailored styles that once dominated this market, the sweater has become a feature for almost every occasion. Hand knit and bulky for everyday wear, bejeweled and beaded for use at the most

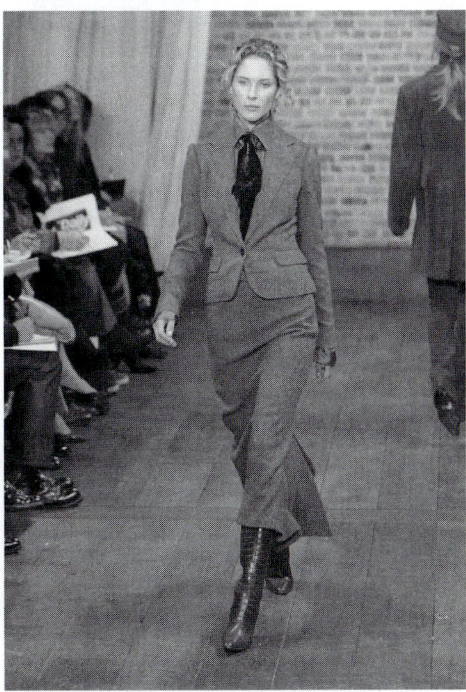

Figure 8.5 Chic suits are a departure from the traditional.
(Courtesy of Fashion Syndicate Press.)

formal events, and intricately detailed with artistic and creative patterns, this market has never been better or larger.

Most designers such as Ralph Lauren and Donna Karan have expanded their collections and feature a full complement of sweaters and other knitwear items. These include a wealth of individual pieces that range from everyday to special-occasion knitwear.

Swimwear

Once a functional product only, swimwear gained its fashion reputation when companies such as Rose Marie Reid and Cole of California gave it a new look in the 1950s. With styling that was as inventive as that demanded by other segments of the women's fashion industry and with fabrics, color, and trim that showed a new enthusiasm, a different life began for the swimsuit (Figure 8.6). It was no longer classified as the "bathing suit" with that single connotation. It was formed into a fashion item with pizzazz and glamour. Lamé, metallics, laces, velvets, and sequined lycras joined the more traditional fabrics, and the assortment significantly grew. As with other fashion entries, the swimsuit's styling and fabric use changes to meet the demands of the market.

To give it the ultimate fashion image, many swimsuit manufacturers have entered into licensing arrangements with apparel designers who style the lines and affix their signatures to them. In some cases, these renowned designers do not create the styles, but assign their development to assistants. The designer name helps sell the goods.

Rainwear

Once worn only during inclement weather, the raincoat has become a fashion apparel product that transcends different seasons and uses. In fact, it is often referred to as "all-purpose" outerwear. Many women have chosen to replace the traditional cloth coat for winter and spring wear. Constructed with interlinings that are removable, as demanded by changes in temperature, this type of coat is the choice of many women.

The industry comprises two segments, one that produces the traditional models, as in the case of Burberry and Aquascutum, and the other that regularly changes its styles, colors, and fabrics as frequently as fashion dictates.

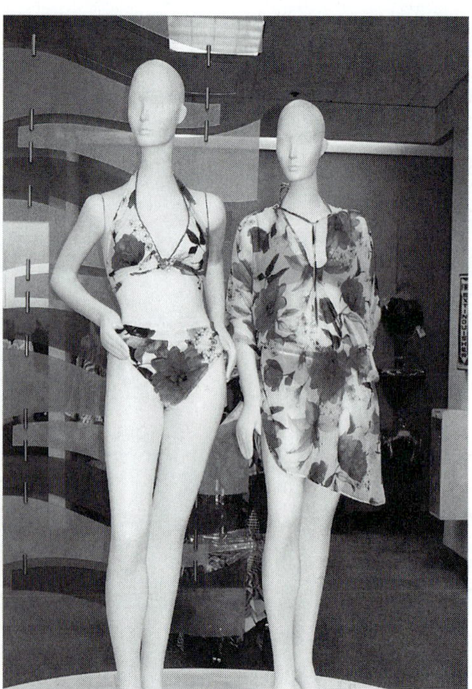

Figure 8.6 Swimwear and matching cover-ups are typical of many collections.
(Courtesy of Ellen Diamond.)

Pants

When American women took their places on factory assembly lines during World War II, not only did they perform the jobs that once belonged to their husbands, sons, and lovers, but they also adopted the factory style of dress. Wearing coveralls or pants and shirts, which provided both comfort and convenience on the job, women soon began to carry over that mode of dress for casual occasions.

Manufacturers, believing that there was a market for such products, developed lines of pants. Immediately, they were eagerly accepted by many women who wore them in place of skirts. The rest is history!

Today, pants are worn everywhere. Whether it is the casual type for shopping and everyday wear, or the dressy, festive styles for special occasions, pants remain a favorite among women.

The product lines come from a variety of places. Typically, sportswear collections at every price point include pants along with their other items. In those offerings, they are teamed with jackets, sweaters, and blouses that make up complete ensembles (Figure 8.7). Of course, they can be purchased separately to meet the consumer's needs. Some pants manufacturers produce only trousers in a variety of fabrics and silhouettes.

Blouses

Until the 1970s, blouse manufacturers played an important role in the fashion industry. In recent years, many of those companies have expanded their operations to include other "separates" in their lines. Few devote their businesses strictly to the blouse.

The popularity of the business suit has fueled a resurgence in the need for blouses. In industries such as banking, finance, and law, where suits are the traditional requirement, the obligatory blouse has become ever more important.

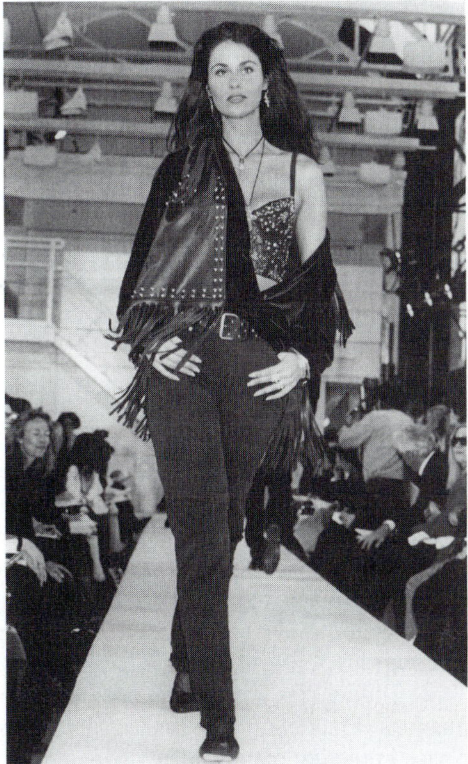

Figure 8.7 Pants are teamed with high-fashion tops to create sophisticated ensembles.
(Courtesy of Education/PH College, Donna Karan.)

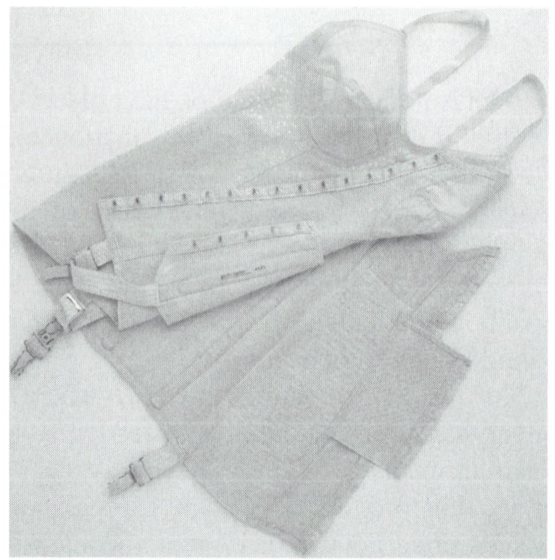

Figure 8.8 This corset, designed in the 1930s, was typical of its time.
(Courtesy of Dorling Kindersley Media Library, Liz McAulay.)

Innerwear

Garments worn beneath dresses, suits, and other clothing were not recognized as a separate product classification until recently (Figure 8.8). Also known as *intimate apparel*, **innerwear** was once hidden away in lost corners of department and specialty stores. Since the 1980s, however, when Victoria's Secret began to merchandise a variety of intimate items in a romantic manner, innerwear became an important classification and moneymaker in women's fashion.

Designers of other apparel have also helped to bring a freshness and uniqueness to this merchandise. When Calvin Klein first introduced a line of boxer shorts, it opened the doors to a new acceptance of intimate apparel. Not only used underneath garments, many items have become fashion products that are worn on the outside. This became extremely popular when Madonna introduced the bustier into her act. This fashion was adopted by her devotees all over the world as standard dress.

Maternity Wear

Not long ago, pregnant women were left behind in terms of fashion apparel. They often resorted to choosing larger sizes in regular clothing while they could and then made the transition into lackluster maternity wear. As we see in the stores and advertisements that feature this merchandise, today's offerings are as fashionable as other women's apparel. This occurrence was attributed to the fact that many women worked well into their last weeks of pregnancy, making the need for stylish clothing a necessity.

Jeans

Once primarily used as functional, rugged pants for heavy-duty occupations and activities, jeans emerged in the 1970s as a fashion product. The traditional Levis, Lees, and Wranglers gave way to more exciting fashion designer jeans that featured such names as Calvin Klein and Pierre Cardin. Soon after the enormous acceptance of this "new" product, which became a status symbol with the designer's logo or name on the outside of the back pocket, other companies began to move their efforts into this arena. Denim was now adorned with leather and metallic studs, and prices soared. Jeans are now worn for most every occasion and by every group.

Today, "fashion" jeans coexist with the likes of Levis, each appealing to different markets (Figure 8.9). The lines are ever-growing in size and style and occupy more and more space in retailer merchandise mixes.

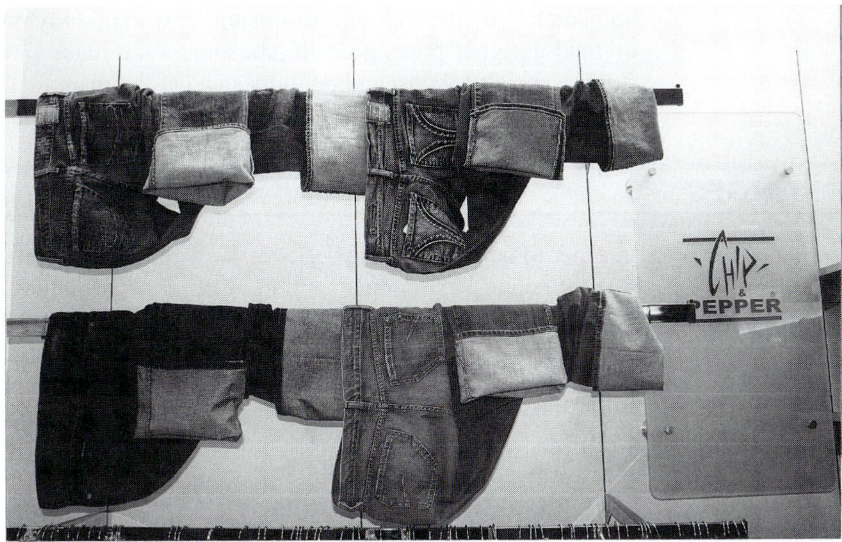

Figure 8.9 Today's jeans run the gamut from the traditional to the very chic.
(Courtesy of Ellen Diamond.)

Bridal

At every price point from the inexpensive ready-made dress to the haute couture creation that has virtually no price limitation, the bridal gown has been successfully merchandised for generations. Where young woman have sacrificed in many ways, it is often the purchase of the wedding gown that entices them to spend endlessly.

The industry is relatively small, but the styles produced cover every conceivable shape and silhouette. Using the most extravagant tulles, laces, silks, satins, and brocades, the results can be spectacular (Figure 8.10).

Designers like Vera Wang, considered by many to be the doyenne of the bridal industry, produce custom-made dresses for an elite clientele. Their designs are generally copied

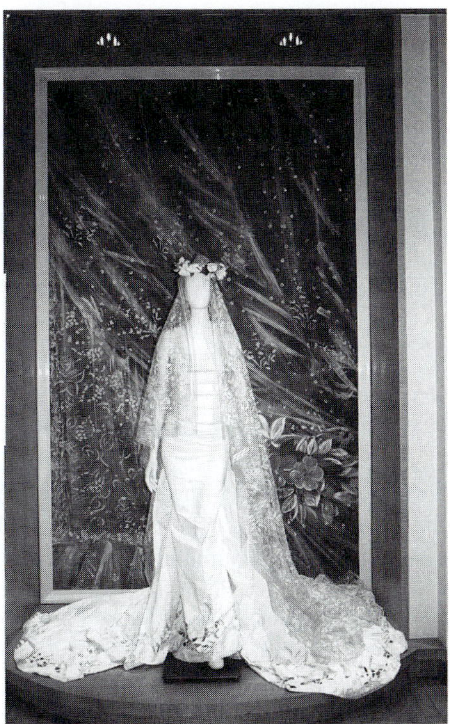

Figure 8.10 Bridal gown designs range from traditional to contemporary.
(Courtesy of Ellen Diamond.)

immediately by the waiting manufacturers who quickly produce replicas at a fraction of the original designer price. Sales to consumers are made through special areas in department stores, specialty shops, and boutiques and at the manufacturers' own premises.

SIZE RANGES

In order to better serve the needs of the women's market and eliminate the need for extensive alterations, the industry offers different size ranges. In the 1950s, the main game in town was the missy sizes that generally ranged from 10 to 18, with a minimum of junior size collections.

Since then, the women's market has responded to consumers by offering different size ranges that address such characteristics as height and proportion.

Misses

Also referred to as *missy*, the **misses size** offering is for the fuller-figured and longer-waisted customer. Manufacturers usually restrict their production to five sizes in the range, with most featuring a run from 8 to 16. Some manufacturers of misses sizes extend their lines and produce garments in sizes as small as 2 or 4, with others featuring size 18.

Juniors

Although many consumers consider the term *junior* to describe a younger customer, this is not technically the case. In sizes, the **junior size** garment is one that is proportioned to fit the slimmer-hipped, short-waisted figure. Because younger people often possess these basic characteristics, the producers of juniors generally manufacture garments with a more youthful appeal for this size specialization.

The sizes are odd-numbered and range anywhere from 1 to 15. As do the misses manufacturers, those that make juniors also limit their size ranges. Typically, the most popular range begins at 1 and extends to 11.

Petites

Short women always had problems when it came to buying clothing before **petite sizing** became popular. They had to buy juniors or misses sizes and have them altered to fit their bodies. Not only did this provide an inconvenience to the customer, but the expense of the alteration increased the price of the garment.

Today, women who are 5 feet 4 inches or shorter find scores of manufacturers who produce apparel tailored to their measurements. The success of this size range is evidenced by the fact that many designers and manufacturers of misses and junior lines often produce the same garments in petite.

Women's

Although the word *women's* is used in the fashion industry to describe all of the product classifications associated with females, it is also used to describe the range of sizes for the largest, fullest figured female of average height. **Women's size** availability usually ranges from 14 to 24, with some manufacturers adding a 12 and others extending the line to include 26.

The major complaint from the wearers of women's sizes has been the lack of styles that were indicative of the fashions of the times. The needs and desires of the customer hadn't been properly addressed by the producers who merely decided by themselves what the fullest-figured women should wear. Dark colors and simple lines generally made up most of the collection.

Today, the image of the large-size market has changed. Designers of the more traditional sizes now offer their collections in women's sizes and have reaped the benefits of such action. Retailers like Lane Bryant, which specialize in large sizes, have also changed their merchandise mixes and feature all types of silhouettes and colors for their clienteles.

Half Sizes

The **half sizes** range also targets the fullest female figures, but they are shorter than those who wear women's sizes. They are not only shorter but short-waisted and might be considered as the heavier versions of the junior petite market. Their sizes generally range from 12½ to 24½ with some manufacturers featuring 26½.

Tall Sizes

Women of above-average height once had difficulty finding clothing to fit them. Although the tall woman wears a regular misses size, the lengths in that range were inappropriate.

Today, in **tall sizes** that range from 8T to 20T, women 5 feet 8 inches and taller can find every type of merchandise available to them. Specialty shops and online resources have sprung up, and many department stores have now opened tall-size departments.

SILHOUETTES, STYLES, AND DETAILS

To better understand women's markets and better serve the needs of those consumers, industry professionals ranging from merchandise managers to sales associates must have a working knowledge of design elements that comprise the garments. Women's clothing design comprises basic **silhouettes,** or shapes; **styles,** the characteristic appearance of the garments; and **details,** the individual parts that make up the garment's structure.

Silhouettes, styles, and details do not change, but their popularity and acceptance at a particular time make them part of the fashion scene. Every garment passes through the stages of the fashion cycle, beginning with its introduction, then moving through a period of growth, then onto the maturity stage, and ending with a decline in sales. The length of time that each style's popularity lasts is difficult to predict or measure. Some have endured for years and have become **classics,** whereas others have quickly moved out of popularity in a matter of a few months. Those with extremely short-lived acceptance are called **fads.**

Designers of women's apparel and accessories adapt, manipulate, and alter all of the basic elements that make up the product. By doing so, designs of distinction make their way into the marketplace to be judged by consumers who will either buy them or reject them.

Silhouettes

Although scores of different styles are produced and marketed every season, each is constructed along a basic shape or outline. They are the **tubular silhouette,** whose lines are straight; the **bell silhouette** that features a bouffant form and emphasizes the woman's bustline and hips; and the **bustle configuration** that accentuates the back of the garment.

It is the creative ability of the designers that takes these three basic shapes and transforms them into individual styles. It might be the uniqueness of the fabrics, unusual trim, or just detailing, such as collars and necklines that makes each silhouette take on its own look.

Styles

Basically, a style is the characteristic appearance of the garment that distinguishes it from all others. In the fashion industry, the term is used not only to describe the appearance of the complete garment but its elements as well. A pleated skirt, for example, is often referred to as a style.

The following is a compilation of some of the popular styled dresses, skirts, coats, jackets, pants, and blouses that have enjoyed fashion success. It should be noted that while some are not considered fashionable today, they have had success during some periods and will more than likely become important again.

DRESSES AND SKIRTS

A-line. When the skirt portion of the dress barely hugs the waistline, skims the hips, and flares to the hemline. In a skirt, the waistband is fitted, and the hips are merely skimmed by the fabric.

Blouson. When the bottom of the blouse portion of the dress is loosely gathered at the waistline and "puffs up," making the waistline invisible.

Chemise. The epitome of the tubular look, it is straightlined and void of a waistline. During the most popular period of its acceptance, in the late 1950s and early 1960s, it was called a *shift*.

Dirndl. A waistline of a full-skirted dress or separate skirt that features "gathers."

Empire. Instead of placing the waistline at its usual place, it is inserted just below the bust.

Gored. A full skirt that is made up of individual panels that are narrow at the top and wide at the bottom.

Jumper. A sleeveless dress that is worn either with a blouse or by itself.

Peplum. A style that uses a straight or flared piece of material that is attached to the waist and extends to the hip.

Pleated. Dresses or skirts that feature folds of material that are either pressed or stitched into place. The width and construction of the pleats vary. "Knife pleats," for example, are narrow and fold in just one direction, whereas "box pleats" are generally wider and fold in two directions.

Princess. A form-fitted torso and full skirt that is made of angular-shaped gores without the incorporation of a waistline.

Shirtwaist. A dress whose bodice resembles a man's shirt and skirt that is either straight or flared.

Trapeze. An exaggerated version of the A-line shape.

Trumpet. A form-fitted skirt that flares out like a trumpet at the knees.

Tunic. A sleeveless or sleeved garment that extends to the thigh and is worn over a skirt.

COATS AND JACKETS (FIGURE 8.11)

Blazer. A basic single- or double-breasted jacket fashioned after a man's sport-suit jacket.

Bolero. A short jacket that features curved bottom sides at its hemline.

Car coat. A three-quarter-length style worn over pants.

Cardigan. A collarless jacket buttoned down the front.

Chesterfield. A single- or double-breasted coat or jacket that has as its distinguishing feature a velvet collar and flap pockets.

Duffel. Also known as a toggle coat or three-quarter jacket, it is made of a sturdy material such as melton and uses wooden toggles and loops for its closure.

Mandarin. A coat or jacket that has been adapted from the Chinese. It is generally made of brocade fabric and is characterized by a small stand-up collar, wide sleeves, and off-center, loop-type closings.

Norfolk. A hip-length, sport jacket generally constructed of tweeds or Shetland materials and featuring a box-pleated front and patch pockets.

Raincoat. A coat that was originally produced to be worn during the rain. It has become popular today as an everyday coat, replacing the traditional spring coat. Its stylings range from the classic single- or double-breasted to those with a contemporary design flare.

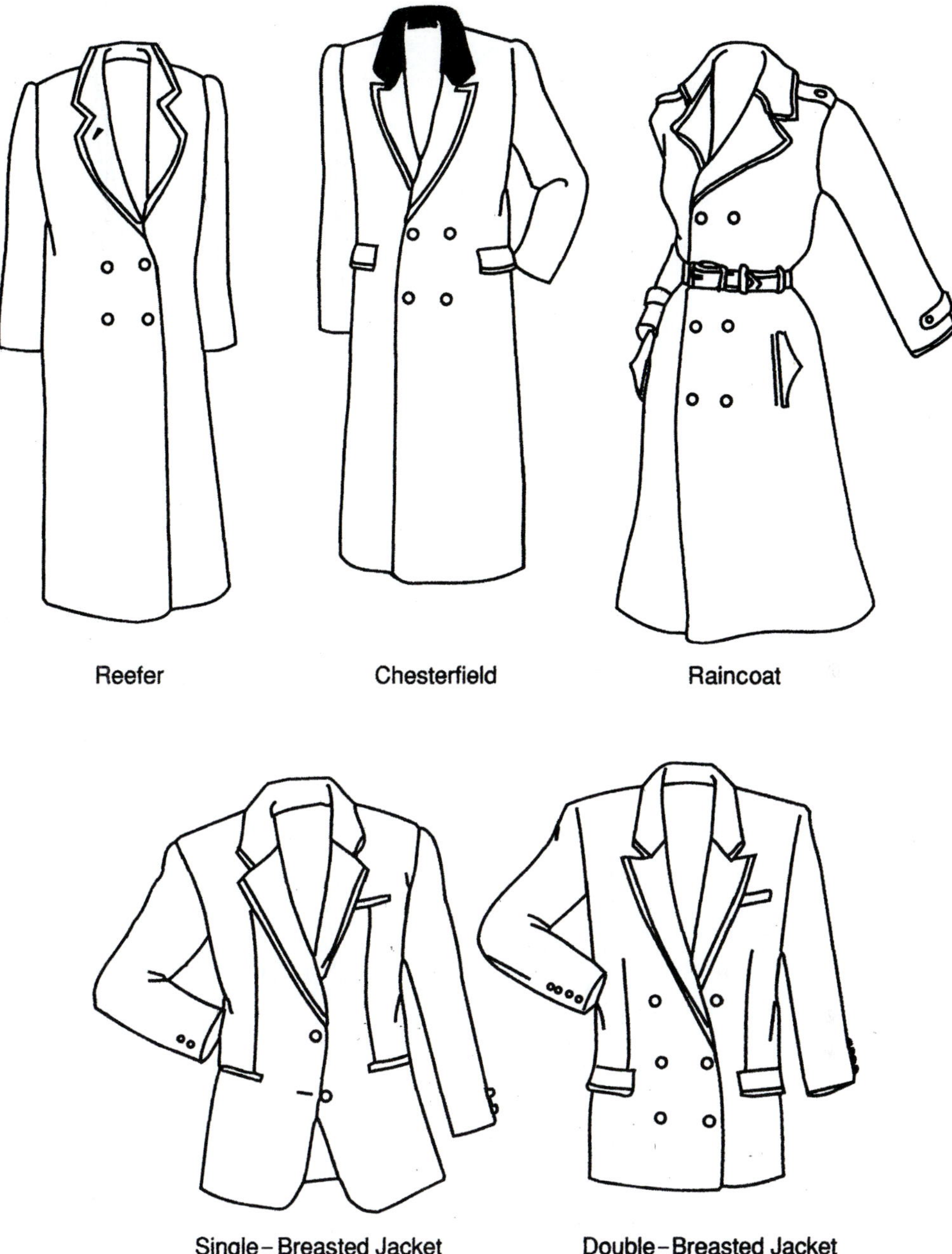

Figure 8.11 Selected coat and jacket silhouettes.

Redingote. A coat that is paired with a matching dress. It often uses a cutaway front that enables the dress to be shown.

Reefer. A princess-line coat.

PANTS (FIGURE 8.12)

Baggies. Loose-fitting pants that achieve their fullness from the "gathers" at the waistline and tight fit at the ankles.

Bell-bottoms. Narrowly fitted at the hipline with a flare beginning at the knee and extending to the shoes.

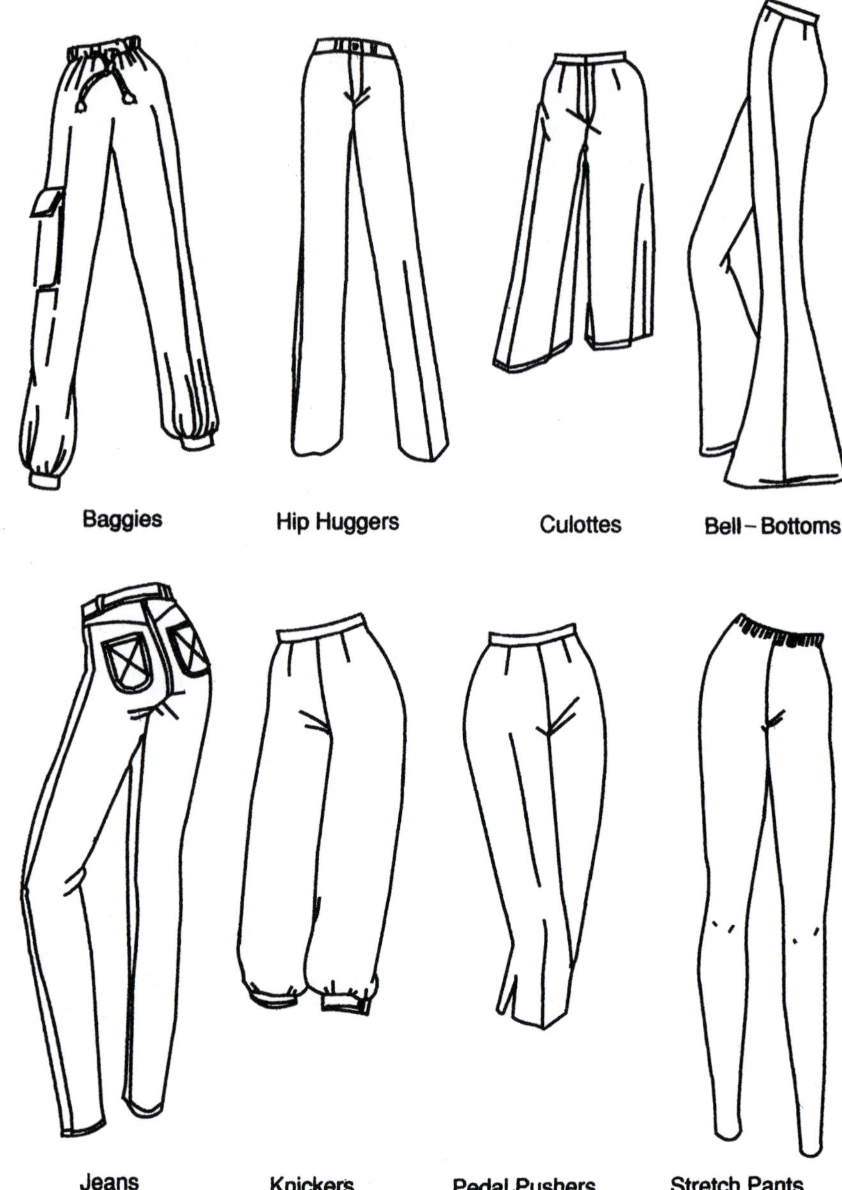

Figure 8.12 Selected pants silhouettes.

Culottes. Short pants that give the impression of a skirt.

Hip huggers. Pants that begin below the waist and hug the hips.

Jeans. Predominantly made of denim and originally featuring western styling.

The designer craze in the 1970s introduced jeans that featured more detailing and displayed the designer's name on the back pocket.

Jodhpurs. Riding pants that are tucked into boots.

Knickers. Short pants that are gathered just below the knee and feature a band or elastic that hugs the leg.

Pedal pushers. Pants that fall just below the knee.

Shorts. Pants that end anywhere from the thigh area to below the knee.

Stretch pants. Made of an elasticized or knitted material, form fitting, and often using a strap under the foot to hold them in place.

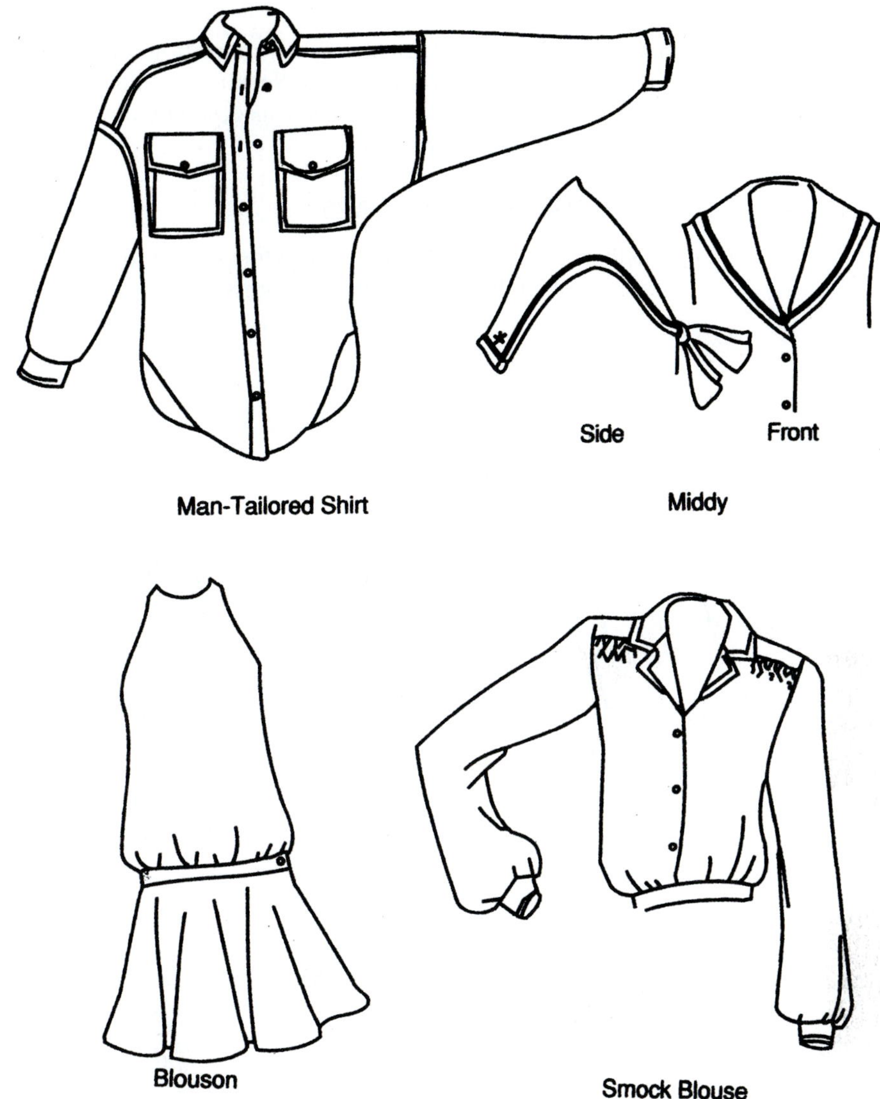

Figure 8.13 Selected blouse silhouettes.

BLOUSES (FIGURE 8.13)

Blouson. A loose-fitting style that uses elastic or a drawstring at the waist to form "gathers."

Camisole. Originally used as a lingerie cover-up of the bra, now also worn separately as a garment. Generally, it has two narrow straps that extend over the shoulder.

Man-tailored. A shirt that resembles a man's dress shirt with button-front closings and either "barrel" or French cuffs.

Middy. Copied from the sailor's uniform, featuring a low waist, long sleeves, and a squared collar on its back.

Polo. A knitted shirt with half sleeves.

Smock. A loose-fitting shirt that features a "yoke" back and full gathers or "smocking" that extends from the yoke, giving it its fullness.

Tank top. A sleeveless, loose-fitting top.

T-shirt. A collarless, knitted shirt.

Details

A unique neckline, imaginative sleeve insertion, or inventive closure are details that help distinguish one style from another. Necklines, collars, sleeves, cuffs, and trim are just parts of the finished product. When each successfully augments or complements the others, the result is a complete garment.

NECKLINES AND COLLARS

Whether it is a simple collar or neckline or one that is intricately featured, this part of the design is often the focal point of the dress, suit, coat, jacket, or blouse (Figure 8.14).

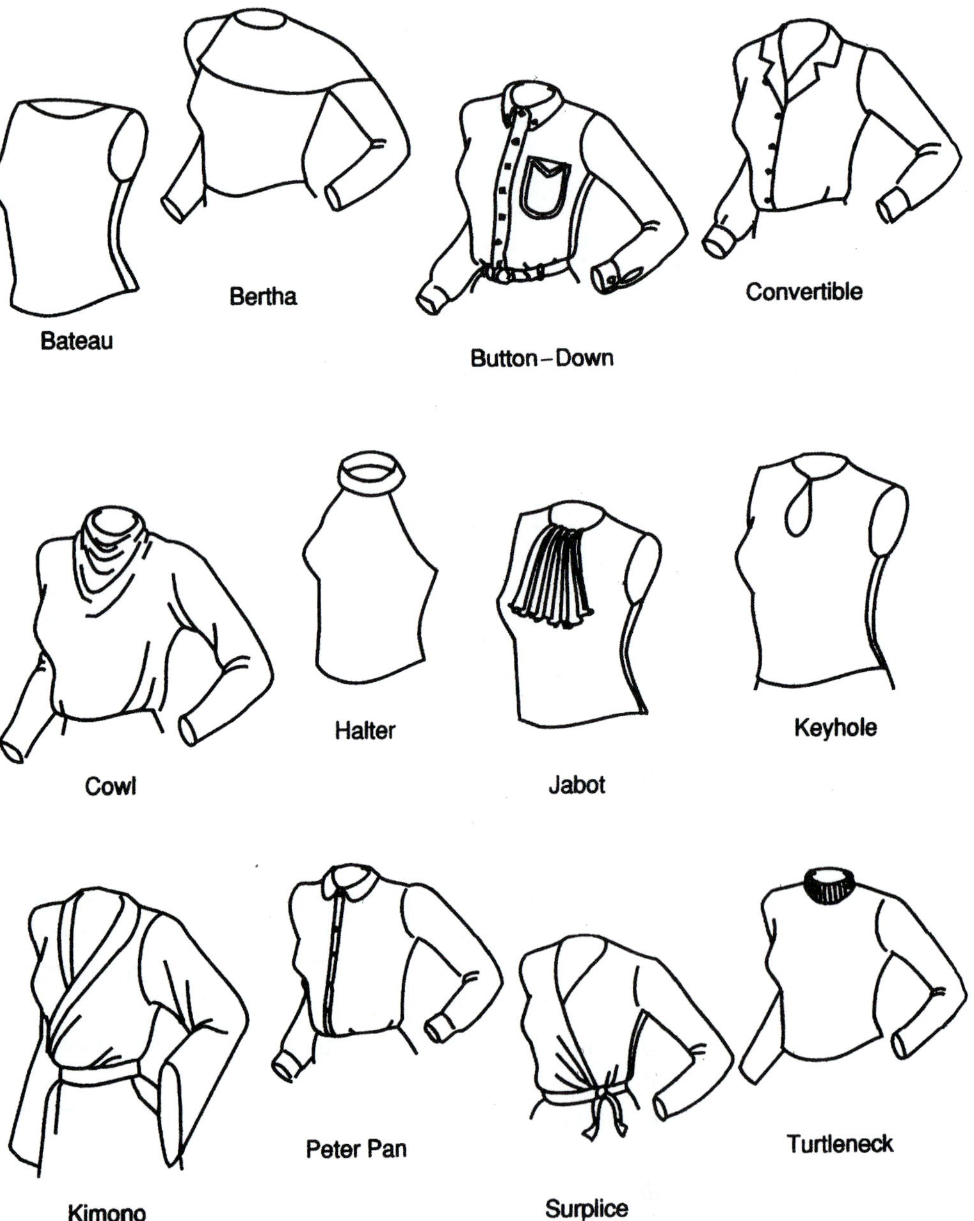

Figure 8.14 Selected necklines and collars.

Bateau. Usually referred to as a "boat" neckline, with an open and wide design close to the neck.

Bertha. A large collar that resembles a cape, which extends from the neck and covers the shoulders.

Bow. A strip of fabric that is either attached at the neckline or made removable with the use of buttons or snaps; sufficiently long to be tied into a bow.

Button-down. Traditionally used in "preppy" or "Ivy League" styles, a collar that features two small eyelets or openings through which buttons on the shirt are inserted.

Choirboy. A large, rounded collar that ends in two points and features two bands of fabric tied into a bow.

Convertible. A collar used either open or closed.

Cowl. A collar cut on the bias or diagonal to permit either front or back draping.

Crew. A rounded neckline, without a collar, that fits close to the neck.

Halter. A backless neckline that is fastened around the neck.

Jabot. A ruffled or pleated extra piece of fabric featured at the neckline.

Jewel. A round neckline that is void of a collar. It is often worn to display a necklace.

Keyhole. An open design that resembles the shape of a keyhole from which it gets its name.

Peter Pan. A small, flat, rounded collar.

Plunging. A low and open neckline.

Puritan. A large, flat, rounded collar.

Sailor. A V front and square back collar, which is adapted from the Navy uniform.

Strapless. Any neckline that is void of straps.

Surplice. A V formed when one piece of fabric is wrapped across another on the front of a blouse or the bodice of a dress.

Sweetheart. A heart-shaped neckline.

Turtleneck. A high neck folded over or turned down.

U-neck. A low-cut, collarless design that forms the shape of a U.

V-neck. A neckline that forms the letter V.

SLEEVES AND CUFFS

From the fullest to the most tapered varieties, sleeves and cuffs may be both fashionable and functional at the same time (Figure 8.15).

Barrel. A cuff, sometimes called a *button-type*, that uses one or more buttons at its closure.

Bell. Sometimes referred to as a *flutter sleeve*; flares into a soft, bell-like shape.

Cap. A short cape design that covers the shoulder.

Dolman. A sleeve design that features a wide armhole tapering to a narrow wrist closing.

Drop shoulder. A sleeve seamed below the shoulder.

French cuff. A double cuff that folds back and features eyelets or openings for the insertion of cuff links.

Leg-of-mutton. Also known as the *Gibson Girl sleeve*, with fullness at the shoulder formed through "gathers" and tapered below the elbow.

Puff. A long or short, full, set-in sleeve that is closed with a tight cuff to accentuate its fullness.

Raglan. A sleeve that extends from the neckline of the garment and drops over the shoulder in one piece.

Set-in. A term used to describe any sleeve that is fitted and sewn into the armhole.

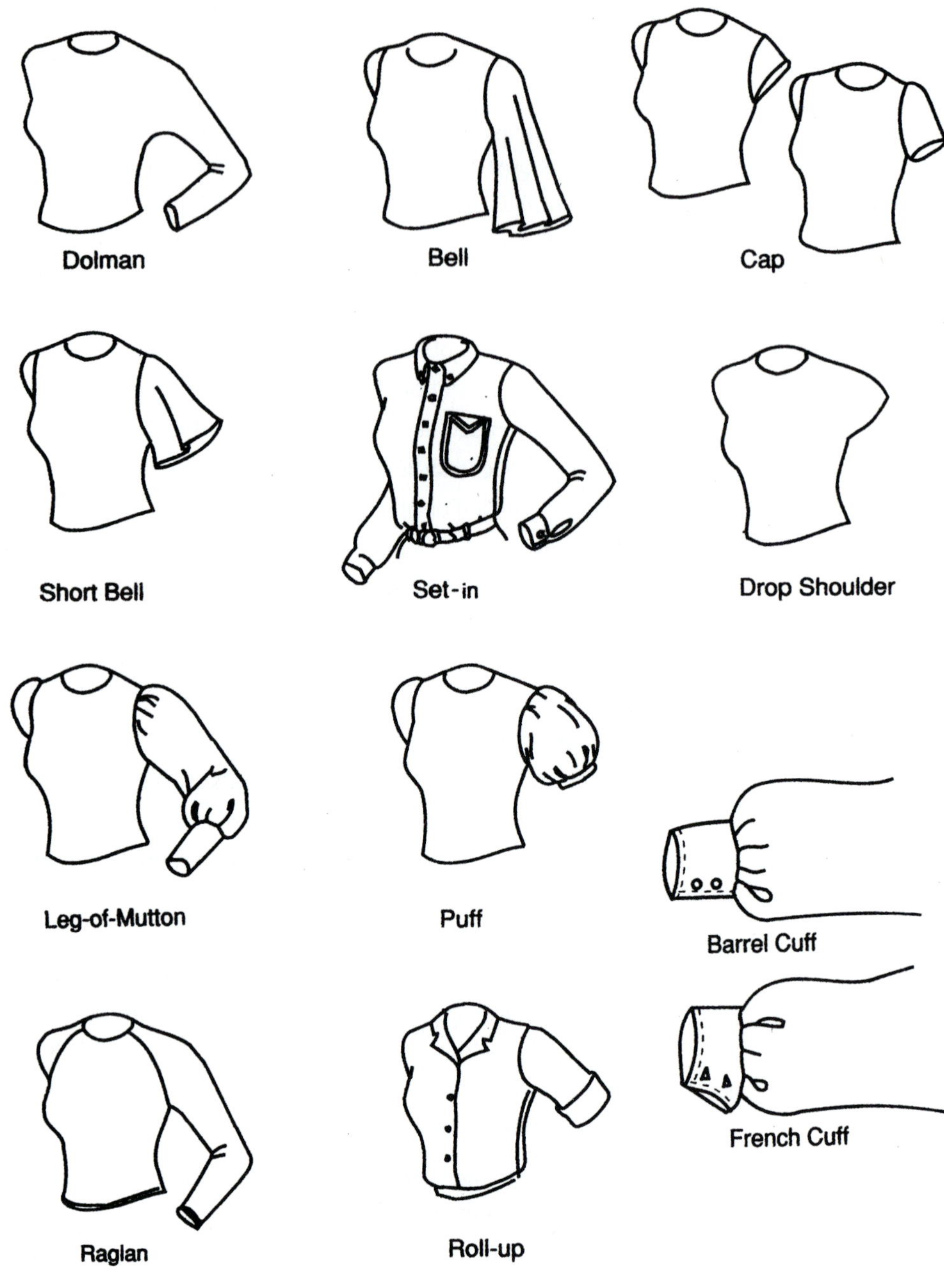

Figure 8.15 Selected sleeves and cuffs.

MARKETING WOMEN'S CLOTHING

The women's apparel market is significantly larger than either men's or children's wear. It changes more frequently than its two counterparts, with as many as six or seven new lines produced each year.

Globally based, buyers for both on-site and off-site ventures regularly comb the various major and regional markets looking for new resources and hot items. In the absence of buyers, retailers use the service of market representatives from resident buying offices and consulting firms to assist them in checking out the pulse of these markets.

To successfully sell women's clothing, the manufacturers and retailers apply numerous techniques and approaches. These include the production of different lines for different seasons, showing and selling the collections, promotional endeavors, and merchandising.

The Seasons

Typically, the women's industry manufactures four or five different lines each year. The number is generally dependent on the individual producer's needs and the target markets, the consumer for whom the merchandise is made. The one season that is not always addressed by some manufacturers is resort wear, which introduces warm weather merchandise for cruises and tropical climates. Only those whose products are at the upper end of the price point scale, such as designer and bridge classifications, consider this a viable time to show a new line. Not only does it give the companies a chance for additional sales and profits, but it also serves as a testing ground for goods that will be produced for the next summer season. Lower-priced merchandise is not appropriate for resort wear because the consumers to whom it is targeted have neither the disposable income nor the time necessary for vacations at this time of the year.

Fall, holiday, spring, and summer are the traditional seasons for women's wear manufacturers. Fall is generally the season in which most businesses expect the greatest amount of profit. It is longer than the others and thus provides the most potential for sales. Fall is also the time for the greatest amount of style and detail change. During this period, designers might attempt a new skirt length or the introduction of a new pants silhouette. Radical changes are often risky and may lead to the demise of the manufacturer that wrongly reads the needs of the market. When a few seasons witness the successful marketing of miniskirts and the next introduces a longer length design, a great deal of concern focuses on the industry and its manufacturers until the style's acceptance or rejection is known. Although fashion, with its excitement and originality, is what the business is all about, innovation and change can often cause irreparable harm to manufacturers and retailers alike. In order to "hedge their bets" against the wrong fashion direction, many designers and manufacturers use the services of fashion forecasters who attempt to predict what lies ahead in terms of fashion.

Holiday is a time when the glitter and glitz surfaces. This brief season generally has its retail selling period concentrated between Thanksgiving and New Year's Eve. Many manufacturers enter this period cautiously by using successful silhouettes and styles from the fall and embellishing them with dazzling fabrics and showy trimmings. In this way, there is some certainty to the success of these new garments. The problem with holiday collections is that once New Year's Day has arrived, the remainder of the merchandise is sacrificed at closeout prices.

Although the arrival of spring generally signals a time for coats to be shed and the heavy garments of winter to be stored away, the uncertainty of the weather causes considerable trouble for manufacturers and their retail clients. It was once a time when lightweight coats and suits were produced in fabrics that were less bulky than those used for fall and winter, but heavier than the ones that would be used for summer goods. Today, spring lines can provide more problems than profit. A significant percentage of female consumers make the transition from winter to summer without stopping to purchase the in-between spring garments. This being the case, the industry in recent years has intentionally neglected the spring season, showing only modified lines of merchandise.

With less importance attached to spring collections, most manufacturers and retailers invest heavily in summer merchandise. The season is longer than ever before, with some lines surfacing in stores, catalogs, and online immediately after the traditional Presidents' Week clearance sales. From then to the end of June, dresses, suits, and sportswear classifications have been joined by swimsuits and active wear. Some manufacturers introduce two summer lines, one for early delivery and one for a later period so that the retailer's inventories will have a fresh look. In the trade, they are often known as summer I and summer II.

Some women's manufacturers such as Liz Claiborne and retailers like The Limited and The Gap, which produce their own lines and subscribe to the "Store is the Brand" philosophy, have instituted merchandising policies that feature more than the traditional four

SHOP-WITHIN-A-SHOP MERCHANDISING

An even greater attempt has been made to separate some women's clothing from others than that used in the merchandise collection method. Couture collections are generally featured in these separate shops. Names such as Donna Karan, Christian La Croix, and Yves Saint Laurent are examples of lines featured in this manner.

Off-Site Ventures

Catalogs and Web sites also have different options in terms of how they present their merchandise to the consumer. Some resort to mixing the offerings according to merchandise classifications, such as dresses and sportswear. Others segment the offering according to label, especially if they are well known. Still others use price points as a means of separating their offerings.

Internet Resources for Additional Research

www.geocities.com/e2davies/brides.html presents a history of the wedding dress.
www.cfda.com is a major fashion trade organization for women's wear.
www.fashion.about.com/od/designeraz/ features a mega list of famous designers.

Merchandise Information Terminology

Bridge collection
Separates
Innerwear
Misses size
Junior size
Petite sizing
Women's size
Half sizes
Tall sizes
Silhouette
Style
Details
Classics
Fads
Tubular silhouette
Bell silhouette
Bustle configuration
A-line
Blouson
Chemise
Dirndl
Empire waistline
Gored
Jumper
Peplum
Pleated
Princess
Shirtwaist
Trapeze
Trumpet skirt
Tunic
Blazer
Bolero
Car coat
Cardigan
Chesterfield
Duffel coat
Mandarin coat
Norfolk jacket
Raincoat
Redingote
Reefer
Baggies
Bell bottoms
Culottes
Hip huggers
Jeans
Jodhpurs
Knickers
Pedal pushers
Shorts
Stretch pants
Blouson
Camisole
Man-tailored
Middy
Polo
Smock
Tank top
T-shirt
Bateau
Bertha collar
Bow
Button-down
Choirboy collar
Convertible collar
Cowl
Crew collar
Halter
Jabot
Jewel neckline
Keyhole neckline
Peter Pan collar
Plunging neckline
Puritan collar
Sailor collar
Strapless neckline
Surplice neckline
Sweetheart neckline
Turtleneck
U-neck
V-neck
Barrel cuff
Bell sleeve
Cap sleeve
Dolman sleeve
Drop shoulder
French cuff
Leg-of-mutton sleeve
Puff sleeve
Raglan sleeve
Set-in sleeve
Regional market
Seventh Avenue

EXERCISES

1. Choose one of the basic silhouettes used in women's clothing and find styles that represent it. Fashion magazines such as *Elle, Harper's Bazaar, Vogue*, and *Glamour* regularly feature photographs of many items from which you may choose.
   Select five different styles that use this basic silhouette and discuss how each one has been enhanced by its designer to make a unique creation.
2. Visit a large department store to determine the manner in which it features one product classification. If dresses are used, for example, indicate the specific departments that house dresses and the concept in the merchandising of each.
3. Select the name of a sportswear manufacturer from the many labels or "hand-tags" used to identify it. Contact one of these companies to determine the specific seasons they produce their collections and why they were selected.

Review Questions

1. Before the 1880s, which women had fashion merchandise available to them?
2. What is the definition of a *bridge collection*?
3. What has accounted for the enormous expansion of the active sportswear classification?
4. Which two designers helped launch the sportswear industry into the prominence it now holds?
5. For what reason has the rainwear industry been able to expand its sales volume?
6. Explain the reason for the quick acceptance of pants as traditional women's apparel.
7. Which retailer is given credit for the popularity and growth of innerware?
8. Discuss the change in the status of jeans from practical pants to those that enjoyed fashion status.
9. How did designers immediately "tell" consumers about their labels?
10. In what ways do misses and junior sized clothing differ?
11. What is the difference between women's and half sizes?
12. What are the three basic silhouettes on which all dress designs are based?
13. How does an empire waistline differ from the conventionally placed waistline?
14. Define the term *redingote.*
15. In what way can apparel designers enhance their silhouettes without making radical changes to them?
16. What is the difference between a barrel and a French cuff?
17. How does a raglan sleeve differ from one that is set in?
18. What are the traditional seasons in women's wear, and how have some manufactures altered this arrangement?
19. How are small retailers that have neither the time nor money to go to wholesale markets able to see new collections?
20. What is meant by a *store-within-a-store*?

CHAPTER 9

Men's Clothing

After reading this chapter, you should be able to:

- Assess the scope of the menswear industry in terms of its dominant geographical wholesale markets.
- Identify the various clothing classifications that constitute the menswear industry.
- Classify the different sizes and fit categories of menswear and discuss their characteristics.
- Describe the styles, silhouettes, and details used in men's fashions.
- Discuss the methods used in marketing men's apparel and accessories.

Once a severely neglected segment of the apparel industry, menswear, with a wealth of innovative design and distinction, has taken its place as a fashion classification that rivals the women's market. Although in terms of actual size and distribution, it pales by comparison to the magnitude of the women's clothing industry, its importance is evidenced by the number of manufacturers and designers who continue to address clothing for men.

Looking back in the fashion pages of history, it is difficult to find photographs or drawings of men resplendent in finery equal to that worn by women. Although the royal courts of European nations and some of the upperclass gentlemen both here and abroad had an assortment of outfits to fit various business and social occasions, their styles and silhouettes were traditionally shaped or otherwise unexciting.

Women, throughout the decades of the early twentieth century, and even before then, were the mainstays of the fashion designer. The likes of Worth, Paquin, Lanvin, Poiret, Chanel, and Dior were busily engaged in the creation of the latest designs to capture the female audience.

Not until the early 1960s was the male figure discovered (Figure 9.1). Suddenly, men were deemed ready for the "avant-garde" or contemporary stylings that were being abundantly lavished on women. The conventional approach to fashion was augmented by different trouser cuts, jackets of unconventional designs, flamboyant colorations, and fabrics that were not before considered acceptable for men to wear.

As we entered into the early years of the new millennium, men continued to have more and more choices, an advantage once only held by their female counterparts. Scores of designers and manufacturers, as demonstrated by the opening of the new collections and featured on runways all over the world, are devoting their talents to dressing the male figure. While many men's manufacturers and designers create lines exclusively for men, a significant number of women's wear designers have expanded their businesses with the addition of menswear collections. This is often reflected by men and women parading together on the fashion runways.

Today's menswear is a market that features the "new and daring" along with traditional styles, recognizing the fact that men are as individualistic as women in their need for fashion (Figure 9.2). Menswear designers are ready to change their approach to style according to the demands of the market they dress and the dictates of the industries in which many enjoy their careers. One example is the decline in popularity of "casual Fridays," a concept popularized in the 1990s in which men were allowed to opt for less traditional dress on this

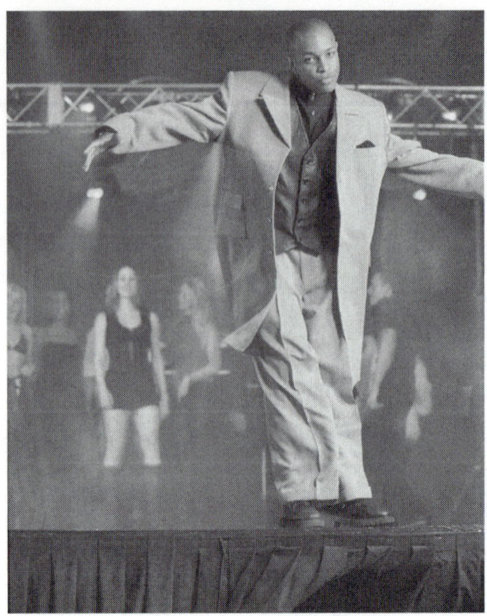

Figure 9.1 This avant-garde suit made fashion headlines in the 1960s.
(Courtesy of Getty Images, Inc., Michael Krasowitz.)

one day of the week. In the early years of the twenty-first century, a return to traditionalism was the order of the day, with more and more clothing manufacturers reemphasizing their **tailored clothing,** a term used to describe suits and coats, and lessening their attention to more casual shapes, fabrics, and colors.

This chapter concentrates on the scope of the menswear industry, the specific clothing classifications, the industry's size and structure, the shapes and silhouettes, the accessories or furnishings that are predominantly male-oriented, and the seasonal nature of the product lines.

Many of the accessories that cut across fashion lines for men, women, and children, such as shoes, jewelry, belts, watches, gloves, hats, fragrances, and trimmings are discussed in the chapters of Section IV.

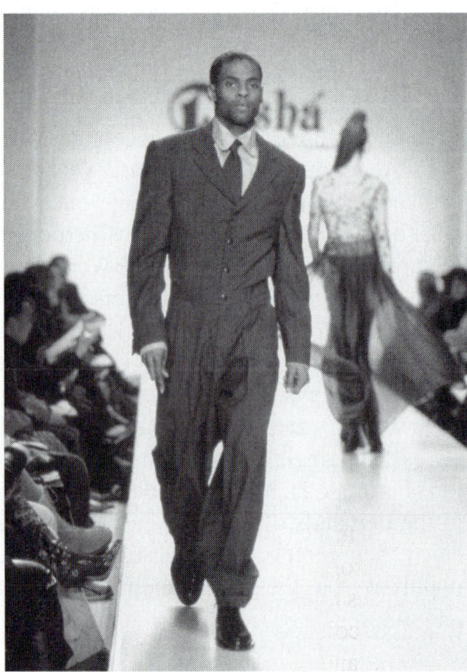

Figure 9.2 High-fashion suits are now featured in addition to traditional models.
(Courtesy of Fashion Syndicate Press.)

SCOPE OF THE INDUSTRY

As in the case of the women's apparel business, menswear is globally based. The markets are numerous, with some centers playing central roles in design, production, and distribution.

The United States plays an overall dominant role in this market. There are more clothing companies based in America than in any other part of the world, with some foreign countries playing smaller, but nonetheless important, roles. Without question, the hub of the menswear industry is New York City, where the hustle and bustle of producers and wholesalers interfacing with buyers during market weeks (the time when new collections debut) make the city hum with excitement.

Clothing, with its fastidious, custom detailing, is readily available in the New York City marketplace as is the abundance of lower price-point merchandise. Merchants may avail themselves of almost any fashion direction that is appropriate for their customers with no need to go to another market. Those, however, who prefer to remain nearer to home for merchandise acquisition might prefer one of the many regional markets. Although there is far less design and manufacturing taking place in these regional locales, many of the industry's leading companies that are based in New York City maintain permanent regional showrooms for their clients. Many menswear firms sell to their customers via the trade exposition route, the largest being MAGIC, which is held in Las Vegas and takes up residence several times a year in vast convention centers and apparel marts. The larger of the menswear vendors use the multichannel route to get their goods to their client base and use a combination of the aforementioned approaches to reach them.

Some of the domestic markets that produce and sell their collections outside of the New York City arena include Los Angeles, San Francisco, Miami, Chicago, and Boston. Mila, Rome, Florence, Paris, Hong Kong, London, and South Korea serve as important foreign markets.

CLOTHING CLASSIFICATIONS

Most of the industry's participants concentrate on a specific merchandise classification such as tailored clothing, formal wear, or active sportswear. A few of the giants, such as the Armani empire, are more diversified in their offerings and have expanded their operations to run the gamut from high-fashion, elegant business suits to jeans and T-shirts in a variety of price points. Some major companies produce collections under a wide range of labels, with each targeted toward a specific market segment. Whatever the approach, the industry is involved in an assortment of product classifications.

Tailored Clothing

This category, sometimes just referred to as *clothing* includes coats, suits, sports coats, and dress trousers (Figure 9.3). It has remained the nucleus of the menswear industry's offerings, although the late 1900s witnessed a relatively brief decline due to the casual Friday concept, because a significant number of men are required to wear such attire for their careers. Although there has been less formality in appropriate attire for business, there are still parameters for men to observe in choosing their wardrobes.

The relaxing of the conventional rules has expanded tailored clothing fashions. Once relegated to the traditional two-button suit, often with a matching vest, the wearer now can choose from high-fashion, double-breasted models, less structured suits, three-button silhouettes that feature "no-vent" designs, or sports coats and pants in a variety of styles, fabrics, and colors. Few companies stay with the rigid confines once dictated by this fashion segment, and they have expanded their lines as the dress codes have relaxed.

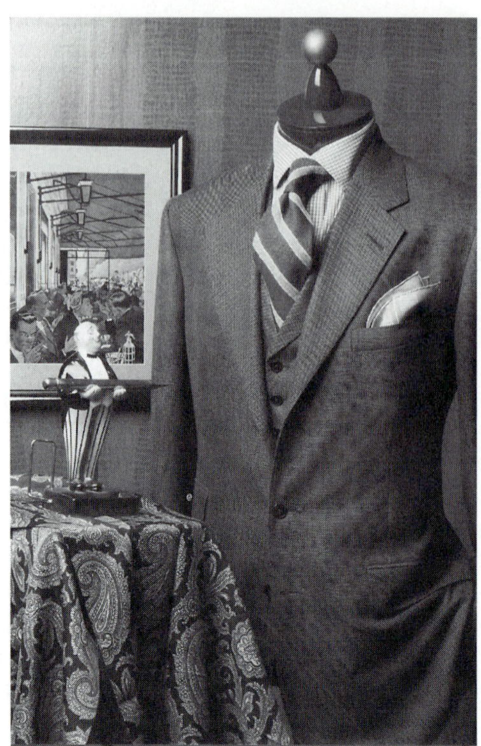

Figure 9.3 This three-piece suit is typical of tailored clothing.
(Courtesy of Alan Flusser Custom Shop, James T. Murray Photography, © 2005.)

Sportswear

From jeans to sweaters, sportswear production and consumption have continued to rise. With the aforementioned relaxing of the rules of dress, a man may opt for a more casual approach when the demands of formality are relaxed. Not long ago, for example, a night at the theater or a visit to a restaurant or club necessitated more structured dress. Business suits were the accepted attire. Today, many men not only dress casually for such social occasions, but they choose other types of clothing.

Jeans, once considered appropriate only for performing more vigorous tasks such as gardening or boating, are now perfectly acceptable for many occasions when worn with a blazer or sweater (Figure 9.4). Calvin Klein, Claiborne, and Levi Strauss continue to widen their offerings to include even greater latitude for the jeans wearer. In addition to the traditional blue with all of the variations, which include acid and stone washing and fading, fashion colors are featured in the product mix.

A visit to any department store, most men's specialty shops, menswear Web sites, and catalogs reveals immediately that sportswear has become a profitable venture.

Active Sportswear

Once relegated to the gym or participation sports, a number of products have become the mainstay of the wardrobes of many men who are definitely not considered active in sports. Jogging suits, tennis outfits, biking shorts, golf clothing, running gear, exercise pants, and tank tops are worn regularly where they once had been considered off limits. Of course, the major revenue-producing product in **active sportswear** is athletic shoes, once referred to as *sneakers*. Their importance, as well as the composition of that industry, is discussed in a later chapter on footwear.

The blending of comfort and innovative styling has made this fashion classification appealing to a large audience. Men perform their supermarket chores in warm-up suits, shop the mall in summer in tennis outfits, have lunch in tank tops and biking pants, or visit friends in golf attire.

Although the target market for such items was originally the younger, slimmer set, it is common today for all ages, sizes, and shapes to wear active sportswear. Retailers that

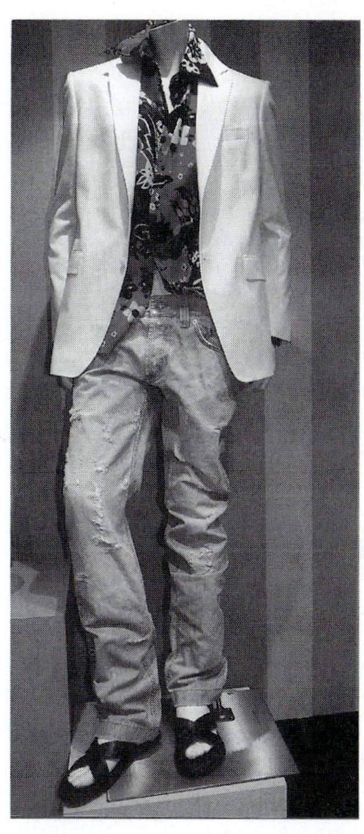

Figure 9.4 A typical sportswear outfit pairs a blazer with jeans.
(Courtesy of Ellen Diamond.)

specialize in larger sizes and tall men's shops, headquarters for conservative dress, and others have joined this trend—and have ultimately increased their profits.

Formal Attire

Although formal attire is considered by many to be part of the clothing segment, its importance in today's wardrobe necessitates its discussion as a separate category.

Formal wear was once only worn by those few men whose business functions and social lives required them to attend galas and other formal functions. The term *formal* meant "white tie and tails," while semiformal indicated wearing a tuxedo. Although the more formal attire was insignificant in terms of men's clothing production, tuxedos were the important components for special evening events.

Today, the **black tie** uniform has replaced the necessity of the traditional black suit (Figure 9.5).

Tuxedos are produced by many manufacturers and designers in a variety of models that range from the traditional suit to the double-breasted model. Unusual fabrics and stylings are often introduced to capture the attention of the man who feels the need to expand his formal wardrobe much the same as he does for his everyday apparel. Designer labels like Bill Blass, Hugo Boss, and Joseph Abboud are all actively involved in this growing apparel segment.

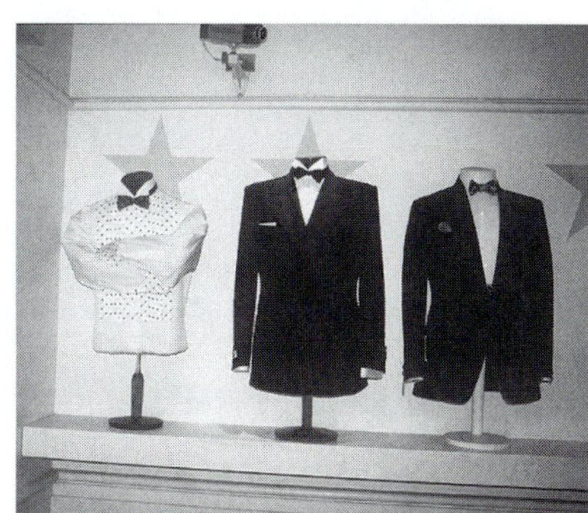

Figure 9.5 "Black tie" often replaces the black dress suit.
(Courtesy of Ellen Diamond.)

Outerwear

This fashion segment usually refers to those garments such as parkas, toggle coats, ski jackets, windbreakers, and any others that are outdoor-oriented. Originally, they were designated for warmth or protection from the elements. The heaviest woolens, corduroys, meltons, and flannels were used in their construction. They were more functional than fashionable.

Today, this category has been expanded to include the brightest, boldest solids and plaids and fabrics that are lighter in weight but, nonetheless, warm. Patagonia, a leader in such clothing, has led the field with numerous new fabrics that provide warmth without weight. The layering of sweaters and shirts have also enabled manufacturers to produce lighter outerwear in denims, twills, and other heavy cotton fabrics. The ability of the textile industry to produce fibers such as Thinsulate, which produces lighter-weight, warm fabrications, has also helped to enlarge the classification's product mix.

Shirts and Furnishings

What was once a product limited to white shirts for business and dress wear and some prints and plaids for leisure time now has no limits. A visit to a major store's menswear department, Web site, or catalogs immediately reveals a merchandise assortment that features almost any color and pattern for career dressing and many fabrics, textures, colorations, and styles for casual attire (Figure 9.6). The plain broadcloth and oxford shirts have been joined by flannels, corduroys, denim, and others.

The success of the shirt industry may be best understood by the names that produce these items. Designers who once spent their time creating apparel for men and women are well represented in the shirt category. Geoffrey Beene, Donna Karan, Ralph Lauren, and Calvin Klein fill the counters along with the standard brands.

The **furnishings** designation is sometimes used to describe items such as bathrobes, pajamas, underwear, hosiery, ties, and braces. As everything else in men's fashion, they too have evolved into a more exciting category. Ties, hosiery, and braces, for example, once basically structured additions or extensions to suits and shirts, are now making tremendous fashion statements on their own, which is discussed in the following section.

Underwear was once thought of as being functional rather than fashionable. Along came designers like Calvin Klein who revolutionized the industry with significant changes.

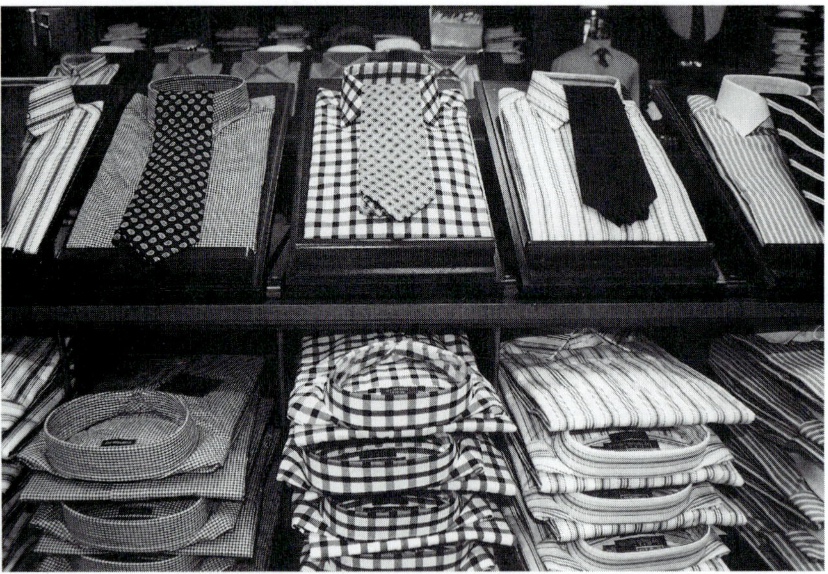

Figure 9.6 The traditional white shirt has been joined by a wealth of patterns. *(Courtesy of Ellen Diamond.)*

The common jockey brief now includes more minimal coverings, and staid, conservative boxer shorts have become a fashion item in fabrics that now include fine cottons, rayons, and silks, and colors and patterns to please almost all males. Boxers, once shunned by younger males, have become for many, the underpants of choice. Along with form-fitting "muscle" undershirts, they have become fashion statements.

Pajama lines have also been expanded to include newer models and fabrics than the traditional fare. With comfort a priority for many men, "ski-types," made of knits, have been added rather than wovens in absorbent materials. Some even make the transition from the bedroom to the informal, outdoor workout.

Accessory Enhancements

Ties, braces or suspenders, and hosiery have finally found a niche for themselves in the men's fashion world. Rather than serving as functional additions to men's dress and casual wardrobes, they have made a place for themselves as fashion "staters." Who has not heard of the "power tie" worn by the industry's movers and shakers?

Many attribute the tie revolution to Ralph Lauren, who, as a salesman in that industry, helped to introduce the wider tie. It immediately took the market by storm and catapulted both Mr. Lauren and the product classification into prominence in the 1960s.

The importance of the tie today has progressed even further (Figure 9.7). The names of Hugo Boss, Donna Karan, Ermenegildo Zegna, and other upscale men's apparel designers grace ties that sell for upwards of $100. The styles range from the more conservative, standard width "reps," which feature the popular diagonal stripes, to the widest, boldest flowers and geometric forms. Along with these models, there is usually an offering of bow ties for the man who wishes to make yet another fashion statement. The bow-tie wearer who considers himself a purist always chooses the type that requires hand tying rather than the ready-made variety that is often found accompanying the dress shirt for formal wear. Although bow tying is difficult for some men to master, those who can are proud of their accomplishment and ready to teach novices.

Socks, too, once hidden under pantlegs, have now entered the fashion foray. No longer limited to basic blacks for dresswear or some subtle coloration for casual attire, the product line has taken on new dimensions. Plaids, argyles, patterns, stripes, and daring colors, in a variety of knits, cost purchasers as much as $35 per pair. They are as carefully selected by many wearers as are the pants and shoes with which they coordinate.

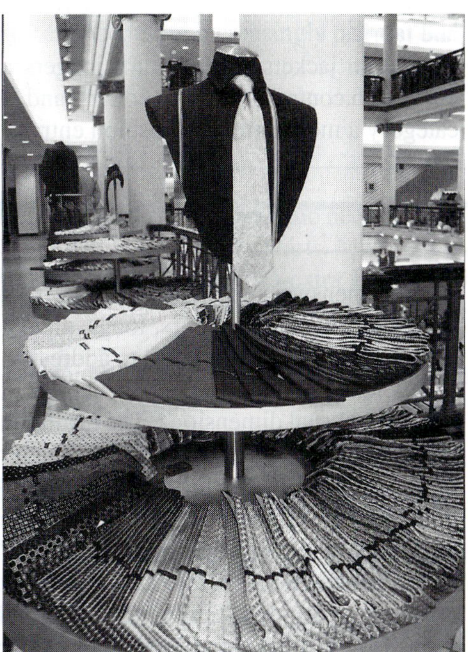

Figure 9.7 Ties have become important fashion accessories.
(Courtesy of Ellen Diamond.)

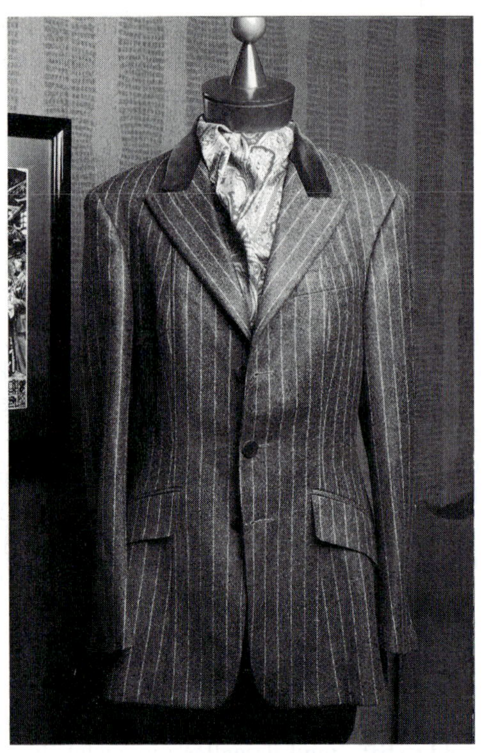

Figure 9.11 The chesterfield jacket features a velvet collar.
(Courtesy of Alan Flusser Custom Shop, James T. Murray Photography, © 2005.)

Ski jacket. Originally designed for the ski slopes and now a fashion item for casual wear. It is made of a variety of lightweight treated cottons or synthetics such as Thinsulate, which provides warmth without weight. Many are lined with down filler for extra warmth. It features a visible or a concealed hood and usually uses a zipper front.

Topcoat. A lightweight version of the overcoat.

Trench coat. Using military detailing such as epaulets and brass buttons on a double-breasted construction; typically produced in water-resistant materials to double as a raincoat.

Tuxedo. A semiformal or black tie suit that is single- or double-breasted with notched, peaked, or shawl collars. The pants are most often the same material as the jacket and feature a satin strip of material on each side.

TROUSERS

Baggies. Softly flaring out from the waistline and either snuggly or loosely culminating at the ankle, the pant is a prime example of contemporary, casual dress. Soft, drapable fabrics enhance the flow of the line.

Bermudas. These short pants, sometimes called *walking shorts*, end somewhere around the knee.

Continentals. The waist is an extension of the narrow pantleg with the absence of belt loops. Fit is achieved with the use of adjustable tabs at the waist.

Conventional. This full-cut, loose-fitting style has either belt loops or an extended waistband and is worn with or without cuffs. Pleated or nonpleated details are used for this style, which is most often featured as part of a dress or sports suit.

Jeans. Adapted from the dungaree work pant, they are usually constructed from denim and feature numerous variations. They range from the narrow, straight-legged, five-pocket style popularized by Levi Strauss to the more designer-oriented models, which include baggy pantlegs, flared bottoms, or anything inventive.

Knickers. Characteristically, they are short, loose pants that gather and fit the leg below the knee. They are sometimes seen on the golf course.

Overalls. Initially a style worn by farmers or construction workers, the pant is extended by means of a panel that fits over the chest. Like jeans, overalls are generally constructed of denim and have become fashionable with the younger set.

Shorts. This shorter version of the Bermuda or walking short ends somewhere around the thigh.

Ski pant. Originally designed for use on the slopes, they are now featured for casual wear, jogging, as pajama and lounge-wear pants, and for physical fitness use. Mostly made of knitted materials, the type dependent on the use or activity, the waist is usually elasticized and the bottom gathered at the ankle.

SHIRTS

Dress shirt. This general style includes men's long- or short-sleeved models, a variety of collars, and different cuff closures. cuts are available in different degrees of roominess.

Formal shirt. Used in conjunction with black tie suits and dinner jackets, the front panels are usually adorned with pleats or ruffles. The shirts are generally fastened with *studs,* small jewelry accessories, at the chest and cuff links at the wrists. Collars are either winged or standard as in the case of regular dress shirts (Figure 9.12).

Ivy League. Constructed of either broadcloth or oxford shirting, the style features a button-down collar, loose fitting, and a barrel or plain sleeve closing at the wrist. It may or may not have a loop at the yoke of the shirt's back panel.

Polo shirt. This knitted, short-sleeved style is detailed with a ribbed collar and sleeve trim.

Sport shirt. This catchall term describes a casual short- or long-sleeved shirt. Sports shirts range from the form-fitting to the loose-fitting variety and are produced in a wide number of fabrics and patterns.

T-shirt. Void of buttons or other closures, it is usually short-sleeved, collarless, and used with any casual pants or shorts.

Western. Dominated by patch pockets, snap closings at the chest and sleeves, and constructed with a yoke back, this style is inspired by the standard dress of ranch hands. It is also called a *cowboy shirt.*

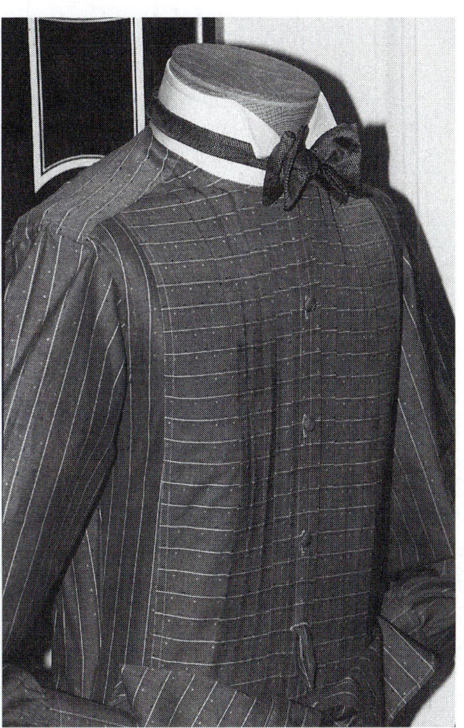

Figure 9.12 The "wing" collar has become a formal shirt classic.
(Courtesy of Ellen Diamond.)

Details

Silhouettes and styles remain constant, but are enhanced by the use of additions, trims, or construction techniques that may be classified as *details*. The seasoned designer is knowledgeable in terms of detailing and uses one or several that may make the final garment distinctively original and functional in design.

Some of the more commonly used details are categorized under three major classifications: coats and suits, trousers, and shirts. Diagrams are shown in conjunction with the descriptions of these details.

COATS AND SUITS (FIGURE 9.14)

Lapels. They are generally peaked or notched. For sports coats, the notch lapel sometimes features an additional tab extension (Figure 9.13).

Shoulders. They range from the natural, which follows the contour of the body, to the padded varieties. The padding might be slight, as in the case of traditionally cut coats and jackets, or exaggerated, as used in many European-cut models.

Pockets. Three categories are generally used that serve as functional devices or mere embellishments. Patch pockets are usually reserved for sportier or casual garments and are plain, tucked, or accented with flaps. Flap styles, with concealed pockets, are mostly used for business-type suits and are either placed horizontally on the coat and suit or on the diagonal. A sleeker look is achieved with the use of insets where the pocket opening is discreetly placed and the actual pocket is on inside of the coat or suit body.

Vents. Suits are detailed with center vents or two side vents, or they may be ventless. Coats are either single-vented or ventless. Center **vents** six to ten inches from the garment's hem are the most commonly used types. Side vents are usually deep-cut, about eight or more inches, and are used in more contemporary models. **Ventless** detail is used for European-cut suits. This style does not allow for the extra room needed for many typical male figures.

Various types of stitching, suede patches at the elbows, buttons, tabs at the base of the sleeves, prominent zippers, toggle closings, epaulets, piping, seaming, and other details are added to make the basics more distinctive.

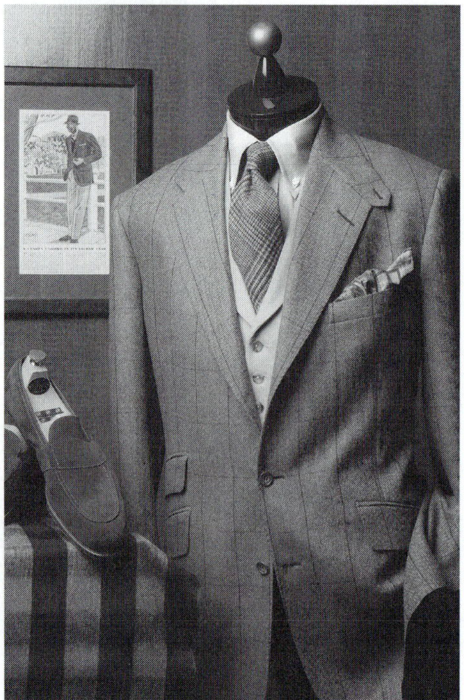

Figure 9.13 A notched lapel adds an additional tab foil for extra fashion flair.
(Courtesy of Alan Flusser Custom Shop, James T. Murray Photography, © 2005.)

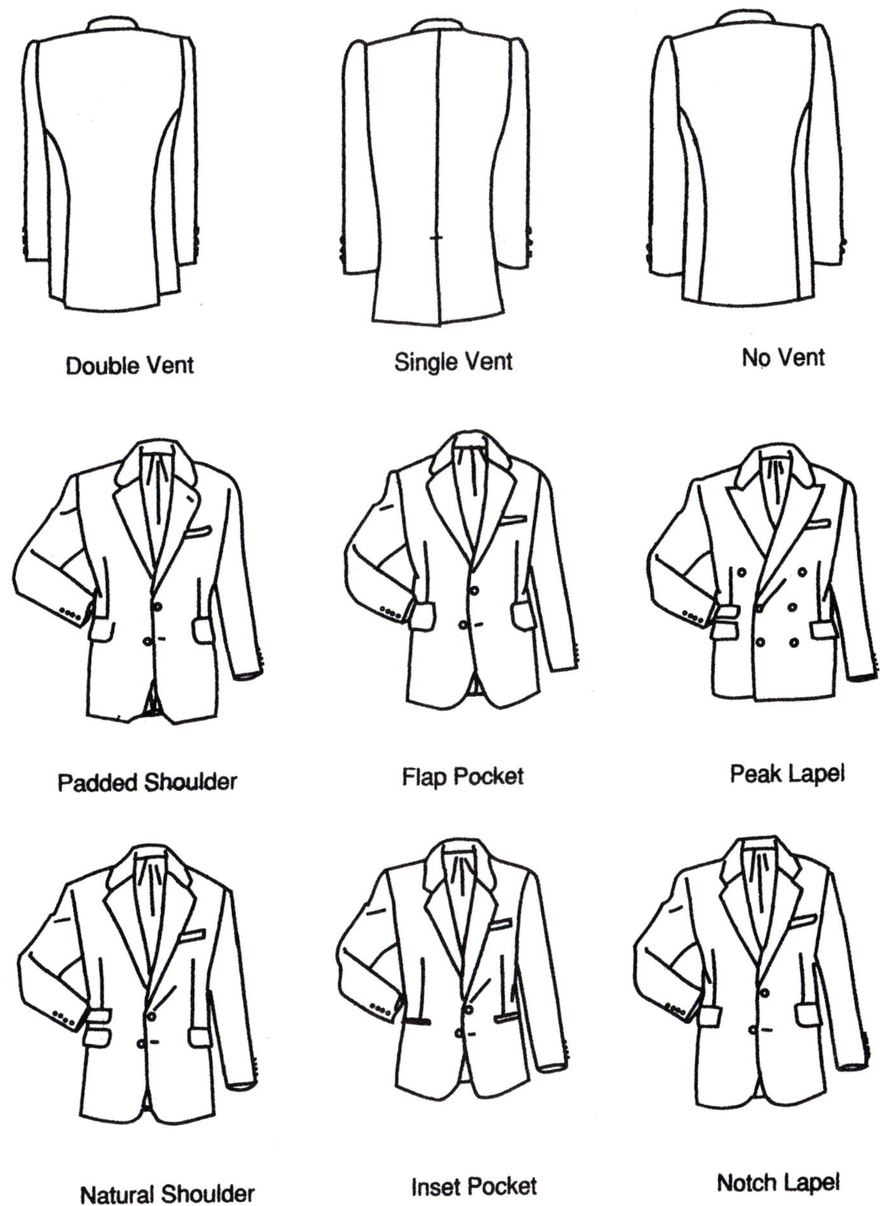

Figure 9.14 Selected jacket details.

TROUSERS (FIGURE 9.15)

Pockets. Many are similar to those found in coats and suits, but others are also used for both decoration and function. The scoop variety is slightly rounded, the patch comprises an additional piece of fabric, and the set-in is concealed save for the welt and slight opening.

Hems. Pantlegs are either horizontally hemmed, diagonally hemmed, or are cuffed.

Plain front. The fabric is void of pleats and conforms closely to the midsection.

Pleated front. Single, double, or triple pleats provide for additional room at the midsection and also add a fashion emphasis.

Belted. Loops are provided for the belts.

EXERCISES

1. Visit the shirt department of a specialty or department store to observe this season's offerings in the dress shirt category. Using this information, prepare sketches or take photographs of each style that dominates the current field. Another option would to use the pictures of a major retailer's catalog. These illustrations should then be mounted on construction board and augmented with newspaper and magazine advertisements that feature similar models.
2. Prepare an oral report on the wholesale men's markets. Be sure to include the major wholesale locations as well as the regional offices. Information about these geographical locations may be secured by researching such periodicals as DNR and other trade papers, all of which are generally offered in libraries. Another means of research is to use the Internet. By logging onto a search engine such as **www.google.com,** or **www.askjeeves.com,** you should be able to find the information you need.
3. From various consumer magazines such as *Esquire* and *GQ*, gather photographs of one of the current season's trends. For example, you could concentrate on tailored clothing, formal wear, casual attire, active sportswear, or accessories. Mount each photograph on a presentation panel and present your findings to the class.

Review Questions

1. Why is New York City the major wholesaler in the United States?
2. What is meant by the term *classification*?
3. List the major menswear classifications and briefly describe the products that fall within each.
4. Discuss why formal wear has become a mainstay in the wardrobes of many average men.
5. How has "tie merchandising" changed and why?
6. Define the term *braces.*
7. Differentiate between regular, short, and long men sizes. What are the measurements for each?
8. In what way does *athletic cut* differ from the *regular* size in men's suits?
9. Why are men's sport shirts generally sized from small to extra large and dress shirts more specifically sized?
10. How have some manufacturers of men's dress shirts "reduced" their size offerings while still addressing the consumer's needs?
11. What does the term *silhouette* signify?
12. Discuss the major differences between the traditional and the European silhouettes.
13. Define *battle jacket, chesterfield coat, toggle coat,* and *safari jacket.*
14. What is the major feature of the Ivy League shirt?
15. What are design details, and what impact do they have on style?
16. Why do some menswear manufacturers subscribe to seasonal offerings other than those that are traditional?
17. In what way does the wholesale market showroom differ from that of the regional trade mart?
18. List two domestic trade shows and describe their operations.
19. What advantage does the trade show afford the buyer?
20. What is the major European trade show for menswear, and where is it held?

CHAPTER 10

Children's Clothing

After reading this chapter, you should be able to:

- Trace the history of children's clothing from the early 1900s to the present.
- Discuss the state of children's wear manufacturing in both America and foreign countries.
- List and discuss the different merchandise classifications.
- Explain the size classifications in the industry.
- Discuss how children's merchandise is marketed.

Whether it is the runway presentation at a children's trade show, the windows and interiors of today's children's retailers, or Web sites offering children's clothing, the styles featured rival the collections earmarked for adults. The excitement generated by today's children's clothing industry is far different than the products that were available in the early days of the twentieth century.

Photographs of children in the early 1900s reveal that, except for the wealthy, the costumes worn were anything but fashionable. Little girls and boys are seen wearing lackluster, functional apparel that was specifically made for them by their mothers or outfits that were cut down and remade from their parents' discards. Only the wealthy had the financial resources to spend on fashionable clothing, most of which was custom-made.

Yesterday's children were quite different from today's younger generations. Decisions on most things, such as clothing, were made by their parents. If one were fortunate to get something new to wear, the selection was made by the adults.

Fast forward to today's playing field! A newfound independence has surfaced with the immense offering of television directed at children's audiences (Figure 10.1). Successful programming continues to influence the styles and fashions that are made available to this generation. Even the smallest toddlers react to the fashions worn on the screen. By the time they are of school age, many are making their own clothing choices.

Because the children's market is made up of so many different age groups, from infancy to preteens, the offerings are quite diverse. Some manufacturers focus on specific age markets, whereas others cover the full range.

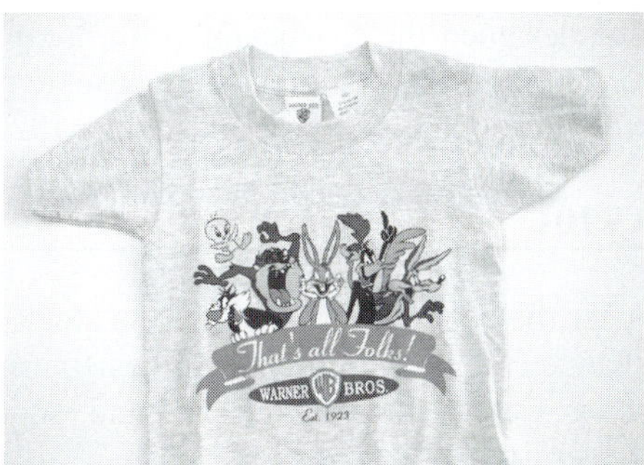

Figure 10.1 Cartoon characters are extremely popular in children's fashion.
(Courtesy of PhotoEdit, Michael Newman.)

FASHION HIGHLIGHTS FROM THE 1900s TO PRESENT DAY

Before 1900, children's fashions were restricted to mini versions of adult attire. The clothing designs for children echoed the tastes and needs of their parents. Early in the twentieth century, however, there was some indication that fashion would begin to play a more important role in dressing children.

Each decade saw the introduction of new fashions. Some reflected changes in attitude and mores, others included protests of the times, and still others were based on events that captured the public's attention.

1900s

As a carryover from earlier times, children's fashions were still confined to copies of what adults wore. Because both men and women were greatly influenced by the Victorian and Edwardian eras and their costumes reflected these periods, children's clothing followed suit.

1910s

At the beginning of this decade, formality in attire still reigned. There was, however, a trend to a more relaxed and less confining mode of dress when styles influenced by the movement westward started to appear. In 1915, Levi Strauss introduced denim **coveralls** that were both durable and functional. Little did the people of those times realize that denim would later resurface and serve fashionable as well as functional purposes.

During the same time, the United States Rubber Company produced a shoe that combined canvas uppers with rubber soles. These were the original **Keds** that are still worn by people of all ages today. At the time, the product was considered a functional shoe like the coveralls with which it was worn. It has become a mainstay for both athletic endeavors and as fashion apparel accents.

1920s

After emerging victorious from World War I, the nation reached out to newer fashions. Much of the industry's production would still mimic the styles of their parents; however, more relaxed silhouettes were becoming the norm.

The major innovation of the decade was the flapper dress worn by both women and young girls. For the flapper silhouettes to be properly worn required a radical change in undergarments. Those that were previously appropriate were too bulky for the new style. The Carter Company, a leader in today's children's fashions, introduced short, cotton-knit undergarments that better suited the new dresses.

Children were treated to other denim styles that were popularized by the early Levi Strauss coverall. In 1921, OshKosh B'Gosh, still an important children's wear manufacturer today, introduced overalls for boys that resembled the ones worn by their fathers; soon after, Lee designed the first jeans to use a zipper-fly front. Boys wore baggy, tweed pants that ranged from shorts for the younger set to full length for those in their preteens. Knickers, too, were fashionable for boys during the 1920s.

1930s

After the economic disaster of the stock market crash, the early 1930s saw little at first to change fashion. Children's clothes continued to echo their parents' wardrobes. The flapper styles were a thing of the past and, soon, older girls emulated their mothers by wearing longer, leaner dresses.

Child stars and movies began to influence fashion. Little girls preferred dresses similar to those worn by Shirley Temple, perhaps the most famous of all child stars. The major Shirley Temple design featured red and white polka dots and became the favorite of little girls all over the world. For the first time, a major women's swimsuit manufacturer, Cole of California, offered a children's line of swimwear and sports apparel. Children of the upper class sported coats that were trimmed with fox fur.

The cinematic event of 1939 was the opening of *The Wizard of Oz*. It played a role in promoting little girls' dresses. Every young miss was eager to purchase the farm-girl dress worn by Dorothy in the movie.

By the end of the 1930s, a new style was emerging in Europe. Children's close-fitting ski jackets and pants were introduced, bringing a fresh look that combined both fashion and function.

1940s

Although the United States was deeply involved in World War II, there was a continued fascination with Hollywood and its famous actors. Cowboys rode their horses on the movie screen and little boys' sweaters, fashioned after the ones worn by the cowboy hero of the time, Hopalong Cassidy, became the rage. The western influence started to gain major acceptance in children's fashion.

Buster Brown, the shoe manufacturer, introduced a line of children's hosiery to accompany their footwear as well as a line of apparel. Out of the necessity of quickly dressing children in warm clothing for middle-of-the-night trips to air raid shelters in London and other cities, the "siren suit," better known as the *snowsuit*, was developed. Its popularity soon spread to the United States, where it was accepted by parents as the best protection for their children from cold weather.

1950s

Across the United States, the move to suburbia played a role in apparel design. The look became more relaxed, with denim jeans and sneakers replacing more traditional clothing. The fascination with movie celebrities continued to dominate the children's clothing scene. Children's wear was influenced by movie stars James Dean and Elvis Presley.

One of the big success stories came from a new use for felt. Full skirts of that material, emblazoned with large poodle appliqués and worn over full crinoline petticoats, were the rage. The princess line was the shape that was most popular for girl's dresses. Saddle shoes and penny loafers were considered to be the decade's most stylish footwear.

When the occasion called for more traditional dress, boys of all ages were attired in miniature Frank Sinatra clothing that featured a three-button suit and a Tyrolean-styled hat. The boys were dressed as small copies of their fathers.

Some of the specific trends of the decade included mother-daughter dresses from Lanz of California, a heightening of the preference for western wear due to the enormous popularity of the westerns that dominated television, raccoon hats that emulated the one worn by Davy Crockett, coordinated beach sets that were identical to what parents were wearing, and stretch pants that would become increasingly popular with young girls.

1960s

This was an era in which children's wear took on a brand-new look. Fashion trends were influenced by the Kennedy White House, its occupants being younger than any who had preceded them, and the Beatles, who brought new British fashions to the United States.

At the beginning of the decade, mother-daughter dresses were the rage. The styles were simple, following the designs created for the First Lady Jacqueline Kennedy and her daughter, Caroline. The famous suit silhouette of President Kennedy became a favorite for men across the country, with boy's replicas soon following.

Television made an impact on clothing for boys and girls. Patty Duke's princess dress was quickly adopted as the party dress for preteen girls; *Leave It to Beaver* inspired casual dress for boys; and *The Monkees* television show introduced the eight-button, Edwardian-style shirt that was embraced by the boys' wear market.

With the arrival of the Beatles in the United States, boys' clothing took on a new turn. Not only did the Fab Four introduce the "mod-look" in apparel, but most young boys wore their hair longer and fashioned it after the cut favored by the entertainment world's new sensations.

Bell-bottom pants were introduced in 1968, and their popularity lasted well into the following decade.

1970s

This was the decade in which synthetic fabric replaced natural fibers, double knits became popular, and new standards of dress allowed girls to wear pants to school instead of dresses.

Bell-bottoms, now wider than ever, were joined by flared pants and hip huggers as the decade's most fashionably correct pant silhouettes. Various types of denims worn with midriff tops combined for one of the most successful children's styles.

Designer names, once reserved exclusively for the apparel worn by men and women, were introduced to the children's market. Through licensing arrangements, famous designer labels such as Pierre Cardin would be found on a wide range of clothing for the youth of America.

Again, television had a major impact on the designs of the day. This time it was the popular *Brady Bunch* that influenced fashion. Printed shirts worn with denim pants augmented with vinyl belts for the boys and maxi-dresses for the girls were worn by children of all ages.

John Travolta's *Saturday Night Fever* introduced the three-piece polyester suit that would immediately take the young men and boys' market by storm.

By the end of the decade, designer jeans would again stir new approaches to fashion. First introduced by such names as Gloria Vanderbilt and Calvin Klein for adult styles, the fashion spread to children's wear. Where denim was once regarded as appropriate functional, casual attire, it would now be accepted as the right choice for numerous social occasions. This crop of jeans became status apparel, with the names of the designers featured on the outside of the garment for everyone to see. Not only did denim take on a new meaning, but the designer emphasis significantly increased the prices to new heights.

1980s

The eighties were a time when prosperity abounded in the United States. Children's wear business soared to new heights, as baby boomers met with significant monetary success and had families that the industry would target.

The advent of MTV provided new entertainers on whom children's fashions could focus. The styles sported by such performers as Michael Jackson and Madonna were quickly translated into apparel that the younger generation happily embraced.

Manufacturers and designers of men's and women's collections now entered this new arena with collections that featured complete assortments of apparel. Names like Boston Traders, J. G. Hook, and Ralph Lauren successfully filled the market's needs. Others, including Liz Claiborne, so prominent with adult designs, could not find their right niche and closed their children's divisions.

The three-piece polyester suits of *Saturday Night Fever*, which were so popular with boys in the 1970s, were replaced with the unstructured silhouettes featured in *Miami Vice.*

The entertainment world still strongly influenced the inspiration of fashion design. The success of *The Teenage Mutant Ninja Turtles* in the movies, on television, and in comic books transferred into significant wealth for the manufacturers who were licensed to produce products depicting the *Turtle* characters. At the close of the decade, *The Little Mermaid* film proved to be a licenser's dream, as manufacturers capitalized on the success of the film with a large number of thematic products.

By the close of the decade, items such as cargo pants, jams, denim overalls, Spandex bicycle shorts, miniskirts, leggings, Capri pants, and athletic shoes, once reserved for the gym, were the choices of the young.

1990s

As the last decade of the twentieth century began, there were many carryovers from the 1980s. Kids chose athletic footwear styles for almost every situation from such companies as Nike and Reebok. The phenomenon continued throughout the decade.

Bell-bottoms were again introduced, but their success was nowhere near that of earlier times. Of course, they still took their place as one of many pant silhouettes.

Casual wear included jeans and sweatshirts, which bore the names of professional teams and colleges, as mainstays. Baseball caps were one of the most important accessory items throughout the decade, with many boys and young men sporting them backwards on their heads.

Once again, blockbuster movies played a major role in children's design. Both *Beauty and the Beast* and *Aladdin* served the industry well.

As the decade grew closer to the end, there was a return to emulating adult clothing. Designers such as Ralph Lauren and Tommy Hilfiger took the children's market by storm with a wealth of products that were identical copies, logos and all, of their parents' clothing. Many retailers who made their marks with adult apparel expanded their empires with entries that were exclusive outlets for children. The Gap expanded through GapKids and Baby Gap, Talbots with Talbot Kids, and The Limited with Limited Too. These retailers also followed the lead of the aforementioned designers who used many of their adult styles and silhouettes as the basis for children's collections.

2000s

With the new millennium, children's wear still captured the attention of the apparel and accessories industries. Jeans continue to play a dominant role for the young female set, being worn with everything from sweatshirts to dressy tops. Jeans, while still featured in a number of shapes, began to feature a lot of "jewels" and embroidery. Frayed denims also gained popularity.

Baseball caps remained more important than ever, as did the wearing of athletic shoes that often passed the retail price of $150.

At this point in time it is still too early to predict what the highlight of this market will be for the decade.

MERCHANDISE CLASSIFICATIONS

The categories of children's fashions may be broken down in any number of ways. The classifications most frequently used by professionals in the field are those chosen by *Earnshaw Publications,* the magazine of the children's wear industry. Most of the classifications include both boys' and girls' items in every range of sizes. Some, such as dresses, naturally represent only the girls' market.

Jeans

The single largest classification is the jeans category (Figure 10.2). Made of denim, the silhouettes range from the straight leg variety to others that include bell-bottoms and flares. Most of the styles feature fly-front closures. For small children, the waistband is often elasticized. Although denim is the sole fabric used for jeans, recent technology has given this rough, durable fabric new looks. Processes such as acid washing, tie-dyeing, and stone washing have added variety to traditional jeans. Embroidery and other enhancements have made jeans more fashionable than ever before.

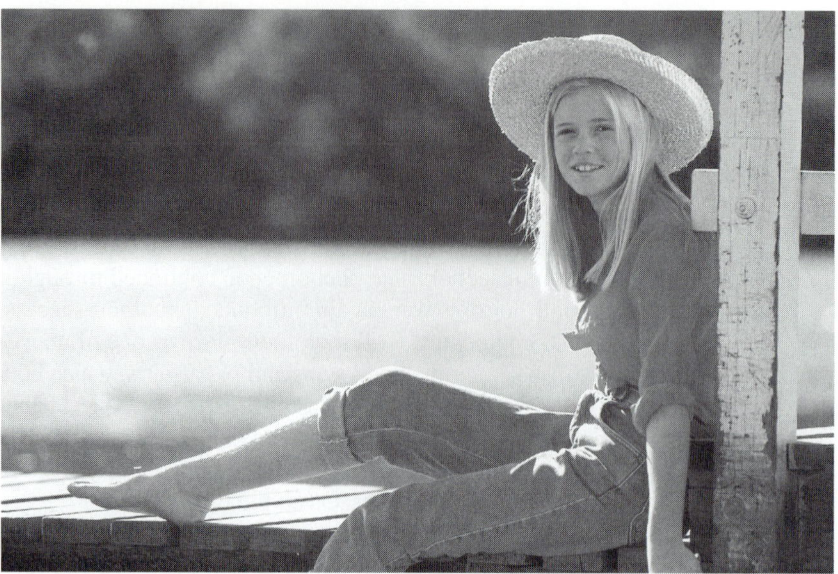

Figure 10.2 Jeans are among teenagers' favorite apparel.
(Courtesy of Photolibrary.com, Trevor Worden.)

Outerwear

The range in this group includes coats, parkas, baseball jackets, ski jackets, and snowsuits.

Coats. A wide range of styles feature lengths anywhere below the knee. They are available in a variety of weights from the heaviest woolens to water-resistant cottons and blends used for raincoats.

Parkas. This three-quarter length outergarment usually features an attached hood and **toggle closures.**

Baseball jackets. A design copied from the outerwear worn by professional baseball players, these children's jackets are usually made of flannels or meltons that use two contrasting colors in the design. Many styles are exact duplicates, logos and all, of the various baseball teams. From time to time, the jacket is produced in leather.

Ski jackets. Originally used as standard wear for skiing, they are favorites for regular casual dress. The major feature is warmth without weight. Once produced in nylon, other fibers such as Thinsulate have given these styles even greater warmth and less weight than before.

Snowsuits. They are produced in a variety of styles. Most are one-piece and feature zippers for easy access. A variation on the snowsuit is the **bunting,** which uses a pouch bottom instead of two pant legs. This is primarily designed for infants. Some buntings may be rezipped into pant legs.

Swimwear

The products simulate those worn by adults. They come in a variety of styles for boys and girls. The boys' designs are either the loose-fitting types that resemble shorts and are available in short or longer versions or the tight-fitting versions that are fashioned after the preferred style of serious swimmers. Girls swimsuits are either one- or two-piece. They feature snug-fitting silhouettes, "boy" legs, or ruffled skirts.

Interest in swimwear has increased in recent years with the introduction of patterns that echo children's favorite television or movie characters.

Sleepwear

The variety mostly concentrates on one- or two-piece pajamas and nightgowns. Small children's styles usually feature such favorites as Snoopy or Barney. The most popular pajama

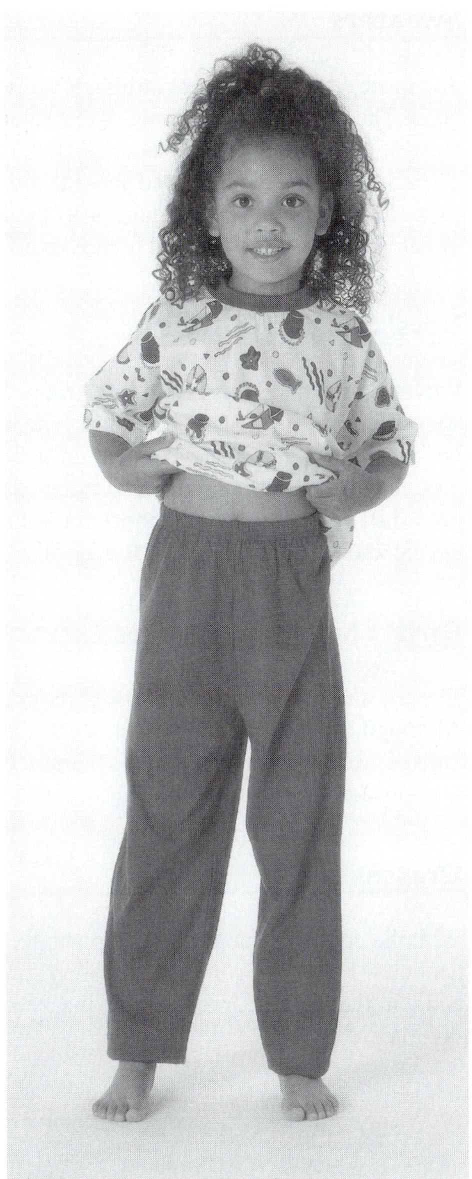

Figure 10.3 Little girls often prefer two-piece pajamas that feature unique prints.
(Courtesy of Dorling Kindersley Media Library, Susanna Price.)

style for boys resembles skiwear, with snug-fitting elasticized waists and ribbed bottoms for cold weather and shorter styles for summer. There has also been interest in boxer shorts with matching tops as alternatives. Little girls also wear pajamas (Figure 10.3), but their older sisters often prefer nightgowns.

Bathrobes are part of this classification and come in a variety of materials that include velour for warmth, terry cloth for absorbency after a bath, and lighter weights for other times.

Underwear

The majority of children's underwear is knitted. Babies and toddlers wear sleeveless T-shirts in either all-cotton, which provides the most comfort, or blends of cotton, nylon, and polyester, which provide absorbency plus additional durability.

Preschool children wear sleeveless shirts or T-shirts over their underpants. Little girls' styles usually use some ruffling or trim to enhance the basic designs. Little boys' underpants are usually of the **brief** variety and feature popular cartoon characters.

Older children continue to wear the styles worn as preschoolers, with patterns reflecting their favorite television or movie characters.

Sweaters

The basic styles are either cardigans, which have button closures, or those that slip over the head. The sleeve lengths range from sleeveless to full length. The necklines are generally crew or collarless, turtlenecks or mock turtles, or collared in a variety of designs.

Sweaters are knitted and serve the wearer by providing warmth to the body. The fibers used range from the finest gauges to the bulkiest varieties. Either machine or hand-made, sweaters come in wool, wool blends, man-mades, cotton, and linen.

Boys' Shirts and Tops

Woven shorts and knits are in this group. Most of them are knitted and come in a variety of styles. They are primarily the T-shirt types or the polo variety with small collars. T-shirts have become the number one element in a boy's shirt wardrobe since the industry began to produce patterns that featured famous cartoon characters and logos of athletic teams. The polo shirt is mainly used for more formal occasions. The woven shirt has lost a great deal of appeal and is used only when the social occasion demands it.

Girls' Shirts and Blouses

As with their male counterparts, girls may also select from wovens and knitted varieties. Although girls wear more woven shirts than do boys, the market has significantly shifted to knits. The designs range from the plainest crew necks and turtlenecks to the fanciest trimmed versions.

Dresses

With the continued popularity of pants for most occasions, the use of dresses has somewhat declined. However, some size groups still show interest in dresses (Figure 10.4). Specifically, in the infants' and toddlers' markets and the preteen category, dresses have remained favorites.

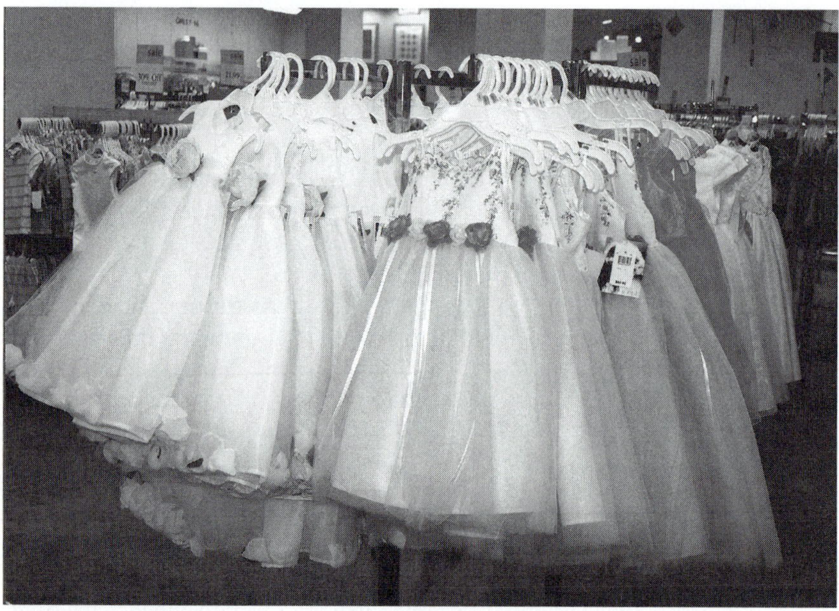

Figure 10.4 Party dresses are big sellers for special occasions.
(Courtesy of Ellen Diamond.)

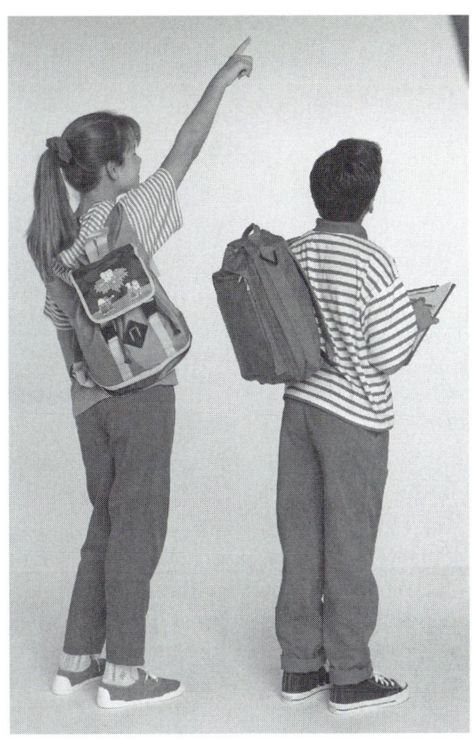

Figure 10.5 Boys and girls often carry backpacks to hold their books and school supplies.
(Courtesy of Dorling Kindersley Media Library.)

Boys' Dresswear

A relaxation of dress standards has seriously affected boys' dresswear, which includes suits, sports coats, and pants. The acceptance of a pair of jeans topped with a knit shirt has caused this decline in more formal boys' wear. Where dress pants and woven shirts for schoolwear and a suit or sports coat and dress slacks were traditional for social functions, the less rigorous dress codes have caused erosion in this market.

Accessories

There has been considerable interest in children's accessories. They include belts, hair ornaments, handbags, hosiery, hats, and jewelry. Along with these traditional elements, the backpack has become a standard for school-age children. It is both functional and fashionable (Figure 10.5). Children of all ages, from five-year-olds to those who attend high school, may be seen wearing these bags to school.

Children's accessories received a boost when many licensing arrangements permitted the use of Disney, Warner Brothers, and other cartoon characters to be emblazoned on the various items.

SIZE CLASSIFICATIONS

Whereas adult size categories are determined by the heights and weights of the wearers, children's sizes are generally classified according to age; that is, children pass through different size ranges as they enter each chronological age. The smallest sizes are categorized as infants' clothing and the largest is preteen for girls and student or youth sizes for boys.

Infants

Newborns and young infants wear sizes that are designated according to months. The smallest **infant size** is three months and progresses at three-month intervals until twenty-four months. Although age is specifically used as the barometer in this classification, the infants'

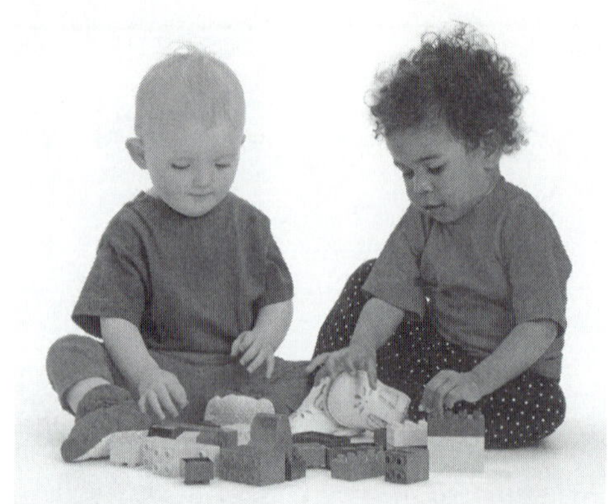

Figure 10.6 Toddler outfits are made to fit over bulky diapers.
(Courtesy of Dorling Kindersley Media Library.)

actual length and weight are also important in the choice of a particular size. Large newborns and extremely small six-month-old children might wear the identical size. Individual sizes merely focus on the typical weights for each age.

Toddlers

When the infant sizes no longer fit, the next classification produced is the **toddler size.** Small children from ages of about one to two and a half who have been crawling for a while and are beginning to walk generally graduate to this size range. The sizes range from 1T to 4T, and the styles usually have a fullness in the pants that easily fit over bulky diapers (Figure 10.6).

Children

Clothing in this category ranges from about 3 to 6X for girls and about 3 to 7 for boys. These **children sizes** are targeted toward preschoolers who have shed their diapers and young school-age children. Children from ages three to six usually stay in this size range. Because the diaper is no longer needed, most trousers feature narrower or slimmer silhouettes.

Girls

Sizes 7 to 14 are earmarked for girls six years and older. Typically, regular girls' sizes are on the narrow side. In addition to the regular size range, **chubbies** are also offered for fuller-figured youngsters.

Boys

These sizes are the counterparts to the girls' classification. They begin at size 6 and go up to 20. Because there is such variation in boys' shapes, this category is subdivided into three classifications. Regular is for the average size boy, slim for the thinnest, and husky for the chubbiest.

Preteen

Having outgrown the size range worn for many years, girls of about ten to twelve years of age move into the **preteen size** category. The sizes range from 6 to 14. Because those in this market are no longer satisfied with the styles they have worn for so long, a radical change in design takes place (Figure 10.7). Preteen clothing mimics the styles of teenagers, but in shapes that are proportioned to fit their less-developed bodies.

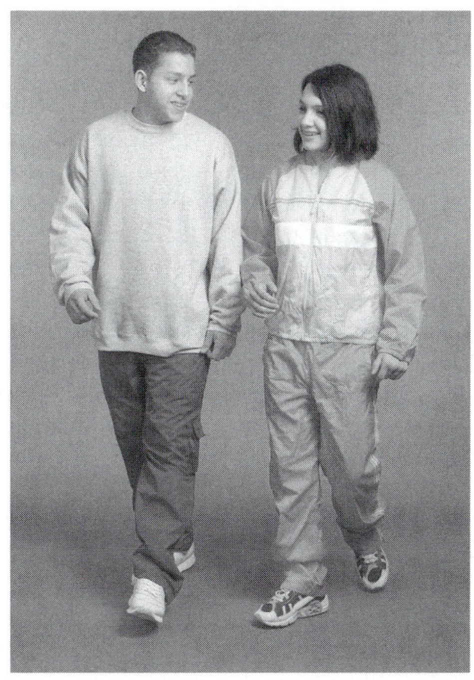

Figure 10.7 Preteen girl and youth sizes generally feature comfortable sports attire.
(Courtesy of Prentice Hall School Division, Bill Burlingham.)

Youth

The boys' counterpart to preteen is known as **youth** or **student sizes.** They are fashioned for boys who have outgrown size 20, but have not developed enough to wear traditional men's sizes.

STYLES, SILHOUETTES, AND DETAILS

The various shapes that make up the children's markets, and the trim that embellishes each design, somewhat mimic those found in their parents' clothing. Jeans, for example, use the same silhouettes, as do their trimmings. If one looks at the men's T-shirt market, the boy's entries are quite similar, down to the teams' logos emblazoned on them (Figure 10.8).

In fact, when an adult's style is popular, it is often copied into children's styles. Even the coloration is the same for adults and children. Thus, for a familiarization of these different styles, silhouettes, and details, review those in the men's and women's categories.

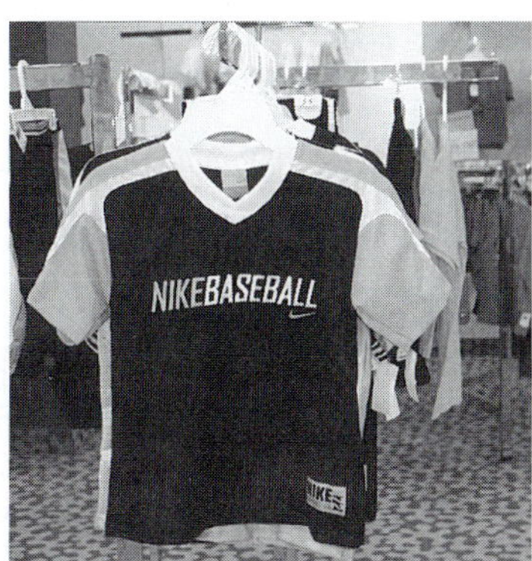

Figure 10.8 The sports logo is a popular detail on clothing for the children's market.
(Courtesy of Ellen Diamond.)

MARKETING CHILDREN'S WEAR

The children's wear industry is the smallest of the apparel markets. There are few major players in this industry, with the earliest dating back to the 1890s.

Many companies specialize in a specific type of clothing and size classification, whereas the offerings of others cut across different size ranges.

The industry typically offers two major collections each year, with some introducing a third for holiday and resort. The larger manufacturers maintain permanent showrooms for their lines, whereas others are grouped together in the offices of manufacturer's representatives. The largest of these producers maintain branch offices in regional markets across the country.

In addition to these showrooms, many children's firms use the trade show route to sell their products. Throughout the world, buyers congregate during children's wear market weeks to view the new offerings. At the typical trade fair, producers from around the globe set up booths that feature their merchandise lines.

Among the major trade shows are the International Kids Show; Mode Enfantine, a French exposition; Modaberlin, a show that features children's clothing and accessories along with men's and women's lines; and Pitti Immagine Bimbo, a Florence, Italy, entry.

In addition to the display of each manufacturer's lines, most of these expositions feature fashion shows to show the buyer the next season's direction and seminars that assist both manufacturers and retailers with future merchandising plans.

Although the showrooms and trade shows are used successfully in marketing children's wear, not every retailer visits them to make purchases. To reach that group, many companies call on potential customers at their retail locations. The companies' trading areas are divided into regions or territories to which sales personnel are assigned.

To call attention to their merchandise assortments, many manufacturers use trade publications such as *Earnshaw* and *Women's Wear Daily,* which have special sections devoted to the children's market, to show new merchandise to prospective customers. Some use consumer periodicals such as *Parent* magazine to entice consumers into asking for the merchandise at their favorite stores and Web sites. Cooperative advertising is often used to entice certain merchants to feature specific items. In these situations, the manufacturers contribute 50 percent of the cost of the retail advertisement.

A significant shift in marketing in the children's wear industry has occurred in recent years. Some independent manufacturers still sell their lines to retailers, but several companies now engage in **vertical marketing.** That is, they are the manufacturer and retailer of their own collections. The Gap, through its GapKids and Baby Gap lines, OshKosh B'Gosh, and others create their own products and market them in brick-and-mortar outlets, catalogs, and Web sites directly to the consumer. This has taken a toll on the depth and breadth of the traditional marketing of children's wear.

With this approach, it makes the typical distribution of children's wear more competitive than ever before. Only those that market their products carefully may be left to get a share of the business.

Internet Resources for Additional Research

www.lovetoknow.com/top10/kids-clothing.html lists the top ten children's Web sites and how to reach them.

www.histclo.hispeed.com/photo/photopubus.html lists the most important children's wear publications.

Merchandise Information Terminology

Coveralls
Keds
Bell-bottom pants
Toggle closures
Bunting
Briefs
Infant sizes
Toddler sizes
Children sizes
Chubbies
Preteen sizes
Youth/student sizes
Vertical marketing

EXERCISES

1. Prepare a report tracing the history of children's wear prior to the 1900s. Along with the report, drawings of the typical styles of the times should be mounted on foam board. Information may be obtained by using a search engine or through visits to the library.
2. Visit a children's department in a department store and a Web site of a specialty retailer that features children's clothing. For each one, determine the following:
   - Price lines
   - Size ranges
   - Merchandise assortments
   - Manufacturers featured
3. Visit a major children's brick-and-mortar operation to assess the proportion of merchandise produced domestically and offshore. For each product classification, determine the percentage of each.

Review Questions

1. What were children's fashions like in the 1900s?
2. When were the first denim products offered for children, and which company was responsible for their introduction?
3. In what period was the first canvas shoe combined with rubber soles, and what were they called?
4. What was the major dress silhouette for girls of the twenties?
5. Who was the first child movie star to influence girls' fashions?
6. Name the famous movie of 1939 that influenced the girls' dresses for the next few years. What specific dress style became popular because of this film?
7. In the 1940s, what theatrical trend in film influenced apparel worn by boys?
8. Discuss how felt was used as a popular fabric in the 1950s.
9. What name was given to the clothing styles worn by the Beatles in the 1960s?
10. How did licensing affect the children's market?
11. Who initiated the change of status for jeans in the late 1970s?
12. What fashion did John Travolta popularize in *Saturday Night Fever* for boys?
13. Discuss some of the fashion trends that were popular at the close of the twentieth century.
14. How has denim apparel expanded from the practical apparel for which it was originally intended?
15. What is a *bunting*?
16. What "signature" do children's pajamas use to attract the attention of the wearers?
17. What phenomenon helped make children's accessories important?
18. On what is the infant size typically based?
19. How do preteen styles compare with those of teen styles?
20. Discuss vertical marketing as it relates to today's children's wear distribution.

SECTION FOUR

Wearable Accessories and Enhancements

CHAPTER 11

Footwear, Handbags, Luggage, and Belts

After reading this chapter, you should be able to:

- Identify the various component parts of shoes and boots.
- Discuss the concept of lasting and its importance to proper shoe fit.
- Explain how shoe designs are transformed into patterns.
- Describe the manufacturing processes of shoe production.
- Identify the various types of footwear styles.
- Outline the procedure for proper footwear fitting.
- Discuss the handbag industry and identify its various styles.
- Explain the importance of belts as fashion accessories.
- Discuss the different factors that should be considered in the purchase of luggage.

As well-dressed men and women are being catered to in prestigious shoe salons bearing such names as Salvatore Ferragamo, Gucci, Cole-Haan, and Bally, other fashion enthusiasts are steadying themselves on one foot in flea markets as they contemplate the purchase of a pair of shoes. In both of these totally different environments and in others such as department stores and specialty stores, consumers are shopping for footwear to enhance their apparel. Even off-site ventures such as the catalogs and Web sites are becoming important places for those willing to "buy without trying."

While shoe sales continue to increase, only in rare instances are shoes central to the purchase of apparel.

Although the spectacular runway shows herald the apparel creations of designers everywhere, significantly less attention is focused on the shoes and boots that enhance and augment the clothing. Only rarely does a footwear style generate long-lasting life that seems to come to life over and over again. Carmen Miranda, a diminutive Latin American musical star of the 1940s, achieved greater physical stature with outrageous **platform shoes.** The craze immediately captured the attention of women all over the world, and every decade seems to reintroduce the platform shoe. Courreges, who helped transform couture from the traditional to the more avant-garde, gained international attention with his go-go boot designs that accompanied the miniskirts of the 1960s. These footwear fashion innovations are among the few that have achieved distinction. Humans began constructing shoes to protect their feet around 10,000 B.C. The industry today has grown to produce more than 7 billion pairs of shoes annually. Although function remains a concern of the manufacturers and wearers, the business is primarily fashion driven.

While shoe brands like Joyce, Naturalizer, and Selby are giants in the industry, their style designers never received the attention or acclaim afforded their counterparts of apparel design, and they have remained in the background as the unsung heroes of their companies. Since the early 1980s, however, the industry has rapidly expanded with designer names that were once found only on men's and women's clothing labels. Recognizing that powerful

half-sizes in an array of different widths and colors. Thus, a particular man's shoe that is available from sizes 8 to 12, in widths from AA to DDD, and in black, brown, and cordovan requires, for one of each size, an order of forty-eight pairs. To make certain that a sufficient number of pairs will be available to accommodate the consumer, more than one pair must be ordered in the more popular sizes, resulting in minimum orders for at least 100 pairs of a style. This not only requires a significant outlay of capital by the retailer, but must also provide for considerable inventory space. It is not unusual for the end of the season to arrive to find the retailer left with hundreds of **broken sizes** that must be sold. Because of the difficulty in shoe merchandising, the initial markups taken are generally greater than that of other fashion items.

No matter at which level of the shoe industry one participates, it is imperative to develop a complete understanding of the product, including its component parts, production techniques, and styles. Through total comprehension, sellers will be better prepared to serve the needs of their customers.

Shoe Component Parts

The shoe is composed of three main parts; the upper, the soles, and the heel.

The **upper** basically consists of three pieces: the **vamp,** which covers the toes and the front portion of the foot and includes the shoe's **tongue,** and the two **quarters,** which encompass its back portion (Figure 11.3). More complicated styling could add additional pieces to the upper.

The **sole** is actually more than one layer, consisting of the **insole,** which lies on the inside of the shoe, directly below the foot; the **midsole,** another layer lying between the insole and the outsole; and the **outsole,** the outermost layer of the sole, which is thicker than the others to withstand the wear of friction caused by contact with the ground.

Heels, or **bottoms** as they are often referred to in the manufacturing process, come in a variety of styles and heights and are the last parts to be added to the shoe.

The assembly of these components may be achieved in a number of ways, each of which is discussed later in this chapter.

From Concept to Construction

Shoe designers, or *line builders*, a name used in the industry to describe the creators of the product, are responsible for styling. As is the case with the designers of apparel and other accessories, their inspirations come from a variety of sources. They listen closely to fashion forecasters who predict, sometimes as early as a year in advance, what trends will be favored

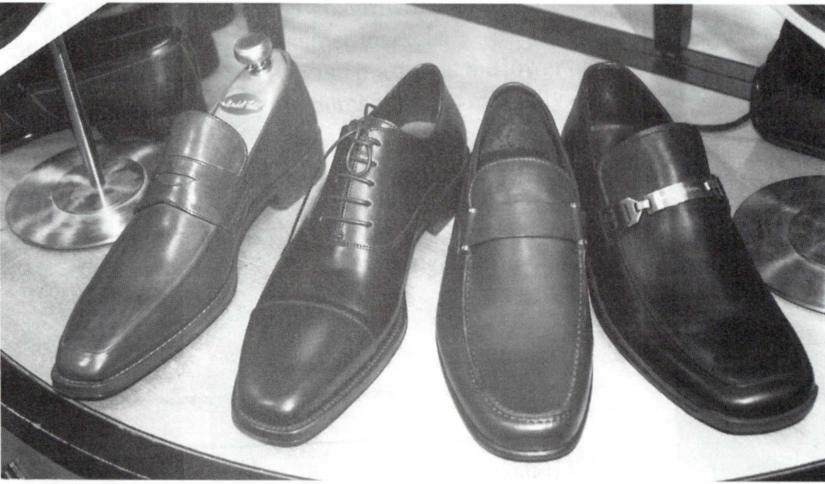

Figure 11.3 Shoe uppers are either laced or made to slip on the foot. *(Courtesy of Ellen Diamond.)*

in the companion industries such as clothing and sportswear, indicating which shoe styles might complement the designs. They may also be inspired by a theatrical production or the desire to revisit a period in fashion history. Line builders often rely on their own original creative genius.

Although fashion plays a dominant role in footwear design, it should be understood that comfort and utility are also of considerable importance. In the enormous market of athletic shoes, for example, fit and comfort are key ingredients that have been enhanced in recent years with the addition of designer touches that embellish the numerous styles. Colorful accents and ornamentation have taken the utilitarian product and moved it to center stage in terms of overall market share in the footwear industry.

Although the designer performs the creative task, he or she generally works in conjunction with both the merchandisers who assess the needs of the marketplace and the production team that translates the styles into wearable models.

The route from the original concept to the finished product involves many stages, including developing the designer *last*, translating the designer last into the production or development last, making the pattern, manufacturing the *dies*, cutting the materials, fitting or stitching, *lasting*, assembling the remaining components, *bottoming*, and finishing. Some construction is so complicated that more than 200 individual operations are involved from beginning to end.

DEVELOPMENT OF THE DESIGNER LAST

After the design has been hand sketched or accomplished with the use of a CAD (computer-aided design) system, a form, or **last,** must be created on which the model shoe will be constructed. Each last embodies the style, size, and fit characteristics that will make up the finished shoe. The **designer last** is most often sculpted from wood by skilled craftspeople. After the last has been examined and the decision has been made to go ahead with the style as part of the line, it is then transformed into a production or development last.

CREATION OF THE PRODUCTION OR DEVELOPMENT LAST

A separate last is needed for each style in every size and width that will be produced. If there are 50 specific size and width combinations, for example, fifty individual lasts must be produced.

Typically, the production last is mechanically built from polyethylene logs that are placed on duplicating lathes that copy the designer's original last. With the use of the CAD system, engineers can then produce a flat representation of the last that will be used for making the patterns.

PATTERN MAKING

The objective of pattern making is to represent the three-dimensional last as a flat surface. There are many parts to a shoe, each of which must be made into a perfectly accurate pattern to ensure a problem-free final product. The pattern parts include the uppers, linings, insoles, outsoles, heels, and any other functional or decorative pieces.

The patterns may be created by using one of several methods. One popular option begins with wrapping the last with strips of adhesive tape that are then pencil marked to indicate the key design and reference points. The tape is then cut along the design lines and peeled away from the last and flattened onto pattern paper, where each piece is then traced and finally cut. At this point, many companies grade the patterns needed for the various shoe sizes. Once this has been completed, cutting dies must be manufactured.

DIE MANUFACTURING

To cut through the many layers of material needed to make the shoe, cutting **dies,** similar to cookie cutters, are made. Sharp steel strips are bent around the various paper patterns to form individual dies for each part of the shoe.

CUTTING

After the dies have been completed, they are used to cut the materials. The dies are positioned over the materials and, by means of a press, cut through one or more layers. With

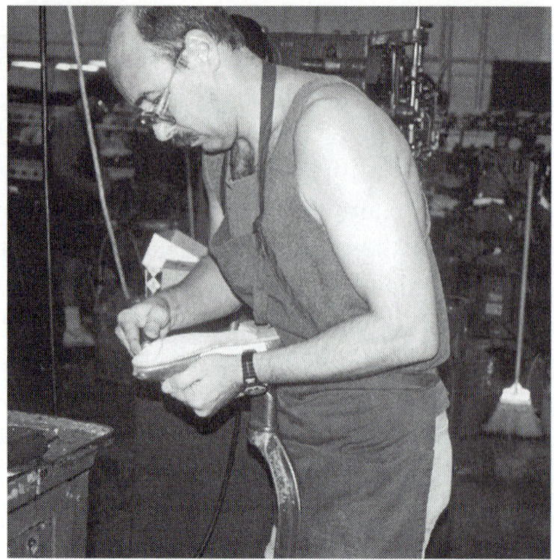

Figure 11.4 The shoe is fitted on the last to make it conform to the desired shape.
(Courtesy of Ellen Diamond.)

leather, cutting is usually done one at a time to avoid imperfections. Man-mades, on the other hand, may be cut in layers because they are uniformly produced in factories. Where leather is cut by individual craftspeople to make certain that material use is optimized, man-mades may be cut by means of automated cutting systems that significantly speed up the process.

FITTING OR STITCHING

The largest number of individual operations is performed in the **fitting room** where all of the individual parts are sewn together. For example, the vamp lining is attached to the vamp, the quarter lining applied to the quarter, the quarter sewn to the vamp, and so forth. As many as sixty individual procedures are accomplished at this stage, including stitch marking, which helps to accurately position the upper and other components; skiving, to reduce the thickness of the leather where needed; **doubling,** the placement of fabric interlining between the upper and lining to improve comfort; eyeleting, punching holes through which laces will be inserted; and stitching, which may be either functional or decorative or a combination of both.

LASTING

In the **lasting** room, the fitted upper is pulled over the last in a series of operations that makes the upper conform to the shape of the last (Figure 11.4). At this point the final upper takes the shape of the shoe. A number of different lasting techniques are used, depending on such factors as the quality of the shoe and its function and appearance. Each technique involves closing the heel area first and then the top section, and finally closing up the sides (Figure 11.5).

These lasting techniques are among the most common:

- **Goodyear welt** joins the upper and sole to secure a firm attachment and a smooth insole. The construction is unique in the formation of two seams in the attachment of the shoe bottom. The first is a hidden chain-stitched inseam that holds the welt, or narrow strip of leather, upper lin-

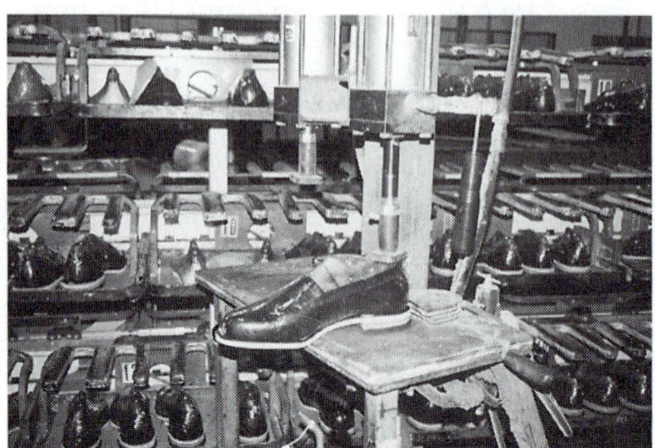

Figure 11.5 The lasted shoe is fitted with heels through a variety of techniques.
(Courtesy of Ellen Diamond.)

ing, and insole together; and the second is a lock-stitched outseam by which the outsole is attached. It is considered one of the finer methods of lasting.

- **Mackay** lasting is achieved by tacking, stapling, or cementing the upper over an insole that is visible on the inside of the shoe and then attaching the outsole with a chain-stitched seam.
- **Littleway** involves stitching the sole directly to the upper.
- **Cementing** involves the use of adhesives rather than stitching to attach the sole to the upper.

ASSEMBLING REMAINING COMPONENTS

While the upper is being assembled and lasted, various components such as counters, stiffening materials used to strengthen the back part of the shoe; **sock linings,** which cover any stitching during sole attachment; outsoles, the ones that are visible to the eye; shanks, steel pieces that are inserted into the arch of the shoe for support; and heels are being assembled.

Each of these components is needed during a specific time in the production process; therefore, timing is important to make certain that these items are ready when needed.

BOTTOMING

In an area called the *bottoming room*, the lasted upper receives shanks and fillers and is prepared for the outsole to be permanently attached to the upper of the shoe. Then heels are nailed through the insole for strength, essentially completing the shoe (Figure 11.6).

FINISHING

Before the shoe is sent to the packing room to be shipped to retailers, various final operations, collectively called *finishing*, take place. Among those typically used are buffing the bottoms with fine sandpaper to produce a velvety, smooth feel; polishing with wax to enhance the luster of the leather; treeing, which is placing the shoe on the form used in construction to make certain that it was properly shaped; spraying with a lustrous solution that bonds the fibers of the upper materials and preserves and protects the finish; lacing and ornament attachment; and inspection to make certain that the finished product meets the company's standards (Figure 11.7).

After the product is considered ready for delivery to the customer, it is boxed and sent either to a warehouse for storage or directly to the purchaser.

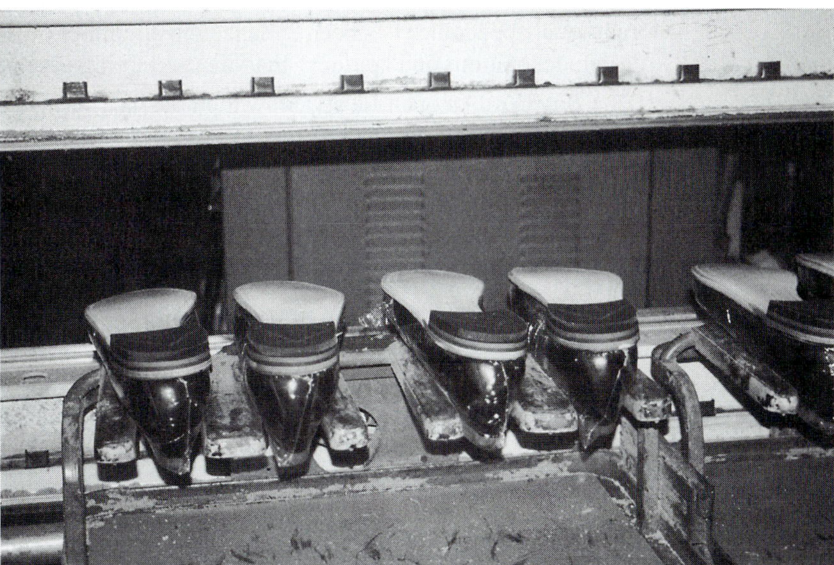

Figure 11.6 Shoes on this assembly line are fitted with heels.
(Courtesy of Ellen Diamond.)

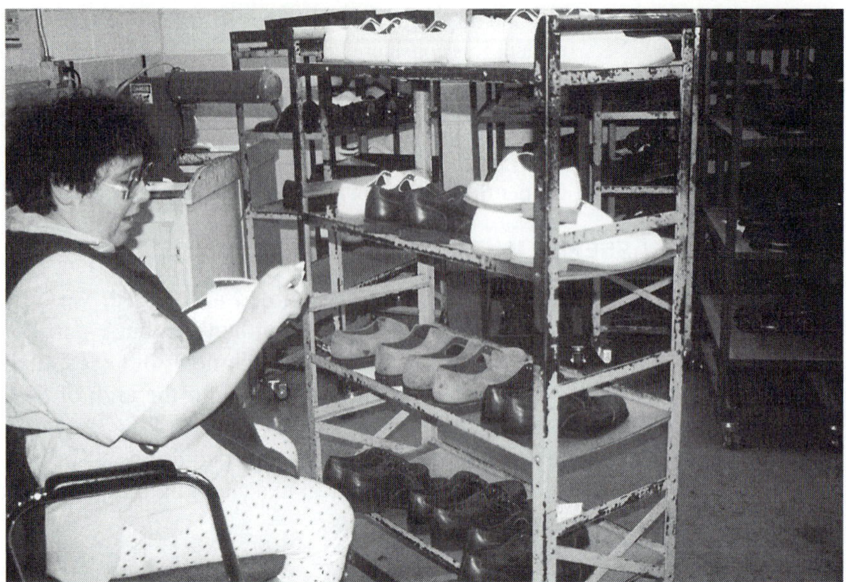

Figure 11.7 Finishes are applied to shoes to enhance appearance.
(Courtesy of Ellen Diamond.)

Styles

Although men's, women's, and children's footwear is available in many styles, the popularity of each is based upon the fashions of the time. They range anywhere from those that are used for physical fitness activities to those that are worn for formal occasions. The following list shows various styles that are traditional favorites as well as some that seem to appear and disappear according to the dictates of the fashion world.

Aerobics. A term used to describe footwear that is used for walking, running, or any moving exercise. These are generally lightweight, leather or fabric constructed, designed to absorb impact to the feet, and equipped with nonskid bottoms.

Bal. A classic close-tied shoe that is generally available in wingtip design, straight tip, saddle (where two contrasting colored leather uppers are used), and plain front.

Basketball sneaker. Available with either high or low sides and in leather or canvas, its traditional appearance has been enhanced in a number of ways, including unusual color and design decorations and "pumps" that are used to increase height.

Blucher. An open-tie style in which the lace stays open at the bottom of the eyelets. It is primarily worn with casual attire.

Boot. A shoe that is extended anywhere above the ankle to the thigh. Initially designed for warmth and heavy-duty activity, it has been adopted by the fashion world and now accompanies any type of clothing (Figure 11.8).

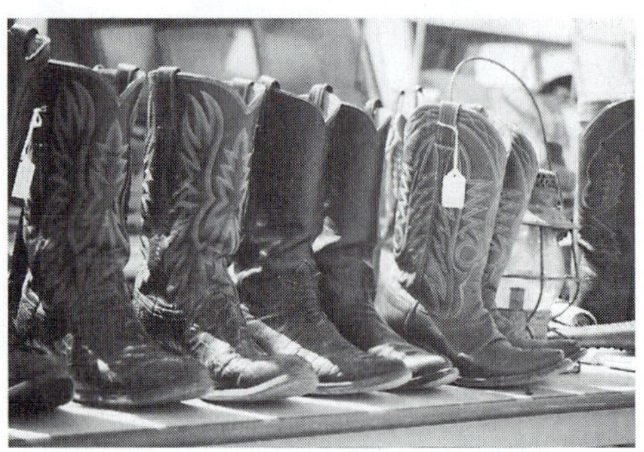

Figure 11.8 Cowboy boots have become fashion mainstays.
(Courtesy of Ellen Diamond.)

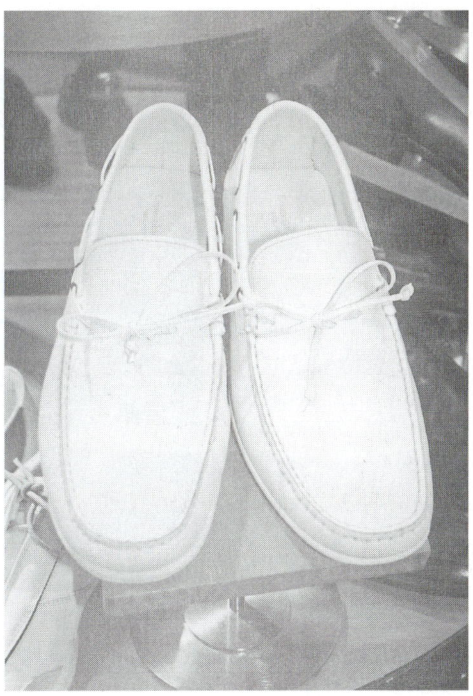

Figure 11.9 Deck shoes are popular for casual wear. *(Courtesy of Ellen Diamond.)*

Brogue. A heavy oxford with decorative stitching.

Buckskins. A blucher shoe made of sueded leather, available in white, tan, and fashion colors.

Clog. A shoe with a heavy platform sole that is made of wood or cork.

Deck shoe. A moccasin that uses lacing through the top and sides of the shoe, has nonskid soles, and is made of canvas or leather. Once relegated to use on boats, it is now a favorite for casual wear (Figure 11.9).

D'Orsay. A women's pump with low-cut sides.

Espadrille. A square-throated, closed-back shoe with a fabric upper and a woven hemp bottom (Figure 11.10).

Ghillie. A low-cut women's shoe that laces across the foot and onto the ankles.

Huarache. A Mexican flat shoe that uses strips of leather woven together to form the upper.

Loafer. A term used to describe any slip-on. It is similar to the traditional moccasin except that it has a sturdier heel and sole (Figure 11.11).

Mary Jane. A woman's or girl's shoe with a strap across the instep and a rounded front.

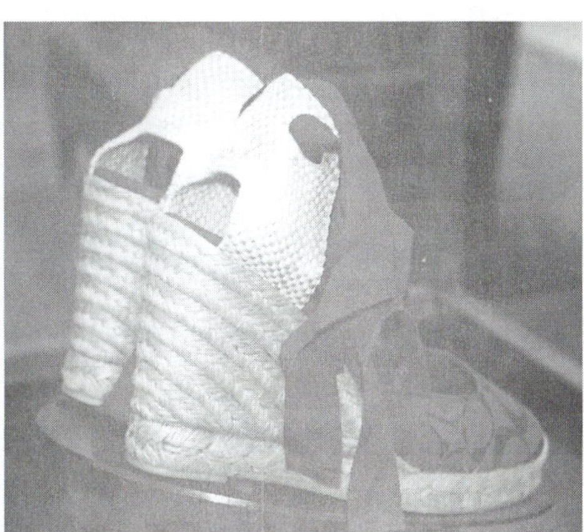

Figure 11.10 This high-fashion espadrille features a woven, hemp platform. *(Courtesy of Ellen Diamond.)*

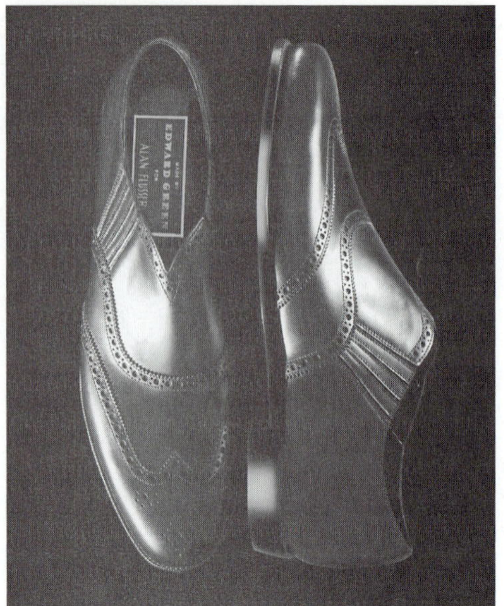

Figure 11.11 This loafer has been designed for dress wear.
(Courtesy of Alan Flusser Custom Shop, James T. Murray Photography, © 2005.)

Moccasin. A shoe construction whereby a single piece of leather is used for the upper, extending all the way under the foot. Generally, attached soles are made of harder leather. It is closed with heavy seaming that is often sewn by hand.

Mule. A backless slipper.

Oxford. A low shoe that features laces over the instep.

Pump. Low-cut shoe with seamless head-to-toe design.

Saddles. Shoes that feature a piece of leather extending from the shank over the throat of the vamp and upward to the quarter on both sides. It often uses a material that contrasts with the rest of the shoe.

Sandal. One of the oldest forms of footwear that traditionally features a sole with straps.

Sling back. A pump with a strap across the back.

Slipper. A shoe worn at home.

Sneaker. A canvas or leather shoe that was originally worn for sports activities but has been adapted for street wear (Figure 11.12). Its styles involve lacing across the instep, and it comes in various heights.

Spectator. A term used to describe a shoe with two contrasting colors that usually has a wooden or stacked heel.

Thong. A sandal that uses a piece of material to slip between two toes (Figure 11.13).

Wedgie. A shoe with a heel that extends from the back of the shoe to the ball.

Western boot. A calf-high boot with a wooden stacked heel and a pointed toe.

Wingtip. An oxford with a stitched tip shaped like a wing.

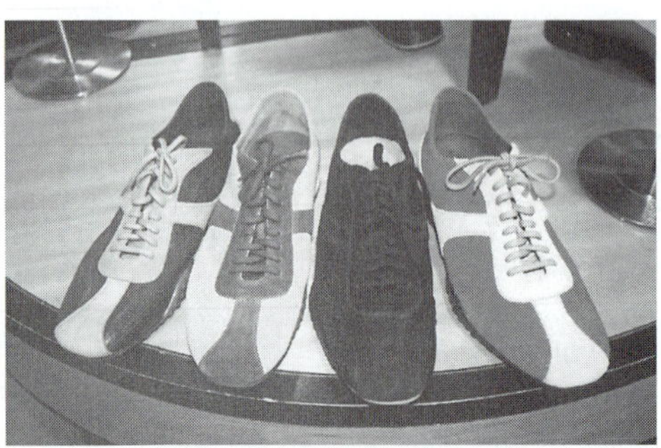

Figure 11.12 Ordinarily worn for sports activities, today's sneakers are fashionably correct for street wear.
(Courtesy of Ellen Diamond.)

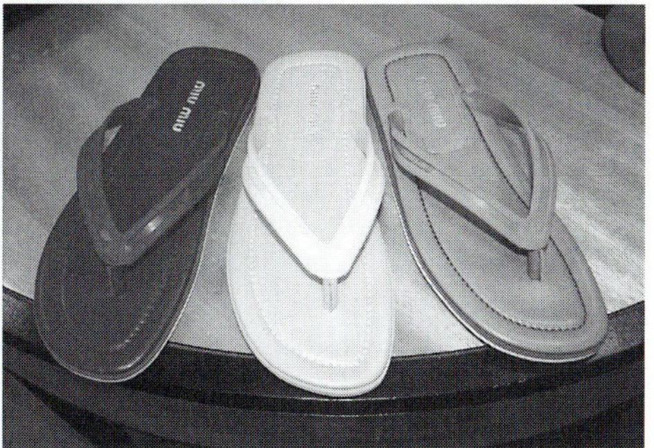

Figure 11.13 Thongs are worn for a variety of activities and occasions.
(Courtesy of Ellen Diamond.)

Judging the Fit

The first attraction to the shoe or boot is generally style, color, or fabric. However, proper fit is necessary to bring comfort to the wearer.

To make certain that the fit is appropriate, these rules should be followed:

1. Feet should be measured in the standing position; if one foot is larger than the other, the larger foot should be used to determine size.
2. Measurement should be made from the heel to the ball of the foot, not the toe, to ensure the best fit.
3. The thickness of the hosiery should be considered during measurement because thick socks will increase the size. It is always best to wear the same hosiery during the try-on time that will be worn with the shoe.
4. The time of the day the shoe is fitted should be considered because the foot swells later in the day.
5. The toes should be wiggled to make certain there is between 1/4 and 1/2 inch between the longest toe and the front of the shoe.
6. Both shoes should be tried to assess fit because often one is larger than the other.
7. A few steps should be taken to judge slipping and comfort.
8. If the shoe pinches the foot or feels loose, another size should be tried.

Caring for Footwear

With the cost of shoes and boots continually increasing, several simple rules should be followed to extend their usefulness.

1. They should be rotated in the wardrobe. Although the foot naturally perspires and leather absorbs the moisture, time is needed for drying out.
2. **Trees,** preferably made of cedar, should be used to help the shoes dry to their original shapes.
3. Leather footwear should never be stored near a heat source because this will dry the leather too quickly. Natural drying is best for the product.
4. New footwear should be polished before the first wearing, which not only will protect it but will make future polishing easier.
5. Polishing should be done with the application of small circles of paste or cream, followed by brushing, then by polishing with a fine, soft cloth.
6. Heels and soles should be regularly checked to make certain that they are not worn down past the point of repair.

HANDBAGS

Once considered primarily for its function, the handbag is now an extremely important part of the fashion business. Not long ago, the industry took its cues from apparel designers and shoe manufacturers and created products that would enhance or coordinate the designs of

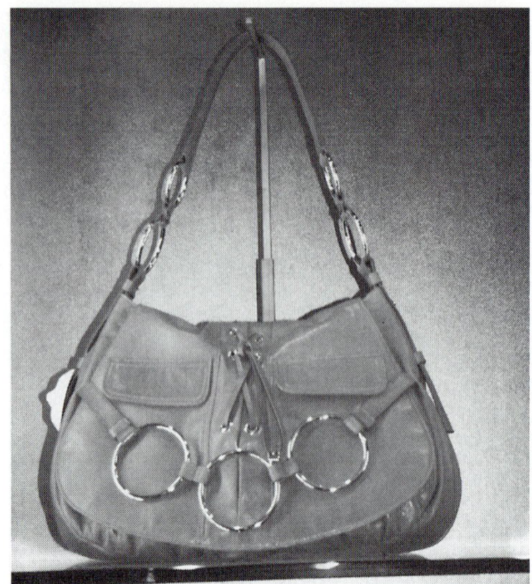

Figure 11.14 A shoulder strap handbag, embellished with brass rings, makes its own fashion statement. *(Courtesy of Ellen Diamond.)*

both. Today, although the clothing design often signals the need for specific types of handbags, this alone is not the motivation for the industry to produce its wares (Figure 11.14).

The nature of the industry has radically changed from one that was unheralded in terms of designer names to today's environment in which designer labels are as important as they are to apparel. During the 1970s, much attention was focused on the handbag when the Cardin and Dior signatures started to appear on the bags themselves and not merely on the inside labels. It was a time when the famous LV logo was displayed on a vinyl collection and customers flocked to purchase the bags at prices that began at $200. Today, this same signature logo is still drawing significant attention from shoppers around the world.

Still recognizing the importance of the designer label, handbag manufacturers, which once were more concerned with styling than making their names recognizable to the consumer, are much involved in licensing agreements with renowned fashion names. The name of Liz Claiborne and others grace a wealth of the handbags being offered for sale by retailers in their brick-and-mortar outlets, catalogs, and Web sites.

The designer handbag phenomenon also continues to expand by way of many marquee labels including these products along with their other wares. Prada, for example, one of the world's upscale "names," markets a collection of handbags that sells for upward of $1,000 along with shoes and apparel for men and women.

Public acceptance of these designer labels in handbags has become so vital to many fashion retailers that they have set aside separate departments in their stores that exclusively feature individual names such as Louis Vuitton, Fendi, and Prada. To give even more recognition to these designer handbag collections, some, such as Gucci and Louis Vuitton, have their own retail premises that feature only their products.

Still, comparatively inexpensive handbags account for much of the industry's sales volume. With modestly priced imports coming from offshore producers, retailers are merchandising these products on "main floor" counters, in their catalogs, and on their Web sites. Rounding out the handbag market are the counterfeits of the famous models sold by street vendors and flea markets around the world.

Component Parts of the Handbag

Using as few as three or four parts or as many as thirty, the most important components are the frame, the body over which the design is constructed; **gussets,** side panels that allow for expansion; lining, which covers the construction stitches or glues for a neater look; handles of varying lengths and materials; and closures such as buckles, zippers, locks, clasps, snaps, and drawstrings.

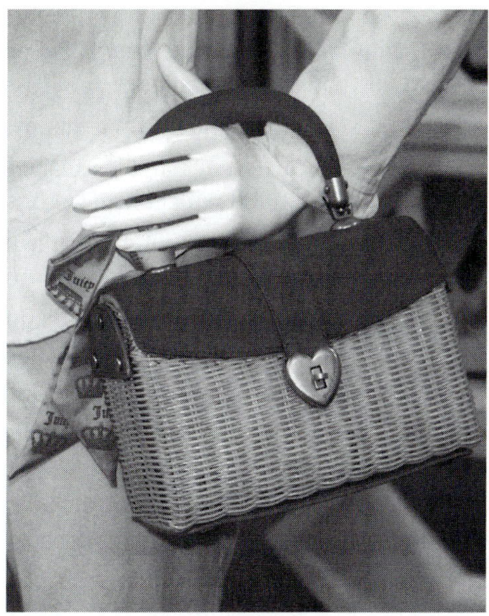

Figure 11.15 Straw and fabric handbags are popular in summer.
(Courtesy of Ellen Diamond.)

The outer materials used to cover the construction include leather, which still dominates the market; vinyl; plastic; fabrics than range from canvas for casual wear to brocades for evening use; Lucite; straw; and metallics (Figure 11.15).

Ornamentation may be in the form of metallic logos such as the one used to identify the Chanel collection, synthetic stones, appliqués, flowers, beads, fringe, or tassels.

Construction

As in the case of other fashion merchandise, the designer initiates the process with a design on paper that has been hand-rendered or computer generated. Then, a sample is prepared in a material such as muslin or felt and is fitted with any closures or ornamentation. After the decision has been made to go ahead with production, patterns of all of the parts are developed.

The patterns are then used to cut the individual pieces. In the case of leather, each part is individually cut so that the craftspeople can carefully avoid scars and markings inherent in the leather. The actual cutting may be accomplished with a sharp knife or by means of dies that stamp out the pieces in cookie-cutter fashion. For fabric handbags, **die stamping** may be used to cut many pieces at a time, thus reducing the cost of construction.

The pieces are then assembled by machine or by hand and made ready for the stiffening materials that will be inserted between the body of the bag and the lining to provide support; stays, plastic strips that will hold the body in shape; or fillers, often made of foam, which give the product a softer feel.

The body of the bag is then fitted to the frame and made ready to receive the handles, closures, and ornamentation.

After the bag has been completed, it is inspected and made ready for shipment to the merchants. Some bags are individually boxed, whereas others are bulk packed, the determining considerations being price, quality, and material.

Styles

As in the case of other fashion accessories, styles fall in and out of favor, with some remaining available as staples.

Some of the more popular handbag styles include:

Box. A square or rectangular-shaped bag made of Lucite, metal, or wood, or a material that covers a rigid surface.

Clutch. A bag that is free of handles and must be held or "clutched" by the wearer. Many manufacturers provide long chain or narrow leather concealed straps that may be used to carry the bag on the shoulder.

Drawstring. A frameless bag that uses a drawstring as its closure.

Envelope. A flat, rectangular-shaped bag that has a flap closure. As in the case of the clutch, it may be fitted with concealed handles or straps for use on the shoulder.

Feedbag. Sometimes referred to as a *duffle*, a large bag that is shaped like a horse's feedbag and carried on the shoulder.

Satchel. Based on the design of a doctor's medical bag. The satchel has a flared, flat, wide bottom and is accented by two handles.

Shoulder bag. Any bag that has a long strap for the carrier.

Tote. Featuring an open top and two strap handles for carrying, a design based on the shopping bag.

LUGGAGE

Once merely a functional item, today's luggage designs are stylish as well as purposefully designed. In addition to some of the designer pieces, such as the Louis Vuitton collection, names such as Tumi have made the offerings as upscale as apparel and fashion accessories, with costs sometimes exceeding $1,000 per item.

With the changes in airline rules, in terms of weight allowances, generally fifty pounds for domestic travel, and seventy pounds for international, the scope of the products have been significantly altered. Even where travelers are willing to spend the extra amounts levied for overweight luggage, some airlines do not allow any bags that cross the established weight limitation. Qantas, for example, does not allow any overweight on its domestic flights, even when the traveler volunteers to pay additional charges.

With the need to reduce weight and the desire for less cumbersome baggage, the industry has responded with lighter-weight luggage and other innovations that have resulted in more choices.

Types of Luggage

Basically, there are two types of luggage in use today. Although hardside luggage is still available, as in the case of leather bags and steel trunks, their popularity is waning. They have been essentially replaced with softside and molded pieces.

Softside luggage is by far the most important type available to the consumer. It has two major advantages, with the most important being its weight. It is extremely lightweight when compared to the hardside and molded varieties. It is also available in a wide variety of colors and patterns, which, if carefully selected, may provide the advantage of easy recognition at baggage claim areas.

Molded luggage features a seamless construction and is durable. Popularized by Samsonite, it offers travelers the assurance of getting to their destination with the pieces in tact. A disadvantage, however, is its inability to expand as in the case of the softside variety.

Styles of Luggage

Within each of the two types of luggage, users may choose from several styles to satisfy their needs. Most manufacturers make their products available as sets, with each piece sharing the same overall appearance, or as individual pieces. For a more economical purchase, the set generally offers the customer better value.

Among the most popular styles are:

- *Rolling tote.* Excellent bags for carrying on the plane. May be carried with the use of the straps or rolled; often has a wide strap on the back that can be easily attached to a larger case.

- *Regular tote.* Similar to the roller, except that it doesn't have wheels.
- *Expandable rollarboard.* Usually measures twenty inches tall and is used primarily as a carry-on, with wheels for easy movement.
- *Expandable rollerboard suiter.* Generally available in twenty-four-, twenty-six-, and twenty-nine inch sizes and used for regular garments as well as to hang suits. Featured are expandable sections that make the piece one to three inches deeper. They have sufficient depth to serve as a base on which a tote may be temporarily attached.
- *Garment bag.* Softly constructed to hold from two to four hanging garments. They feature hooks that may be used to hang the bag in the closet. They fold easily, and many feature handles that may be used for carrying purposes and/or straps for use over the shoulder.
- *Expandable rolling garment bag.* Similar to the regular garment bag, but with wheels for easy rolling and possible expanded with the use of zippers to accommodate up to six hanging garments.
- *Duffle bag.* A soft-sided bag that measures up to twenty-nine inches in length. It may come with or without wheels and/or a strap for ease in carrying.
- *Trunk.* Used on extensive trips to carry large supplies of clothing and accessories. On the outside there are sometimes draws available, and inside are numerous compartments in which small items may be stored. Most are made of steel or some other durable, molded vinyl.
- *Backpack.* A carryall bag that slips over the back with the use of two straps.

Luggage Sets

It is often practical to buy sets rather than a single bag (Figure 11.16). It is especially appropriate for those who travel for periods of a week or more. The price of a set is often better than if individual pieces were purchased, and there is no need to cramp one's belongings into a single case.

Luggage is usually available as two-, three-, four-, or five-piece sets. Typically, the five-piece set features a large suitcase (perhaps something from twenty-six to twenty-nine inches), a garment bag, a duffel bag, a roller carry-on, and a tote. Of course, a wide variety of assortments are produced by many manufacturers.

Purchasing Tips

While many consumers make their decisions solely on price, there are other factors to consider when buying luggage:

- Make certain that *wheeled luggage* is fitted with durable in-line skate wheels that are augmented with ball bearings and durable handles. If the bag is a large garment bag, it should also feature a heavy strap for ease in carrying.

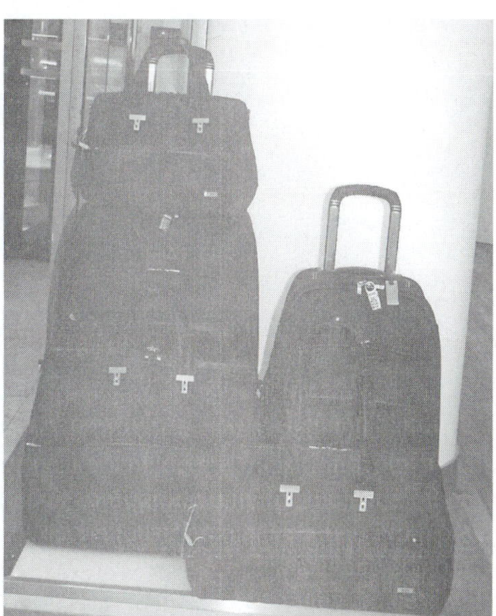

Figure 11.16 Luggage sets offer the consumer many alternatives.
(Courtesy of Ellen Diamond.)

- Select a *duffel* when traveling light is the objective. Available in many different sizes, the *wheeled duffel* is excellent for those who carry a great deal of gear.
- Determine if the bags are the proper size for use on planes and of the best suitable fabric, in terms of weight, so that limits will not be exceeded.
- Assess the number of pockets, mesh bags, folders, and separators to make packing simpler and finding items easier.
- Make certain that there are expansion features to be able to pack larger-than-usual contents.
- Determine whether hard or soft case luggage is best for your needs.
- Evaluate the *denier* of the fabric (a measurement that refers to the fineness of the fabric) and its durability.
- Ensure that the zipper is sufficiently heavy-duty to avoid breaks.
- Choose bags in colors or patterns that will be easy to locate on the luggage carrousel.

BELTS

No longer relegated to use merely as the functional device it once was, the belt now stands on its own as a fashion accessory (Figure 11.17). The domestic industry is primarily centered in New York City and is made up mainly of small producers who serve the needs of two types of customers. They either create their own designs that augment the styles of the apparel market and sell to the retailers, or they provide apparel manufacturers with belts to adorn dresses, sportswear, and ensembles. The offshore market is scattered all over the world, primarily producing lower-priced belts for retail and manufacturer consumption.

This market, as that of handbags, shoes, and other accessories, has reached a status level with the entry of designers who have made their reputations via the apparel route. Logos and signatures of such names as Gucci and Claiborne have helped bring the belt into fashion prominence.

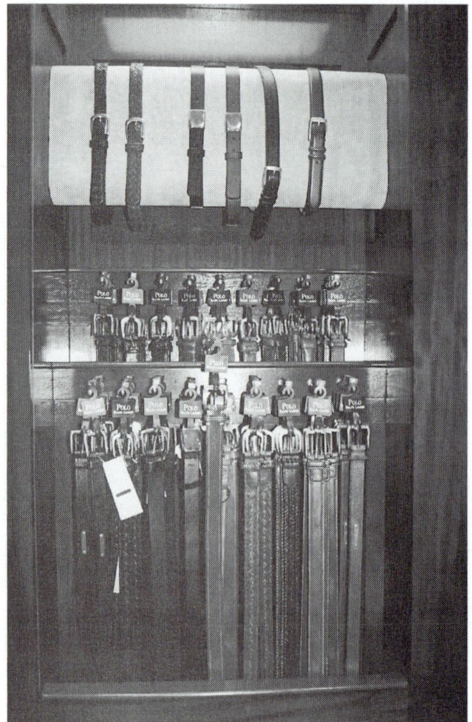

Figure 11.17 Belts come in many styles and are both functional and fashionable.
(Courtesy of Ellen Diamond.)

Construction

Belts are made of a variety of materials, including leather, fabrics, metals, vinyls, and elastic. Their construction is based on the materials used.

In the case of leather, each piece is cut to the desired length and width either by hand or a strap-cutting machine. If the belt requires a shaped design, as in the case of a contour model, a die might be developed and used in place of the traditional machine that makes straight cuts. As in the case of other leather products, caution during cutting must be exercised to avoid blemishes in the leather.

Those belts that are to be backed are done so either by means of a walking-foot machine that sews the two pieces together or by gluing.

Basic fabric belts are constructed in the same manner, except that many materials may be stacked and cut by means of dies, thus reducing production costs.

After the body of the belt has been completed, decorative ornamentation, such as stitching, is applied. Holes, where needed, are then punched, and buckles are inserted and sewn or glued.

Today's fashion world calls for many belts that use nailheads, stones, metallics, and other adornments for leather belts as well as a variety of novelty fabric, Lucite, metal, and vinyl-based belts. Their designs might be ethnic, such as the Native American variety, which uses silver and silverlike materials that are augmented with real or synthetic turquoise stones; bejeweled and laden with a variety of colored stones; or anything that captures the imagination of the designer.

In the case of the cinch belt, which tightly conforms to the body with the use of elasticized materials, or the chain-link metallic, which uses a number of interlocking pieces, construction is simpler than the traditional leather variety. The cinch belt merely requires cutting the elasticized material, sewing its edges, and using snaps or other fasteners for closures. Chain-link types require fastening one link to another to form the desired length and using the excess links to interlock for the fastener. Sashes are the simplest types of belts to produce because they do not require any buckle or formal closure, but only require sewing the edges.

Styles

Some of the styles that regularly serve traditional needs and others that often follow specific fashion trends include the following:

Cinch. Used to accentuate the waistline, generally made of an elasticized material and fitted with a buckle or snap closure.

Contour. A belt that is shaped to fit the contour or form of the figure.

Cummerbund. A wide fabric belt that resembles a sash. It is usually wide in the front and narrower in the back like the type used by men for evening wear.

Link. Chains or metallic pieces interlocked to form the belt. They are made expandable by constructing with elastic.

Rope. A corded model that is wrapped around the waist.

Sash. A fabric that is wrapped around the waist.

Self. Any style belt that is made of the same material as the garment it accessorizes.

Internet Resources for Additional Research

www.inventors.about.com/library/inventors/blshoe.htm traces the history of shoes, sandals, and sneakers.

www.lucire.com/2003a/0415110.shtml traces the history of the handbag.

www.historiccamdencounty.com/ccnews97.shtml provides information about the history of the beaded bag.

www.luggage-net.gb.com/luggage-sets.htm discusses buying luggage in sets.

Merchandise Information Terminology

Platform shoes
Broken sizes
Upper
Vamp
Tongue
Quarter
Sole
Insole
Midsole
Outsole
Bottoms
Last
Designer last
Dies
Fitting room
Doubling
Lasting
Goodyear welt
Mackay
Littleway
Cementing
Sock lining
Bal
Blucher
Brogue
Buckskins
Clog
Deck shoe
D'Orsay
Espadrille
Ghillie
Huarache
Loafer
Mary Jane
Moccasin
Mule
Oxford
Pump
Saddles
Sandal
Sling back
Slipper
Sneaker
Spectator
Thong
Wedgie
Western boot
Wingtip
Trees
Gussets
Die stamping
Box
Clutch
Drawstring
Envelope
Feedbag
Satchel
Shoulder bag
Tote
Softside luggage
Molded luggage
Cinch belt
Contour belt
Cummerbund
Link belt
Rope belt
Sash
Self belt

EXERCISES

1. Select a shoe that you are ready to discard and disassemble it into its various components. Mount each piece on a board and identify it with its technical name.
   Using the visual aid you have constructed, prepare a brief talk outlining the construction of the shoe and the purposes served by each of the components you are displaying.
2. Contact a major shoe manufacturer (their names are readily available in advertisements featuring their lines, and their headquarters are listed on the Internet) to request photographs of the styles they produce. In an oral or written presentation, accompany each picture with the types of apparel with which the shoe is worn.
3. From fashion periodicals such as *Elle*, *Vogue*, and *Harper's Bazaar*, clip photographs of handbags that are being featured for the season. Each photograph should be mounted on a display board and described in terms of its material and use.
4. Collect as many different belts as you can from your own collection and those of family and friends. Each one should be used in an oral report that describes its materials, ornamentation, and uses.

Review Questions

1. Discuss the role played by apparel designers in the manufacture of shoes.
2. Explain why shoe merchandising is more difficult than that of any other fashion product.
3. Which three major pieces comprise the formation of a shoe?
4. Define the term *designer last* and describe how it is generally developed.
5. Why must the last be transformed into a pattern before production can begin?
6. Where are the largest number of individual operations performed in shoe construction?
7. In what way does the Goodyear welt method of lasting differ from the Mackay technique?
8. How are heels fastened to the shoes to ensure strength?
9. Why is shoe rotation suggested to extend the life of the shoe?
10. Briefly describe the difference between the *bal* and the *blucher.*
11. Describe the appearance of the saddle shoe.
12. Which designer names in the 1970s helped bring new prominence to the handbag industry with their logos on the bags' exteriors?
13. Why are gussets used in handbag construction?
14. What is meant by the term *clutch* bag? How do some manufacturers augment the style and make them usable in another way?
15. What material is used in the cinch belt to make it conform to the waist?

CHAPTER 12

Jewelry and Watches

After reading this chapter, you should be able to:

- Discuss the various reasons why jewelry is worn.
- Trace the history of jewelry from ancient times to the present.
- Describe many of the processes used in the manufacture of jewelry.
- Explain the differences among the numerous settings used in precious stones and fashion jewelry.
- Discuss the history of watches and describe the types of timepieces used today.

When the crowned head of the British Empire presides over a royal festivity, her jeweled tiara helps set her apart from other participants. At a ceremonial rite, the Native American chieftain's squash blossom necklace, resplendent in silver and turquoise, often captures the attention of the observer. At fabulous European runway shows, inventive jewelry enhances innovative costumes.

From archeological excavations, we have learned that humans have favored jewels from as early as 20,000 B.C. Long before precious and semiprecious metals and stones were used in jewelry design and production, other materials such as shells, ivory, and wood were crafted into imaginative ornamentation.

Today, jewelry comes from every corner of the world in assortments that range from the rarest and costliest to the five-and-dime varieties. Companies like Tiffany and Cartier cater to the rich and famous with precious treasures that can cost hundreds of thousands of dollars. At the other end of the spectrum, second-hand shops are replete with large collections of baubles, bangles, and beads that suit every shopper's pocketbook and need.

Internationally renowned designers such as Karl Largerfeld, Donna Karan, and Ralph Lauren, who initially concentrated on apparel, ultimately entered the jewelry arena and created masterpieces that ingeniously augmented the costumes worn on the runway. Others such as Elsa Peretti and Paloma Picasso captured the attention of the fashion world with inventive jewelry designs that have remained popular over time.

In comparison with jewelry, watches are newcomers. The earliest varieties first appeared in the late 1700s (Figure 12.1). Although watches are certainly functional products, a look at the elaborate designs of many timepieces immediately reveals a fashion presence. With bejeweled entries that run as high as $100,000 or more, and Rolexes, Cartier's, and Patek Philippes that often cost more than $10,000, more than telling time is on the mind of the wearers.

At the other end of the scale, a reliable Timex can satisfy a functional need for as little as $30, and, for even less, counterfeits and copies of the upscale signatures can easily be purchased at fairs, flea markets, and swap shops. As with jewelry, the offerings are vast, the styles are varied, and the costs are at every price point.

JEWELRY

Many people think of jewelry as an enhancement that merely plays a subordinate, aesthetic role to fashion apparel. Although adornment is, in fact, the major purpose of jewelry, it is not

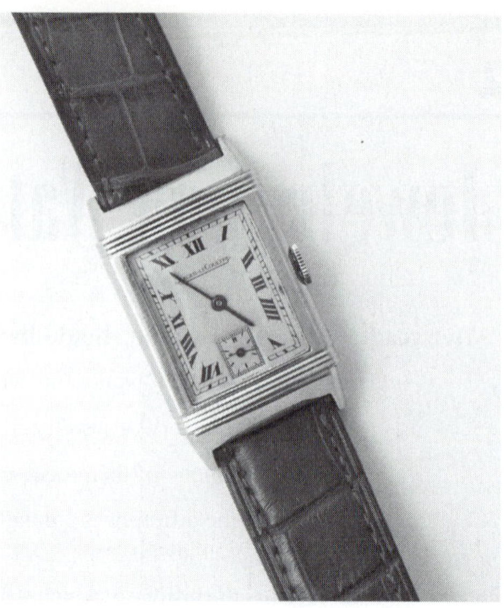

Figure 12.1 Functional timepieces were first produced in the late 1700s.
(Courtesy of Dorling Kindersley Media Library.)

its only purpose. The decorative belt buckle not only provides a fashion statement, but it serves a functional purpose. The ornate pin, while playing a fashion role, also serves as a fastener.

Jewelry has also served more sinister purposes. In medieval times, rings with hidden compartments served as vehicles in which deadly poisons were stored.

As symbolic gestures, various designs have had their places in history. In the mid-seventeenth century in England, funeral rings were worn to commemorate the deaths of the aristocracy. Today, antique shops sell these rings not for mourning purposes, but purely for their artistic nature.

No piece of jewelry has more symbolic meaning than the rings that identify betrothal and marriage. For generations, women have displayed their engagement rings with pride that defies comparison with any other accessory. The wedding ring, from the simplest band of gold to the most elaborate jewel-encrusted varieties, indicates membership in a select institution.

Even religion continues to play an important role in jewelry. The Star of David has been crafted in both realistic and stylized versions in materials that range from precious metals to plastic, wood, and stone. The cross remains a big seller and is often used as a fashion piece.

Pins have routinely identified people's affiliation with fraternal orders, rings have served to commemorate achievements such as graduation from educational institutions, and all kinds of ornamentation have been used for magical and mystical rites. Since the terrorist attacks in the United States on September 11, 2001, lapel pins of the American flag have become symbols of patriotism. From the average person to numerous political figures, the wearing of this "jewelry" has become commonplace.

Although jewelry plays an important role in denoting status, underscoring symbolic meaning, connoting magic, and providing utilitarian function, its use as ornamentation makes it one of the major components of the fashion industry (Figure 12.2).

A Historical Overview

Jewelry has had a meaningful presence in every culture since the beginning of time. From the most primitive designs that used nothing more than common materials to the intricately detailed intrinsic works that used precious metals and stones, jewelry has made its mark in every era.

In all parts of the world, archeologists have uncovered caches of precious rings, pendants, bracelets, and necklaces of gold and stones that were produced by techniques still in use today.

Some of the earliest finds came from Mesopotamia, a region between the borders of Syria and Iran. The Philadelphia Museum houses some of the treasures from that region that feature hammered gold and the semiprecious lapis lazuli stones. Museum shops all over the

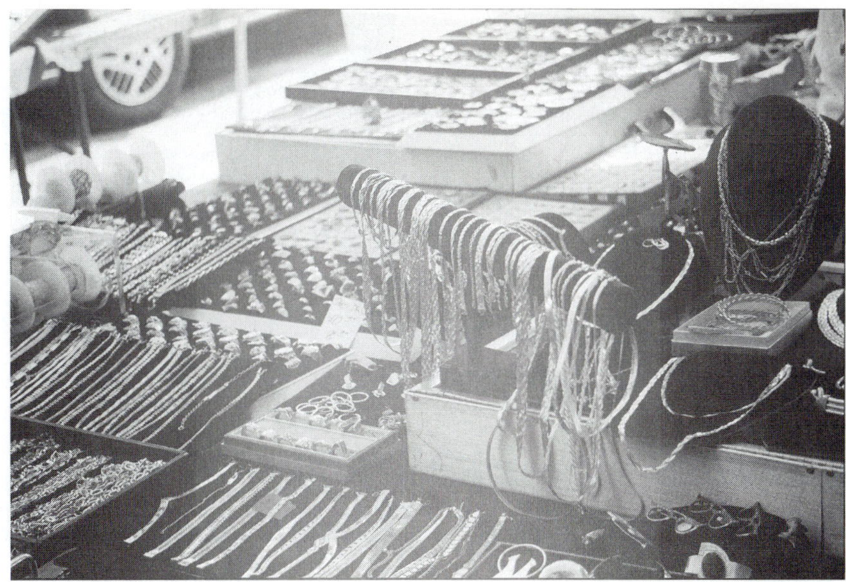

Figure 12.2 Jewelry represents one of the fashion industry's major components.
(Courtesy of Ellen Diamond.)

world feature reproductions of those models, and artists today still draw on these designs to create updated precious and costume versions. The people who inhabited the Mesopotamian region were called *Summarians*, and they produced jewelry in many styles. Most notable were leaf designs (Figure 12.3), abstract flowers, animals, and the symbols that were to become known as the signs of the zodiac.

At about the same time the Summarians were developing their designs (around 4,000 B.C.), Egypt was producing remarkable jewelry. Early metallic engravings and embossing were used in Egyptian designs as were a wealth of stones such as lapis, turquoise, and carnelian. The many gold mines of Egypt offered a wealth of precious metal in which the craftspeople could toil. The jewelry of ancient Egypt featured animal-headed gods and goddesses (Figure 12.4), the eye, the papyrus blossom, and the ankh.

In approximately 700 B.C. Greece, simple jewelry designs were introduced. The offerings were mainly gold or silver or a natural alloy of both precious metals known as electrum. The objects were mainly cast or made of woven chains. The most popular items of ancient

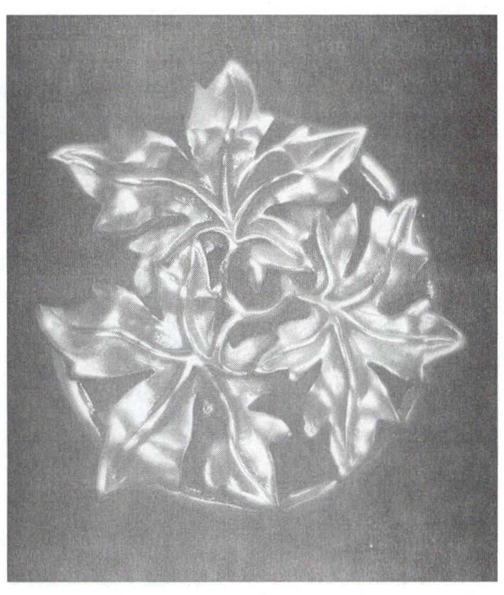

Figure 12.3 Leaf designs date back to the Mesopotamian era.
(Courtesy of Ellen Diamond.)

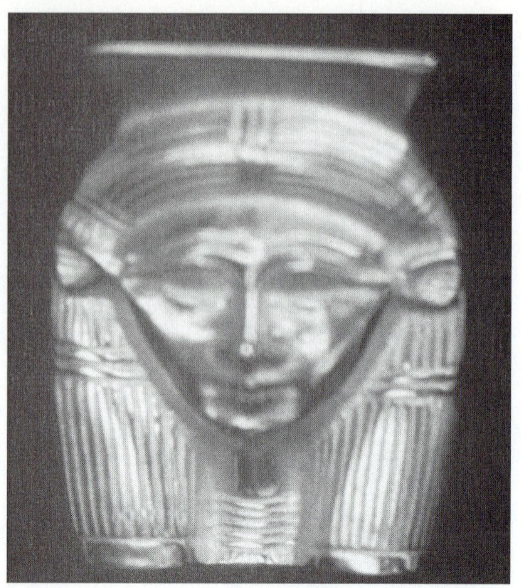

Figure 12.4 Egyptian goddess Hathor was this pin's inspiration.
(Courtesy of Ellen Diamond.)

Greece were earrings. The designs featured animal heads and human mythological figures (Figure 12.5). Later in the Greek era, pendants, pins, bracelets, and rings also came into prominence. In addition to the gold varieties, an enameling technique was developed that permitted color to bead to the jeweler's creation.

The Far East has contributed a great deal to modern-day jewelry. Although some of the treasures from that part of the world date back to 1,000 B.C., it was not until the seventh century that jewelry of that region made its mark. Initially, hair ornaments, rings, and bracelets were made by soldering and hammering. The great period of Chinese jewelry was created from A.D. 960 to 1,279. Hair ornaments remained the major adornments and were crafted from both gold and silver. The forte of the period was workmanship rather than valuable materials, although jade was prominent in many of the creations. Jade has remained the mainstay of Chinese jewelry.

Rounding out the Far East offerings were those that had their origins in India. Since the 1700s, enormous amounts of real and imitation stones have been the centerpieces of the designs. Superstition was often basis of these styles, which have not undergone changes since they first appeared. When metals were significantly involved, they were generally unpolished, leaving the impact of the pieces to the stones they encased. Aside from the traditional necklaces, bracelets, and other items, Indian jewelry concentrated on nose ornaments and toe rings, atypical of other cultures.

Beginning in the early A.D. 300s, European jewelry was centered in Byzantium, Turkey, a sophisticated urban center. High standards and expert workmanship were

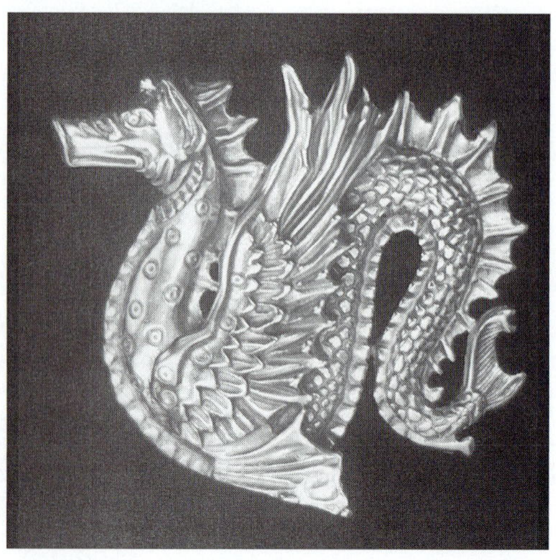

Figure 12.5 The Ketós design is based on a Greek mythological sea monster.
(Courtesy of Ellen Diamond.)

commonplace, with architectural design at the forefront of the styles. Tremendous pendants were held by intricately detailed chains, and colorful enameling played an important part in the creations.

Trade with the Far East during the thirteenth and fourteenth centuries provided Italian craftspeople from Genoa and Venice with materials that would be the basis for elaborate jewels. Gold, silver, and bronze were used to house fabulous diamonds, rubies, and sapphires in necklaces.

During the Renaissance period of the fifteenth and sixteenth centuries, elaborate versions of religious symbols were commonplace. Stylized crosses and other biblical symbols were evident in pendants. Base metals were replaced with gold and silver, and precious stones took a prominent place in jewelry design. The compositions of the time included vast numbers of pictorial subjects such as classical figures. Portraits of rulers and popes were painstakingly carved into intricate designs.

The lavishness of **Baroque jewelry** came into prominence in the seventeenth century. Grand, ornamental designs that reflected the art of the period were evident in jewelry. During this time, faceting was used to increase the brilliance of the stones, and diamonds overwhelmingly dominated the scene. The precious metals were now only used to encase the stones, and the larger the stones, the more important the pieces. Intricate design gave way to a preference for bigger and bigger stones.

The eighteenth century saw the introduction of the Rococo style in Europe that underplayed the lavishness of the Baroque signature. The designs were asymmetrically balanced in mostly pastel colors. Even though **Rococo jewelry** designs were lighter in feeling, they, too, were somewhat elaborate.

At the end of the nineteenth century, neoclassicism, with regard for simple designs of materials like steel, was a relief from the more ostentatious varieties that had come before it. It was the basis for much of the contemporary design we find in today's jewelry offerings.

During Victorian England in the nineteenth century, new technology led to a turn in jewelry production. Rather than using only precious metals, electroplating base metals with thin layers of gold and silver made jewelry an affordable item. Lockets and brooches were popular, and themes of hearts and clasped hands were symbolic of the time. It was a period when jewelry became available for the masses.

The twentieth century afforded wearers **art nouveau** and **art deco** designs. The former's themes were often concentrated on lilies, water, butterflies, peacocks, and women with long flowing hair. The latter avoided the subjects of nature that were evident in Art Noveau pieces in favor of geometric patterns.

No history of jewelry design would be complete without the study of native jewelry. In both Africa and America, native craftspeople made their marks with specific designs.

African jewelry was prominent in Europe in the eighteenth and nineteenth centuries as a result of trade. Gold was either cast or hammered and made into ornamental disks, masks, and human forms. Ivory played an important role in African design, where it was combined with brass and copper.

Native American jewelry, or Indian jewelry as it is commonly called, has a significant place in the industry. Each tribe contributes a specific style that represents its own culture. These include bangle bracelets, necklaces, earrings, brooches, rings, and belt buckles that combine metals with stones. Some of the more typical Native American designs are **squash blossoms** (Figure 12.6), which are necklaces of hollow silver beads embellished with turquoise, and **conchas,** oval silver pieces that are strung together for belts.

Most popular are the Navajo designs that emphasize heavy silver in symmetrical patterns; Zuni, a more delicate style using stones that are inlaid in metal; Hopi, which features a popular technique that joins two layers of metal and cuts a design in the top layer to expose the one beneath; and Santo Domingo, which primarily focuses on beadwork.

Each historical period has brought a distinct dimension to jewelry design. Today's industry draws from these various eras and either reproduces designs as they were originally created or translates the patterns into creations that fit today's lifestyles.

Knowledge of the history of jewelry enables the seller to present a more meaningful discussion on design and helps to make the potential purchaser a better prospect.

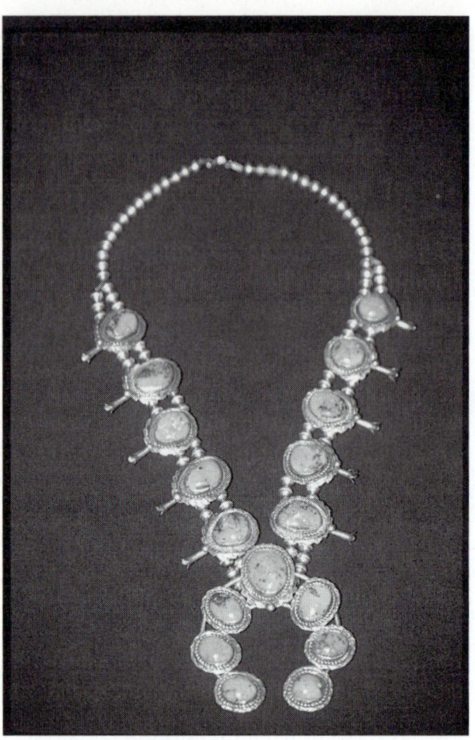

Figure 12.6 The squash blossom necklace features turquoise stones set in sterling silver.
(Courtesy of Ellen Diamond.)

Production Techniques

After the design has been conceived and sketched, it is ready to be transformed into a piece of jewelry. Through the ages, various techniques have been used to for this transformation, including hand crafting, die striking, and casting. Variations of these techniques come at the hands of knowledgeable craftspeople who use their own expertise and ingenuity to create both precious and **fashion** or **costume jewelry.**

Chapter 5, "Metals and Stones," explores the basic terminology related to these materials. Those techniques such as annealing, forging, embossing, and engraving are prominently used in the manipulation and formation of the materials to be used to form jewelry.

Some of the machine and hand production techniques include:

Fusing. By liquefying metal under intense heat, two pieces may be joined without the use of any adhering material. The carefully controlled temperature and amount of heat used contributes to the success of the fusing.

Soldering. The soldering process requires the use of a separate metal that has a lower melting point. The solder must be of the same color and strength of the two metals to be joined so that it will be undetectable on examination. The two pieces to be joined may be held in place by means of wire, steel pins, soldering blocks, or plaster, depending on the type of solder to be used and the size of the piece.

Drawing wire. Many types of jewelry use metals that have been drawn into wires so that they can be used to form different designs. The drawing involves the taking of heavy-gauge wire and reducing it to the desired thickness. The thicker wire is forced through a device called a *drawplate*, which has larger holes on one side and smaller on the other. The thick wire is forced through the wide opening and drawn with pressure until it leaves the other side with its reduced thickness.

Rolling metal. Through the use of a rolling mill, an ingot or heavy piece of metal is transformed into either sheets or wires of any desired thickness.

Metal bending. Metal is often bent by means of square-nosed pliers to achieve specific curves or angles. If the piece of metal is very wide, a machine called a *brake* is used to bend the sheet.

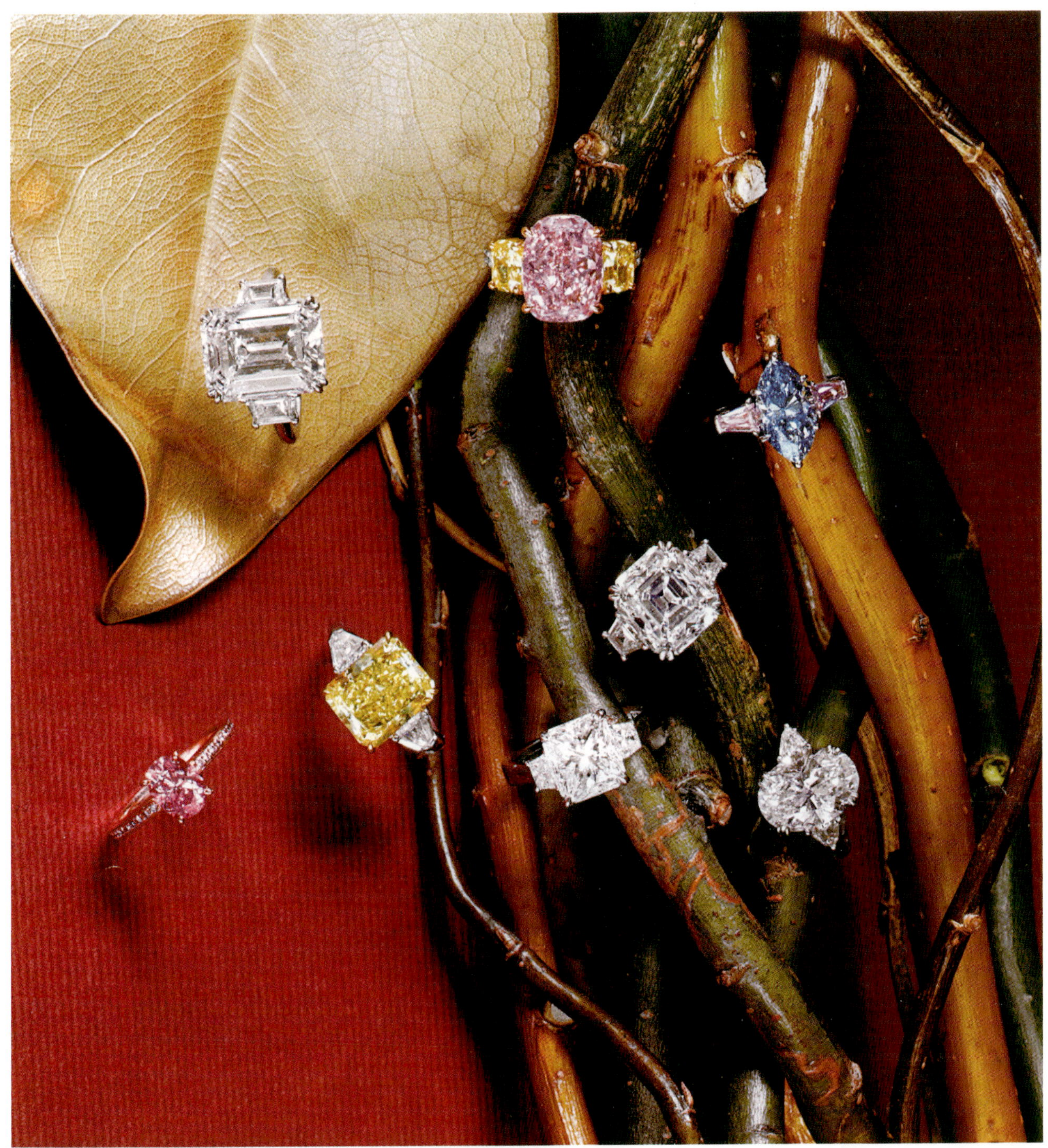

Colored diamonds are adding a new touch of glamour to the precious stone collections.
(Courtesy of Julius Klein Group.)

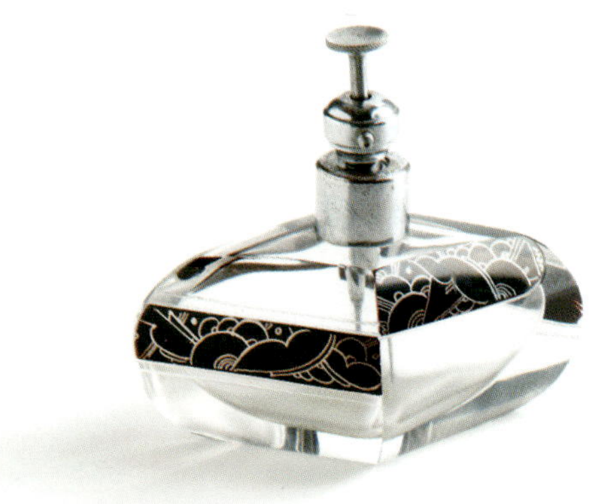

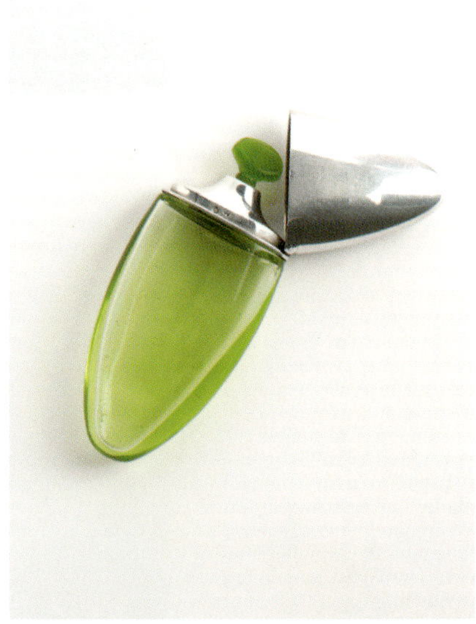

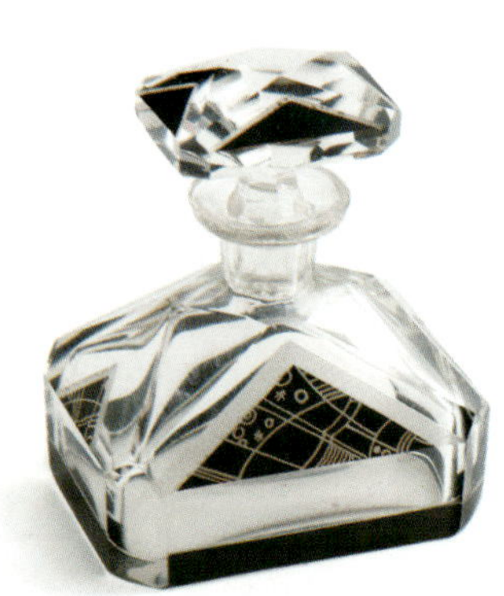

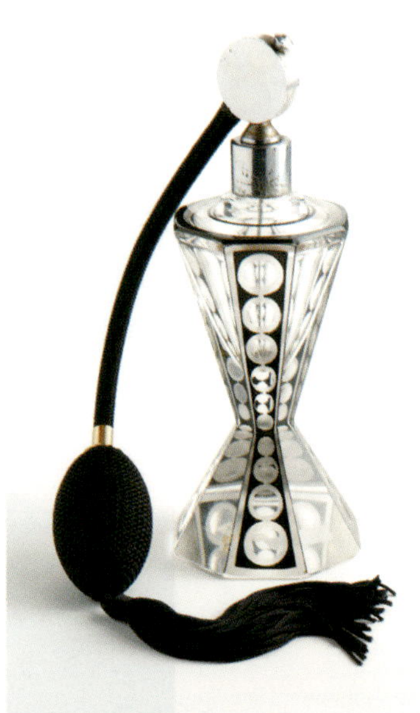

Vintage fragrance containers dramatically enhance boudoir settings.
(Courtesy of Dorling Kindersley Media Library.)

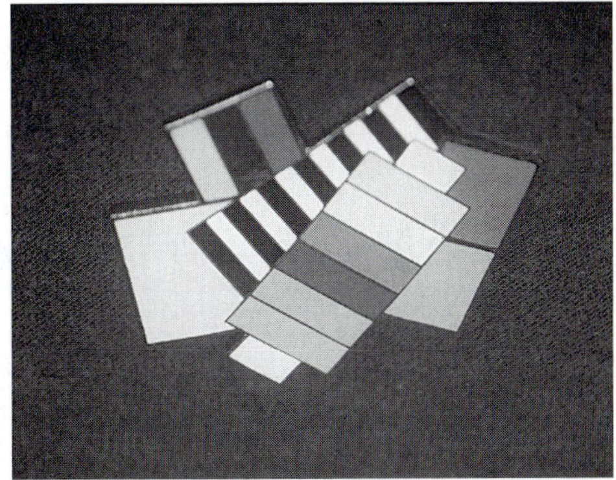

Figure 12.7 This enamel pin was produced by hand cutting.
(Courtesy of Ellen Diamond.)

Repousse. Metal can be formed by this important method. Unlike bending, which merely turns angles or curves, repousse consists of working a flat piece of metal with hammers into a hollow, three-dimensional shape.

Cutting. The cutting process may be achieved with shears that cut through the metal; sawing, when a precise cut must be made; drilling holes, when metal must be cut away; or carving, where the metal may be manipulated through the use of chisels.

Hammering. When a variety of textures is required, different types of hammers may be used to create the desired effect.

Die-striking. When a number of identical pieces must be produced, the metal is shaped with the use of a mold or form. They are placed between the dies and squeezed into shape by means of a hydraulic press at extreme pressures that sometimes reach twenty-five tons per square inch. This production technique results in extremely strong, high-quality settings that are used for rings.

Casting. This process involves making a cast or mold into which molten metals are forced. The mold is then immersed into cold water where it eventually breaks, leaving the newly cast metal in the desired shape. The piece is then cleaned and polished before it is used in the finished product.

Hand manufacturing. When unusual designs, limited numbers, or intricate designs are desired, hand manufacturing is used. It involves one or more procedures already described such as sawing, drawing, hammering, or soldering (Figure 12.7).

Stone Settings

Rings, pins, bracelets, and other jewelry often combine metals and stones. The setting used for a stone is dependent on the value of the stone, its security, and the ultimate price of the finished piece.

There are many different types of jewelry settings. Some of those most frequently used include the following:

The **Tiffany setting** (Figure 12.8) is typically used for stones that are to be prominently displayed without the intrusion of too much metal. It uses four or six **prongs,** or projections

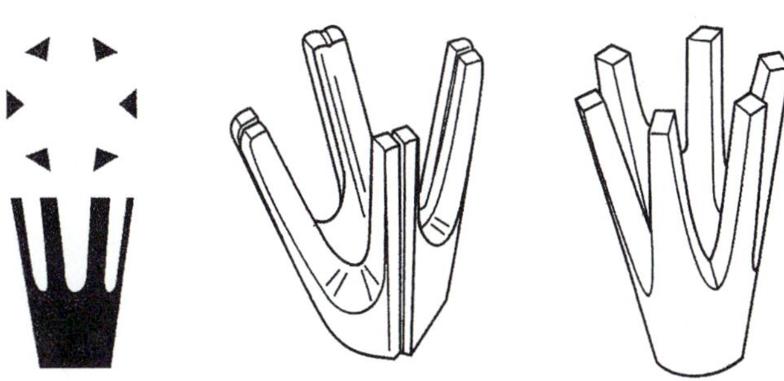

Figure 12.8 Two popular Tiffany settings.

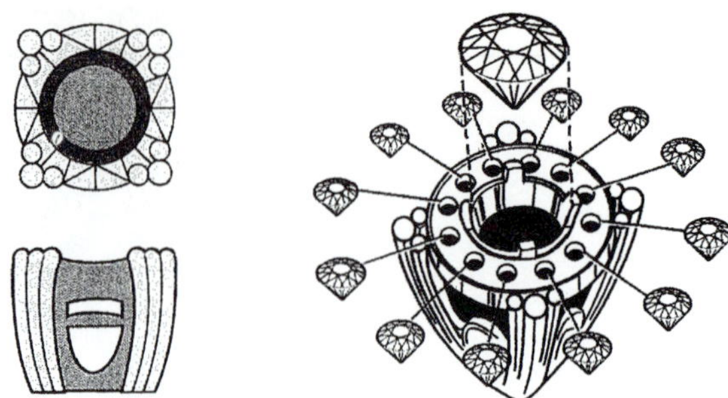

Figure 12.9 Illusion settings.

in V-shaped openings, that press against the stone and secure it in place. It is the most popular setting for diamond engagement rings.

The **buttercup head setting** also uses the prong configuration. It has six prongs that rise from a scalloped base and resemble a flower bud. These forms are generally used for pendants and earrings.

The **illusion head** is used to give the impression that the stone it holds is larger than its actual size (Figure 12.9). It uses a metal border that features a design or texture that surrounds the prongs. This patterned design creates the illusion of a larger stone.

When a number of tightly arranged stones are used to form a closed symmetrical pattern, a **cluster setting** is the choice (Figure 12.10). Generally, six stones are used to surround one in the center, which may be bigger than the others or the same size. For variation, two or more tiers of settings might be stacked one on the other to give the piece a more dramatic effect.

The **pave setting** has extensive blank areas that are tooled into little beadlike surfaces that surround a number of small stones. The area is literally paved with stones and, when featured in combination with the metallic beads, gives the surface a brilliant effect.

In the **channel setting,** the stones are lined up next to each other with no metal between them and set into grooves or channels.

The **bezel setting** holds a stone in place by a rim of metal that goes around its entire perimeter. It is sometimes called a *flush setting*.

In inexpensive rings and other jewelry ornaments, **paste settings** are routinely used. The stones, rather than being held in place by metallic prongs or other projections, are actually glued into the setting. The disadvantage of this type of setting is that the stones often become dislodged and fall out.

Jewelry Styles

Precious and fashion or costume jewelry comes in any number of styles. Each serves a functional or decorative purpose. The popularity of a given style at a particular time depends on the materials used in the manufacture, the dictates of the fashion world, and whether or not it is considered standard, traditional wear. Some jewelry is created expressly for either men or women, whereas some serves both.

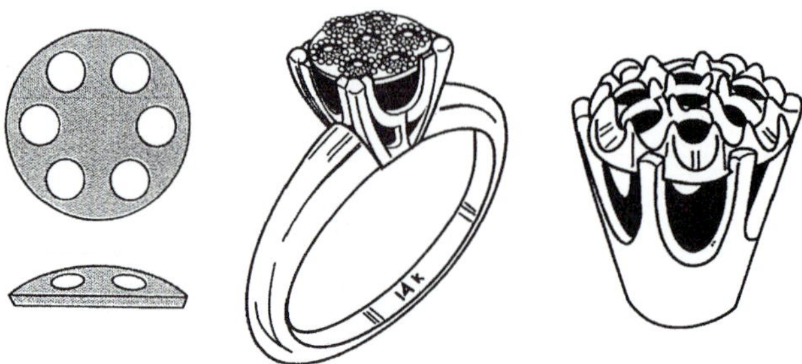

Figure 12.10 Cluster settings.

The following list represents various jewelry styles:

Rings. Bands that are worn on fingers, rings come in many materials and designs. They range from the traditional varieties that are of special significance, such as marriage, engagement, graduation, or signets that contain crests or initials, to the more decorative types such as dinner or cocktail rings that feature an assemblage of precious or semiprecious stones in dramatic arrangements. Often, when fashion is favorably focused on rings, several may be worn on the hand at one time.

Bracelets. Ornaments that encircle the arm or wrist come in **bangle** types, which clip over the hand and onto the wrist, or the flexible varieties, which are constructed of metal links or chain. Charms that offer special meaning to the wearer are sometimes added to the chain or link bracelets. To make the bangle bracelet an easier fit on the arm or wrist, hinges are added to the design. The most expensive bracelets feature diamonds and other precious stones. Contemporary designers generally use a variety of materials such as plastic, brass, wood, colored beads, or glass in bracelet designs.

Necklaces. Available in a number of different lengths and materials, they are worn as decorations around the neck. Traditional precious necklaces may be constructed of diamonds, rubies, emeralds, sapphires, pearls, gold, or silver. The costume or fashion varieties are available in semiprecious stones, metal alloys, beads, or other materials (Figure 12.11). The close-fitting type is the **choker,** which sits snugly atop the collarbone. It might be single or multistranded. Multistranded necklaces that hug the base of the neck are called **bibs.** Longer lengths are called **matinee necklaces** and range from twenty-two to twenty-four inches long, whereas even longer ones are called **opera lengths** and range from thirty to thirty-two inches. *Ropes* are necklaces that are as much as forty-five inches long and may be wrapped around the neck to give the impression of more than one necklace.

Brooches. Ornaments with pin backings are called **brooches.** They come in many sizes, styles, and materials. Typical variations include *lapel pins,* which are used as decorative ornamentation on suit lapels, and *stick pins,* which are usually elongated decorative types.

Earrings. The three major classifications of earrings are categorized according to the manner in which they are affixed to the ears. *Clip-ons* and *screwbacks* grip the ears, whereas the *pierced* variety uses posts that pass through the earlobe and are held in place by means of

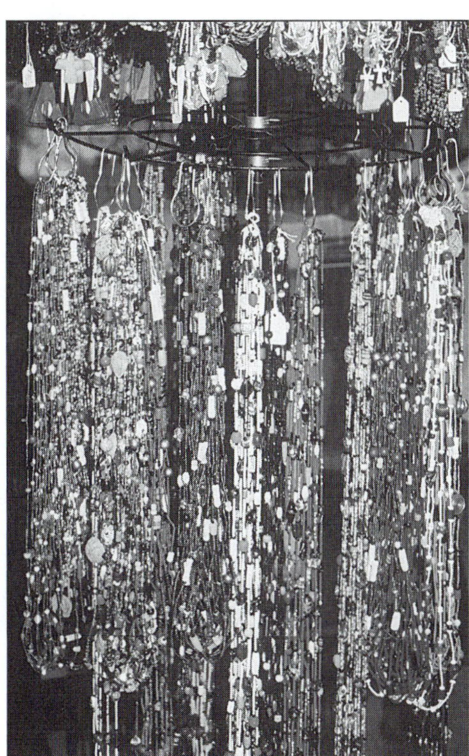

Figure 12.11 These fashion necklaces are strung with many types of beads.
(Courtesy of Ellen Diamond.)

small screws or "clamps." The designs range from the types that fit against the earlobes and are known as *button* or *ball earrings* to those that extend from the lobes and are called *drop earrings*. The latter design often features hoops in many different sizes or extra long styles that are called *chandeliers* because they sometimes resemble miniature, ornate lighting fixtures.

During the late 1980s, the popularity of earrings increased as more and more men began wearing them. Some chose one earring, while others opted for the pair.

Earring jackets. Some earrings are made with holes in their centers so that small studs may be inserted into them. These studs, called **earring jackets,** are often small diamonds or other precious and semiprecious stones that may be changed to suit different needs.

Barrettes. These hair ornaments have clasps into which hair may be secured. They can be used either alone to accent a ponytail hair design or in pairs when braids are worn.

Ankle bracelets. Sometimes called *slave bracelets*, they are usually thin chains that are worn on one ankle.

Charms. These pendants come in a variety of forms and are made of metals, often impregnated with stones and depicting a variety of images. They include animals, hearts, initials, and religious symbols. The charms are generally suspended from a bracelet.

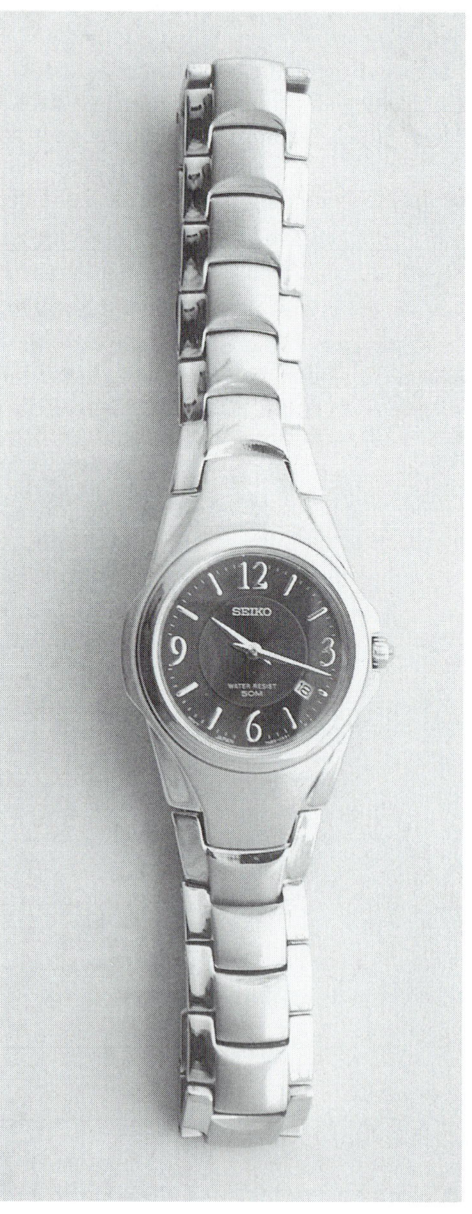

Figure 12.12 Basic watches make fashion statements when adorned with fancy metallic bands.
(Courtesy of Dorling Kindersley Media Library.)

Cuff links. Used with French cuffs, they are designed as cuff closures in place of buttons. The base of the shirt sleeve is produced with an opening through which links are passed and fastened.

Tie clips. These devices clip onto the tie and hold it in place. A variation is the *tie tack,* which is a small device with a post that passes through the shirt and tie and is held secure with a screw backing.

Tiara. This head ornament resembles a crown. It is usually jeweled and worn as an accent to a formal gown. The tiara is a version of the crowns worn by royalty.

Shirt studs. In place of the standard buttons that fasten the shirt's openings, formal shirts are usually designed with openings into which **shirt studs** are inserted. These closures come in a variety of materials such as black jet, jade, rhinestones, and other decorative elements. The appearance of the shirt may be quickly altered with a change of studs.

Watchbands. Serving both functional and decorative needs, watchbands come in many different styles and materials. For sportswear, the band might be made of leather, fabric, or steel links. Dressier watches often use precious and semiprecious stones as well as gold and silver in a wide range of designs (Figure 12.12).

Other jewelry types include *lockets,* which are often heart shaped and may be opened for the insertion of a loved one's photograph; *clasps*, which serve as decorative closings on bracelets and necklaces; *ornamental headbands; slides,* ornaments that are worn on chains that slide up or down adjusting the neck opening; and *hair sticks* that hold ornamental flowers in the hair.

WATCHES

Although we tend to think of watches as functional devices, examination of the many timepieces sold around the world indicates that decorative adornment is still as important as keeping time. One of the earliest watches that is still in existence was designed for the French Empress Josephine in the early 1800s. Although the watch kept time, its extravagant setting in 18-karat gold, enhanced with pearls and emeralds, gave the impression that its significance as a bracelet was greater than its functional ability.

A Historical Overview

Aside from the limited number of watches that were specially made for the aristocracy, watches did not achieve acceptance until the mid-1800s. During that time, Swiss companies began to produce timepieces that were initially designed for use by German naval officers in Berlin. In addition to satisfying the needs of this small group, some of the companies tried to market their watches for the general public. The immediate reaction was disinterest.

During the American colonial period, those who wore watches brought them from England. In the early 1800s, the importation of watches from England was restricted because of the Jefferson embargo. Luther Goddard was an American watchmaker who decided to use this opportunity to begin a watch business of his own. At the start, he produced large quantities of watches with success, but his business was ruined by the lifting of the importation ban. By 1830, English watches were flooding the American market.

During this time the first large-scale watch-producing American business was born. Originally known by a series of other names, eventually it was called the Waltham Watch Company, only to be renamed several more times. After numerous reorganizations and mergers, the American Watch Company was formed. A financier, Royal Robbins, invested a great deal of money in the company and directed its success. Robbins recognized the need for inexpensive watches to serve the military during the Civil War and was able to satisfy its needs. This, coupled with another round of high tariffs on European watches, gave the company the market it needed to maintain a successful business. In 1925, the company changed its name back to the Waltham Watch Company. The company ultimately produced 34 million watches in the United States before it closed its doors in 1957. Today, the name Waltham is still used, but only as a trade name on a Swiss watch.

Watch making is now a world-wide industry. At the high end of the scale are the masterpieces made by Swiss craftspeople. At the other end are poorly crafted imitations, available for a few dollars.

Types of Watches

Beginning with the earliest watches, which required keys to wind the mechanism, to today's quartz variety, which is void of a principal mainspring, the industry now produces several types of mechanisms. They are classified as mechanical, electronic, digital, and quartz.

MECHANICAL WATCHES

Although **mechanical watches** date back several hundred years, they have survived many new inventions of the watch industry. Inexpensive varieties use the pin-pallet technique, which involves metal rubbing against metal. These mechanisms are easily detectable by the loud noises or ticks they make. Although they are modestly priced, they generally lose their ability to keep accurate time after about a year. Their popularity has waned with the introduction of newer techniques that afford the wearer an inexpensive timepiece with better accuracy.

For precision, mechanical watches use **jeweled movements.** The most popular movements have seventeen jewels, although as few as seven jewels are used for less expensive watches and as many as twenty-four jewels are found in special timepieces. The mechanism involves the drilling of tiny holes into which jewels are inserted as friction points. The jewels originally used were rubies or sapphires. Today, most jewels used in watches are synthetics. The use of jeweled movements eliminated the noise associated with pin levers and produced watches that would serve the wearer many years.

The mechanical watches made in Switzerland are considered the world's finest. They are the ultimate timekeepers. Even when subjected to a great deal of physical strain and extreme temperature changes, their accuracy is rated at 99.98 percent, a level unachievable with any other mechanical instrument.

ELECTRONIC WATCHES

The mechanical watch was a successful product for watchmakers all over the world. As production reached enormous proportions in the 1950s, a renowned French watchmaker, Fred Lip, announced an invention to the industry that could seriously affect future production of mechanical watches.

In June 1953, at the behest of the British Horological Society, Mr. Lip was invited to deliver a lecture to the Royal Society of the Arts on his use of a tiny electronic power cell for watches. By 1956, an American organization, the Hamilton Watch Company, was the first to put **electronic watches** into production (Figure 12.13).

Instead of the mainspring barrel used in the mechanical watch, a power cell is used that can last for about a year. A variation of this design was introduced in 1960 that involved the

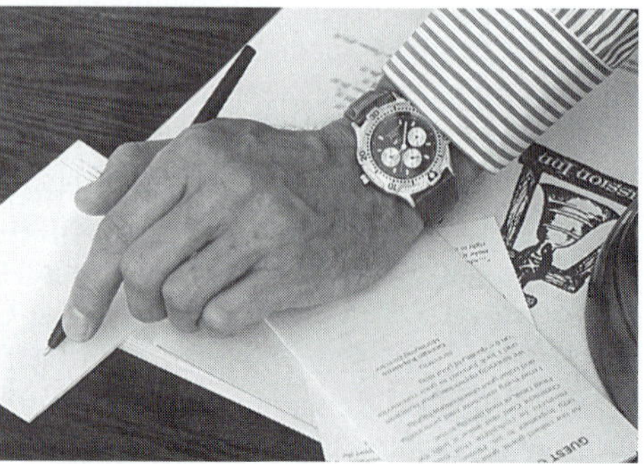

Figure 12.13 The electronic watch has become an industry mainstay.
(Courtesy of Ellen Diamond.)

use of a tuning fork that combined with an electronic circuit to produce an even more efficient timepiece. The Swiss were barely interested in the electronic devices, so Max Henzel, an electronics engineer who was determined to make this new invention a success, went to America to find a company that would be interested in this type of watch making. Bulova refined the new movement and called it the Accutron.

The advantage of the electronic watch is the elimination of the ticking sound, which is replaced with a mild hum, and its ability to keep better time than jeweled movements. In addition, because of fewer parts in its assemblage, it is easier to service.

DIGITAL WATCHES

Instead of the moving parts that are prevalent in the mechanical and electronic entries, a new development revolutionized the industry. By using solid-state components, except for the use of a button, the **digital watch** eliminates mechanical parts. Instead of hands that moved over the numbers of markings to indicate time, the digital watch displayed numbers that indicated the time in hours and minutes whenever the button was pushed.

Swiss manufacturers, fearful of losing their place in the industry, soon began to enter into contractual arrangements with American producers of solid-state components so that they could enter this new phase of technology.

In a matter of a few years, the digital watch industry boomed. For as little as $15, anyone could own a reliable timepiece. In 1982, Swatch entered the market with inexpensive, fashionable watches and quickly captured an enormous share of the industry (Figure 12.14).

QUARTZ WATCHES

With the major changes in technology, the Swiss decided to move full speed ahead in this new era of watch production. These watchmakers established a number of organizations, the main one being Centre Electronique Horloger, known as CEH, to produce a **quartz wristwatch.** At this point, a quartz clock had been popularly produced, but it had to be made smaller for use in wristwatches. In 1967, CEH produced a miniature version of the quartz clock, the quartz wristwatch. It capability as a timepiece was amazing as its accuracy was ten times greater than that of conventional watches (Figure 12.15). Although the Swiss thought they had exclusively captured the quartz market, the Japanese were busy perfecting their own quartz entry. The first company to produce the new watches was Seiko, which marketed its wares all over the world.

The use of quartz crystals enables manufacturers to produce watches that are extremely thin and attractive and keep time that is accurate to two or three minutes a year.

The Japanese quickly rose to the forefront in watch production. With their image of high-quality cameras already gaining worldwide acceptance, the task to foster themselves as quality watchmakers was simple. After a few years, the Swiss caught their breath and also became a major player in the quartz industry. American companies didn't quite market their crop of these watches properly. They believed that with each new advance in technology, people would abandon their old watches for a new model. Unlike other products that lose their popularity when new ones come along, watch wearers expect a great deal of long-term

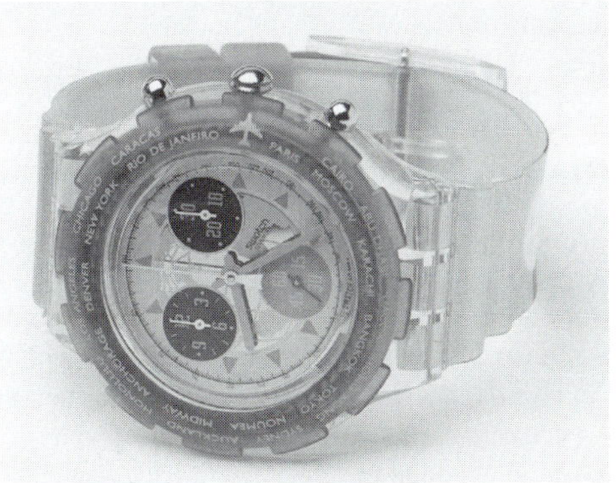

Figure 12.14 The Swatch entered the watch market with inexpensive watches, such as this style. *(Courtesy of Dorling Kindersley Media Library, Andy Crawford.)*

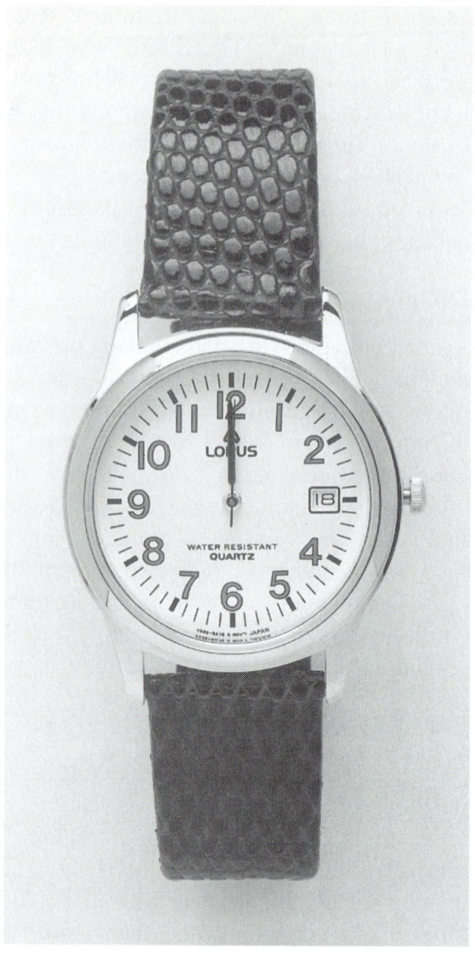

Figure 12.15 The quartz watch has proven to have outstanding accuracy.
(Courtesy of Dorling Kindersley Media Library.)

wear from their timepieces. This marketing miscalculation discouraged them from producing top-quality watches and caused them to lose as a major player in quartz watch production.

Micro circuitry has expanded the watch into a product that keeps more than just time. While the display of days and dates are commonplace in these timepieces, many now act as minicomputers, storing and retrieving such information as telephone numbers, birthdays, and other useful information.

Internet Resources for Additional Research

www.gia.edu/ features a wide range of topics from the world's foremost authority in gemology.
www.gem.org.au/gemmologist.htm explores the role of the gemologist.
www.love-watches.com/History-Watches-Clocks.htm features every important development in the history of watches and clocks.

Merchandise Information Terminology

Baroque jewelry
Rococo jewelry
Art nouveau
Art deco
Squash blossoms
Conchas
Fashion/costume jewelry
Fusing
Soldering
Drawing wire
Rolling metal
Metal bending
Repousse
Cutting
Hammering
Die-striking
Casting
Hand manufacturing
Tiffany setting
Prongs
Buttercup head setting

Illusion head
Cluster setting
Pave setting
Channel setting
Bezel setting
Paste settings
Bangle
Choker
Bibs
Matinee necklaces
Opera-length necklaces
Brooches
Earring jackets
Shirt studs
Mechanical watches
Jewel movements
Electronic watches
Digital watches
Quartz watches

EXERCISES

1. Draw the outline of the upper torso of a female human form and sketch and identify the various lengths of necklaces that may be worn by this figure.
2. Collect four newspaper or magazine advertisements that feature different types of watches. Mount each on a board and describe its features and benefits to the consumer.

Review Questions

1. How long ago did people use jewelry as part of their dress?
2. Does jewelry serve any purpose other than use as an adornment? Explain.
3. Discuss some of the symbolic purposes served by jewelry.
4. Describe the types of jewelry that were discovered in the Mesopotamian region between Syria and Iran.
5. What were the designs of the jewels made in 700 B.C. Greece?
6. In addition to gold and silver, what major precious ingredient is found in Chinese jewelry?
7. Describe the type of jewelry that was popular during the Renaissance period of the fifteenth and sixteenth centuries.
8. Differentiate between *Baroque* and *Rococo* style jewels.
9. During what period was the locket considered an important piece of jewelry?
10. Describe the styles and types of Native American jewelry.
11. Distinguish between soldering and fusing of materials.
12. In what manner do jewelers make thick wires into thinner gauges?
13. Discuss the casting technique used in jewelry production.
14. Describe the Tiffany settings used to hold stones.
15. When do jewelers use paste settings?
16. How do matinee-length necklaces differ from opera-length?
17. What is an earring jacket?
18. When did watches achieve acceptance for purposes other than military use?
19. What is meant by the term *seventeen-jewel movement*?
20. Describe some of the capabilities of quartz watches other than displaying time.

CHAPTER 13

Gloves, Hats, Hosiery, Scarves, Umbrellas, and Eyewear

After reading this chapter, you should be able to:

- Describe the various types of gloves available to consumers.
- List and explain the stages of construction in the manufacture of gloves.
- Recognize and describe various types of hats that have been fashion favorites.
- Explain how hosiery is constructed.
- Discuss how apparel designers made an impact on the scarf industry.
- Differentiate among the various types of umbrella construction.
- Discuss sunglasses as a fashion item.

A man, woman, or child bundled up in the cold might be seen wearing gloves, hats, hosiery, and scarves that immediately imply function over fashion. Although that certainly may be the case, it is not the only reason for such wearable accessories. A look at the fashion world's runways reveal exciting millinery that was created with the same passion as the clothes being shown. In particular, French couturiers have always designed "chapeaus" that brought excitement to these events. Hosiery, too, need not be lackluster. The once practical hosiery, although still dominant in the industry, has been joined by designs that are intricately detailed. A glimpse at the price points of this leg wear will readily show that these are not merely minor enhancements, but items that have been crafted with fashion in mind. The Hermes **signature scarf,** with its price tag of several hundred dollars, carries as much fashion status as a designer dress.

No longer relegated to the hidden corners of retail emporiums, these accessories are visually merchandised front and forward, and are bringing significant profits to their creators and merchandisers.

The roster of designers who, on their own or through licensing agreements, affix their labels to these tidbits of fashion continues to grow. Today, the signature scarf collections bear such designer names such as Ralph Lauren and Yves Saint Laurent. The outrageous hosiery designs of Emilio Cavallini have gained recognition throughout the world and have placed the product in a class with other creative accessories.

Of course, one need not spend extravagantly to enjoy the pleasures of these items. Gloves, hats, hosiery, and scarves are available at prices to fit everyone's pocketbook. Although they might not carry the prestige afforded by the upscale variety, the assortments are varied and fashion worthy.

GLOVES

A look at historical fashion indicates that gloves were important accessories for men and women of the royal courts, beginning with the sixteenth century. In the 1800s, women of the Victorian era chose an assortment of gloves for all occasions. A look back to the 1920s and 1930s shows an increase in the use of the product, and its popularity increased to the

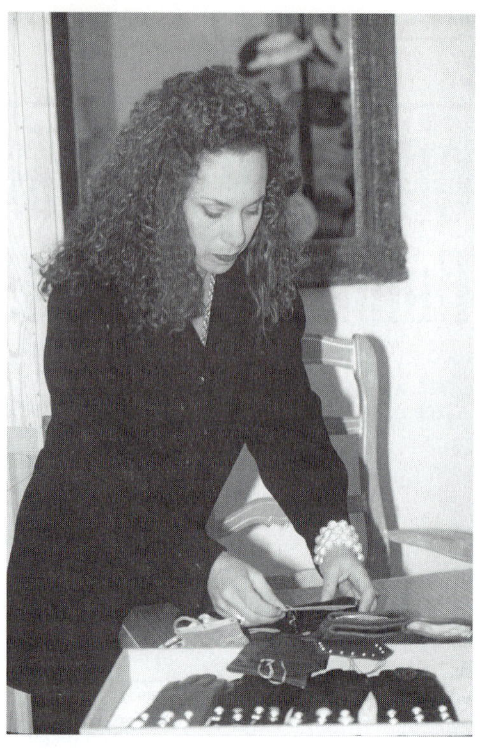

Figure 13.1 Today's glove designers consider fashion in addition to function when creating new styles. *(Courtesy of Ellen Diamond.)*

mid-1970s. At that point, the glove was no longer considered the obligatory companion of apparel, and women, except on the cooler days, shed them.

During the 1980s, the glove industry once again took a somewhat prominent place in the fashion world. Intricately knitted and crocheted designs joined the ranks of the leathers. To give the market a boost, many apparel designers affixed their signatures to glove collections (Figure 13.1).

Component Parts of the Glove

The number of individual parts used in the construction of gloves range from one—for those that are knitted—to four, for leathers or woven materials (Figure 13.2). In the case of the knitted type, the entire glove consists of one piece, made either by hand or machine.

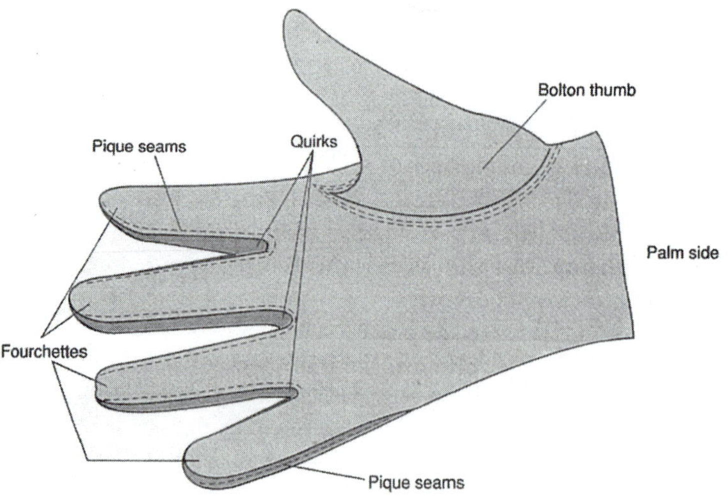

Figure 13.2 This diagram shows the component parts of a glove.

The purpose of the four-piece construction is that it allows for comfort and proper fit. Knits are inherently comfortable because they stretch and easily conform to the wearer's hands.

The **trank** is the rectangular silhouette or shape that constitutes the front and back portions of the glove. To provide room for the fingers, narrow oblong pieces known as **fourchettes** are cut. These inserts may be made of the same material as the trank or different material to provide interest to the design and comfort to the wearer. Sporty gloves sometimes use knitted fourchettes as inserts. To give extra freedom of movement for the fingers, small triangular sections known as **quirks** are inserted. The quirks are made of the same material as the trank. The final part is the thumb. Basically, two types of thumbs are used in glove construction. The **Bolton thumb** bulky and provides freedom of movement for the wearer. Men's dress and sport gloves usually use this thumb, as do ladies' casual gloves. The **quirk thumb** is actually a two-piece component. It allows for a snugger fit and is generally the chosen style for women's dressy gloves.

An additional part is the lining. Some gloves are unlined, as in the case of many knits, whereas others use a wide range of materials. Fur or wool may be the material of choice when warmth is the concern; silk or rayon may be used for sleek, dressier gloves. Linings may be of the **skeleton** type where only the trank is covered, or full where the entire glove is lined.

Glove Construction

In the case of leather glove making, the initial operation involves **taxing.** This is the examination and marking of the skins to determine how many pairs may be cut. The best leather gloves come from skins that have been dampened and stretched to ensure proper fit. Once this has been determined, the cutter is ready to produce the trank. In better-quality gloves, the procedure used is called **table cutting.** This means the craftsperson dampens the leather, pulls it over the edge of the table, and determines the correct shape before cutting the trank by hand. The skill of the cutter ensures that the cut will provide maximum flexibility for the wearer. In less expensive leather glove construction, **pull-down cutting** is used instead of table cutting. This procedure does not use hand cutting or careful manipulation of each piece of leather. It involves the use of a die or outline to form the trank, cookie-cutter style. Once the tranks have been cut, they are piled, one on top of the other, so that the fingers may be slit and thumb holes cut by steel dies.

Assembling the various parts may be accomplished using a number of different seaming techniques. The method selected depends on the cost of the finished product and the desired appearance.

The least expensive seam used in glove construction is called the **inseam.** In this operation, the seams are sewn together on the inside of the glove and then turned inside out. There is no visible seaming when this operation is used. The opposite technique to inseaming is the **outseam.** In this construction, the stitching is done along the edges of the material, exposing the seaming and the raw edges of the glove. In the case of **overseam** assemblage, the raw edges of the materials are seen, with the stitches lapping over them. The effect is used for more casual gloves. When sleek fit and comfort are required, **pique seaming** is the choice. It is the costliest of the sewing methods. It involves the use of a special machine that sews one edge of material over the other, both on the front and back, thus exposing only one raw edge. A variation of this method is known as **half-pique.** In gloves constructed by using this technique, only the seams on the back are overlapped, the remaining ones using the inseam or outseam closure.

In some glove construction, a final step called **pointing,** which involves the application of stitching on the back of the glove. After all of these pieces have been assembled, the gloves are placed on forms and pressed before shipment to the retailers.

Woven fabric gloves use the same stages of construction as leathers, except it is not necessary to table cut them because the fabrics are uniform in terms of appearance and quality.

Knitted gloves require little assembling, because the entire product is constructed of one piece. The only sewing needed is to close the tips of the fingers.

Glove Lengths

Women's gloves come in a variety of lengths ranging from the shortest, which ends just at the wrist, to the longest, which covers most of the arm (Figure 13.3). The lengths are measured in **buttons,** with each button measurement accounting for one inch, starting at the base of the thumb. One-button gloves are the shortest and reach to the wrist, two buttons cover the wrist, four buttons end somewhere between the end of the wrist and the middle of the arm, eight buttons end at the middle of the arm, twelve buttons end at the elbow, and sixteen buttons reach almost to the shoulder.

Glove Sizes

The specific size ranges of gloves depend initially on the materials used. For those that are knitted, manufacturers need not be concerned with the demands of precise fit. Even in the case of woven fabrics, a certain degree of elasticity eliminates careful sizing.

Men's knitted and woven fabric models usually come in S, M, L, and XL. Women's glove sizes are even more restricted with the majority of knits often as one size fits all. The wovens that have a little less flexibility might be produced in the S, M, L range and A for smaller hands and B for larger. Children's sizes are also determined based on the stretch factor.

In the case of leather, sleek fit necessitates a more exacting size range. For men, the standard sizes measure from 7 to 10, with women's sizes available from $5^1/_2$ to 8. Today, the growing number of large and tall-size merchants may stock gloves that exceed the normal run of sizes. Children's glove sizes use age as a factor, as do children's apparel products. The formula for size is half the age of the child. The four-year-old, for example, would wear a size 2, whereas the one-year-old would require a zero. The range runs from 0 through 7.

Styles

There are only a few basic glove styles. The visual differentiation comes from the materials and decorative trims that are used.

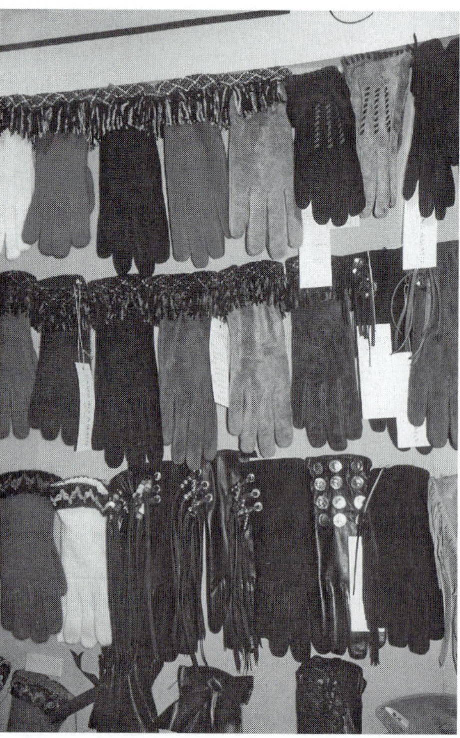

Figure 13.3 Gloves are available in a variety of lengths.
(Courtesy of Ellen Diamond.)

Mitten. The body of this glove separates only the thumb from the rest of the fingers. It is made of many materials and comes in lined and unlined versions. Mittens are particularly easy for children to wear because they require only the thumb to be inserted separately.

Shorty. This two-button glove reaches the wearer's wrist. In leather or woven fabric models, there is generally a side or center opening for easier use. In knitted models, the natural stretch of the yarns eliminates the need for the wrist opening.

Driving glove. Copied from gloves worn by race car drivers, this design has small ventilating holes that provide comfort and additional flexibility for the wearer. They are generally made of soft leather, suede, or fabric, sometimes with knitted palms that allow for a secure grip of the automobile steering wheel.

Gauntlet. The glove has a triangular insert, starting at the wrist.

Mousquetaire. This longer-length glove, used for evening wear, ranges from eight to sixteen buttons. Characteristic of this design is a vertical opening above the wrist that enables the wearer to slip her fingers in and out of the glove without complete removal.

Slip-on. A glove that ends at the wrist or slightly higher on the arm that does not have any fasteners or slit openings.

Care of Gloves

The manner in which one cares for gloves will extend both appearance and function. The type of care, of course, depends on the materials used and the method of construction.

First, when gloves are placed on the hands and ultimately removed, it must be done with care. Tugging on a glove will often stretch it out of shape. The hands must be gently inserted into the gloves and also gently taken out. Gloves, especially leather and vinyl types, should be completely aired after each wearing.

Many of today's glove manufacturers use combinations of man-made fibers in knitted constructions that simplify their care. They are often machine washable and retain their shape no matter how little attention is paid to care. Children's gloves, often mistreated, are produced of these fibers so that they can be laundered many times without the need for special attention.

At the other end of the spectrum are leather gloves. Some require professional dry cleaning, whereas others may be laundered by the consumer. The care label lists how the product should be cleaned. For the washable variety, those made of smooth leather are best laundered while on the hand. A solution of mild, soapy water should be used; when clean, the gloves should be rinsed, removed from the hand, and patted dry on a towel, which will absorb the moisture. Bulkier, hand-washable leathers are generally washed off the hand and finished in the same manner as the smooth variety. To guarantee suppleness, the leather, once dried, should be gently massaged. Some manufacturers recommend that, after washing, the gloves should be placed on plastic forms for drying so that the original shape will be maintained.

Woven fabric varieties usually follow the same procedures as leathers.

HATS

When the film industry chooses ancient Egypt or Rome as its setting for a movie, we are treated to a wealth of millinery that leaders of those periods wore as part of their costumes. Throughout history, most eras demanded that the hat be part of their appropriate dress. One would hardly attend the opening day at the races at Ascot in Great Britain without the benefit of a "timely chapeau."

Although the hat industry has had its ups and downs since the turn of the twentieth century, there were times when millinery was considered a most important part of the fashion industry. In Paris, where haute couture has always reigned, the early decades of the 1900s housed hundreds of milliners. Each performed his or her craft with the same painstaking care

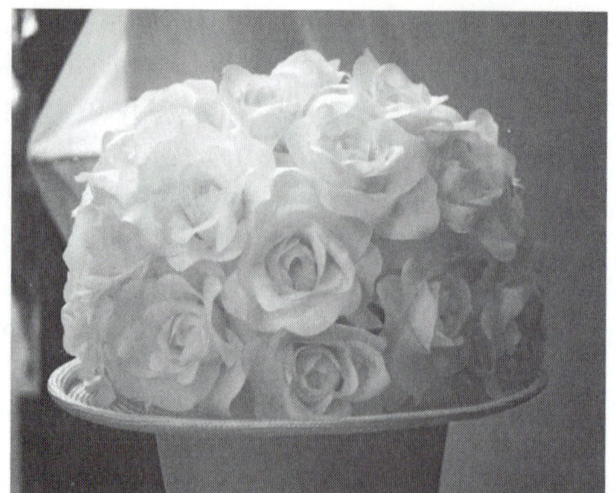

Figure 13.4 The high-fashion hat is still produced for special occasions.
(Courtesy of Ellen Diamond.)

as the creators of custom apparel. Today, with hats nearly as visible as in those golden years, Paris still boasts more than fifty milliners creating original masterpieces that sell for as much as $750 (Figure 13.4).

Hats in the American scene, much like those in France, have also been placed in a lesser role than they once enjoyed. Beginning with the mid-1900s, hats were relegated to few wearers. Men who once had a selection of felt hats in their wardrobes to complement their business attire went hatless. Women, who amassed millinery wardrobes to suit different occasions and needs, also joined their male counterparts and opted to show their coiffures rather than cover them.

Except for the obligatory requirements of religious rites and ceremonies, weddings, funerals, and special situations or when the winds of mother nature warned one to cover up, the hat was dead!

Those hat manufacturers who held on and remained in business are either producing special-occasion millinery or head warmers for women and felt hats for business attire, caps for sportswear, and knitted models for warmth for men. Although it is not typical in menswear, some young executives opted to wear hats as part of their outdoor ensembles.

What has continued to play an important role in headgear is the baseball cap. Today, the vast majority of America's youth has a collection of them that feature college and professional teams as well as the names of cities and states and a wealth of different logos. In addition to the ever-growing departments in sporting goods stores, catalogs, and Web sites, special stores and kiosks such as Lids are in most major malls and airports to serve the needs of the youth population.

One never knows whether or not the popularity of hats will return as a major fashion accessory. Those who are in the business of fashion must be ready for their return and understand their construction and different styles that might again be in vogue.

Hat Construction

The construction of any hat is based on the price of the finished product, the materials used for the body, the decorative trims, and the ultimate appearance.

Inexpensive hats are primarily machine made, whereas the finer, costlier ones require several hand operations.

Before any production can take place, the designer sketches a style, either by hand or with the use of a CAD system, and translates it into a sample. Each design is made up of the body of the hat and the ornamentation with which it is enhanced.

After the model has been evaluated, it is ready for production. Hats that command prices in the $750 range are often one-of-a-kind pieces, which are expressly made for private customers and are totally hand crafted.

Felt hats, the mainstay for men and available in many women's styles, are made by shaping the fabric over **cones.** After repeated steaming under pressure, the body of the hat, known as the **crown,** and the **brim** are formed. After additional steaming and ironing, the brim is ready to be trimmed to the desired width. For inexpensive models, wool or man-made felts are used, whereas the most expensive varieties use fur felt.

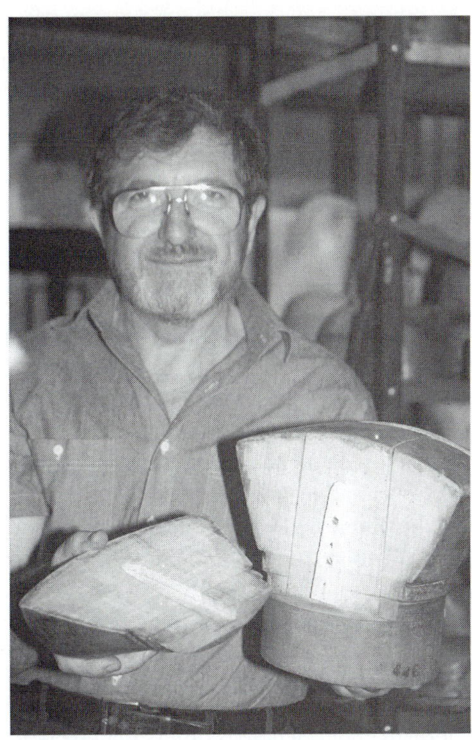

Figure 13.5 Some hats are shaped on wooden form "blocks."
(Courtesy of Ellen Diamond.)

Straw is another industry standard for both men's and women's styles. Some straws are made of woven mats that are shaped on wooden forms called **blocks** (Figure 13.5). Each block is constructed to resemble a particular style. The straw material is then steamed on the block until it takes the shape and form. After it has dried, the item might be fortified with a stiffened material **buckram,** which helps the hat retain its shape.

Another method of straw construction involves sewing narrow strips of straw, one overlapping the other, until the appropriate shape is achieved (Figure 13.6). This method is known as **plaiting** and is accomplished by machine. The plaited material is then shaped on a block and stiffened for shape retention.

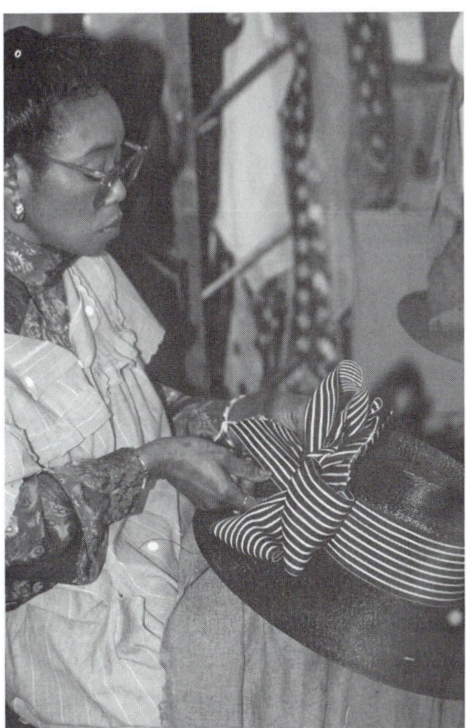

Figure 13.6 A straw hat is trimmed with ribbon for a fashionable look.
(Courtesy of Ellen Diamond.)

Other materials and styles require different construction techniques. In the case of soft fabrics such as velvets or velours, used when an unstructured model is desired, the procedure is much like that used in making a garment. The operator cuts the material to the desired size and shape, drapes it, and sews it into a "soft" style.

Knitting and crocheting are also used for hat construction and may be produced by hand or machine.

Hat Sizes

Men's hat sizes increase in 1/8-inch intervals and range in size from $6^3/_4$ to $7^3/_4$. When less-structured models are produced, such as caps and berets, they are usually available in S, M, L, and XL. The baseball cap generally comes in one size with a band across the back that may be adjusted to fit any head size.

Women's hats are generally offered in a range from $21^1/_2$ to $23\ ^1/_2$. Many also come in the S, M, and L range, especially when the styles are less fitted.

Younger children's models usually coincide with their ages. Infant wear sizes range from newborn to 2. Older children's versions are generally produced in S, M, and L.

Styles

Many different hat models have been in fashion at one time or another. Some are exclusively for one gender, whereas others may be worn by either sex. The following is representative of the available styles:

Baseball cap. A rounded, fitted cap constructed of several *gores*, or triangular inserts and finished with a peak in at the front. Those with five or more stitched rows on the peak are considered of better quality. They are available in colors that are indicative of specific professional or collegiate teams. Variations of the baseball cap are produced in suede. The one-size-fits-all style features an adjustable band in the back.

Beanie. A brimless model made of triangular gores and typically worn for college initiations or "pledging" purposes.

Beret. A soft, unstructured style was made popular by the French. It is worn by men, women, and children and comes in a variety of materials.

Cowboy. A felt hat that is the standard for western ranch hands. It has a high crown and broad brim and is sometimes called a *ten-gallon hat* (Figure 13.7).

Sherlock Holmes. The crown is need of gores, with the front and back replete with peaked, stiffened brims. The most common are made of tweed woolens. The name comes from a fictional British detective frequently depicted wearing the style, also called a *deerstalker cap.*

Derby. A stiff felt hat that has a rounded crown and narrow rolled brim. It is sometimes called a *bowler*.

Fedora. A soft felt hat with a creased crown. It is also called a *Homburg*.

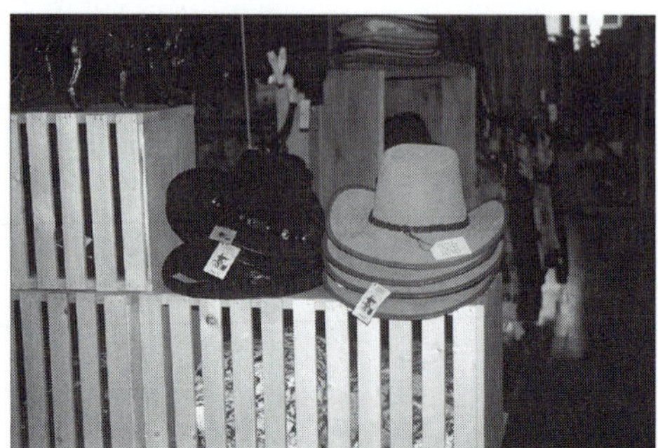

Figure 13.7 Cowboy hats are worn to complete western ensembles.
(Courtesy of Ellen Diamond.)

Panama. A straw hat with a high crown and center crease. It uses the finest straw that has been created through plaiting.

Bonnet. A brimmed hat with a ribbon that ties under the chin.

Cloche. A high-crown, close-fitting hat with a narrow brim.

Gaucho. A flat-crowned felt hat that usually has a rolled, wide brim. A cord, originating from inside the crown, fastens under the chin.

Alpine. Man's soft felt hat with a brim that is turned up on one side. It is also called a *Tyrolean*.

Turban. A soft constructed headpiece that is made of draped fabric that fits around the head.

Top hat. A formal man's hat, usually made of silk, that has a very tall crown and rolled brim.

Tam O'Shanter. A Scottish hat with a round, flat top that is finished with a tassel at the top.

Breton. A woman's hat with a small evenly rolled brim.

Cartwheel. A woman's hat that is large and has a wide, circular brim.

Sailor. A low-crowned hat with a stiff brim.

Nehru. A soft, brimless hat with a creased crown.

Garden party. Wide-brimmed, floppy straw hat embellished with ribbons and flowers.

Ski cap. A knitted hat that usually has a wide, turned-back cuff and is adorned with a pompom on the top.

Picture. A large hat with a floppy brim that frames the face.

Slouch. A soft hat with a center crease and a brim that is turned down. It is often shown as a water-repellent rain hat.

Toque. A woman's small, brimless hat (Figure 13.8).

Hood. A head covering that is usually attached to a coat or jacket and is made of a piece of cloth.

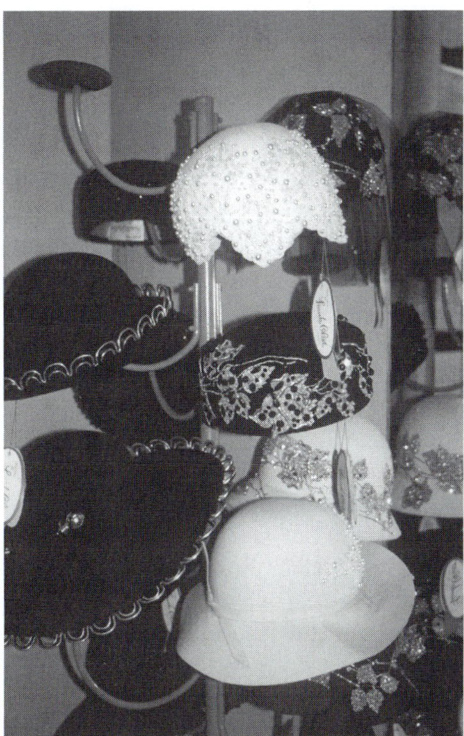

Figure 13.8 Hats of different styles complement fashion wardrobes.
(Courtesy of Ellen Diamond.)

Profile. A woman's hat that features a brim that is up on one side and down on the other.

Fez. A high, cylindrically shaped crown with a tassel at the top.

Care of Hats

The nature and amount of care is determined by the style of the hat and the materials used. Felt and straw models should be kept in boxes and stuffed with tissue paper to help shape retention. The box should be sufficiently large to allow for air space and enough room not to crush the style out of shape. At the end of the season, it is best to have this type of hat professionally cleaned and "reblocked" back to the original shape.

Knitted and other soft hats may be stored on shelves. Some might be freshened through laundering, whereas others might require professional cleaning, as in the case of suede caps. The labels often explain the appropriate care.

HOSIERY

When DuPont introduced nylon as the miracle fiber of the twentieth century, the hosiery producers capitalized on it and it soon became one of the largest segments of the accessories industry. Although leg coverings date back to ancient times, not until the sixteenth century were they adopted by ladies of the royal court as enhancements for proper dress. From that time until DuPont's discovery, the materials used for hosiery construction were cotton and silk.

The leg coverings used were stockings for dresses and skirts and socks for casual attire. The stockings were produced either flat and sewn together with a seam or on circular knitting machines that did not require seaming. They came in a limited number of colors. Some were plain, whereas others featured embroidered designs at the ankle.

To prevent slippage, women wore garters to hold the hosiery in place. In the 1960s, machinery was perfected that would produce **pantyhose,** a one-piece configuration that combined stockings with a panty and eliminated the need for women to wear garters. The new product became so popular that by the 1980s, it significantly outsold regular stockings.

Later developments made pantyhose even more desirable than when this product was first introduced. Manufacturers began to construct the panty portion of the product with materials such as Spandex that helped to control any excess "bulges" and also provided support for the wearer.

Today, most retailers severely restrict their stocking inventories and some do not bother to offer them at all.

In addition to pantyhose, **knee-high stockings** are offered for use under pants. They reach just below the knee; for outward appearance, it seems as though full stockings or pantyhose are being worn. They are popular because they are less restrictive and cost a good deal less than pantyhose or stockings (Figure 13.9).

In addition to stockings and pantyhose, women began to enjoy socks when they embraced pants as an alternative to the skirt (Figure 13.10). Socks of every length became popular, with the major craze belonging to teenagers who worshipped the legendary singing idol Frank Sinatra and wore **bobby socks** to his concerts. That style featured a short sock that had a band that folded over the top. Today, women's socks come in many lengths and materials and are favorites among females of every age. With the less rigorous demands of more formal dress, the sock serves many purposes. It is not only fashionable, but it offers greater warmth than fine hosiery.

Still another form of hosiery that was once widely popular is the **leg warmer.** Not only was it functional as a means of providing warmth, but it also answered a fashion need as well. Worn underneath short skirts or woolen shorts, it has remained a favorite during the winter months in the coldest climates.

Men, like women, wore stockings as far back as the 1600s. They were usually silken, came to the knee, and were held up by garters. They were necessary accompaniments to

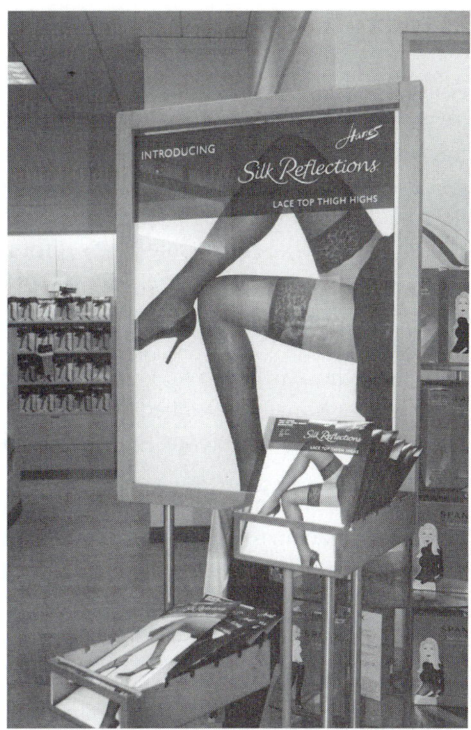

Figure 13.9 "Thigh highs" are an alternative to pantyhose.
(Courtesy of Ellen Diamond.)

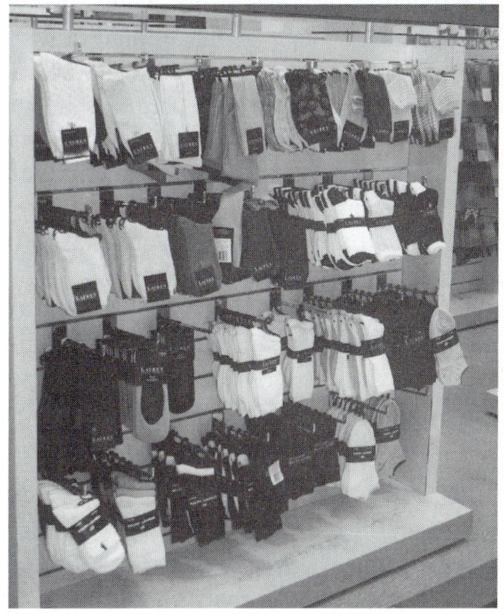

Figure 13.10 Socks come in a variety of styles.
(Courtesy of Ellen Diamond.)

knickers that were worn at the time. When the man's pant leg was lengthened, stockings were produced in shorter lengths. The material of choice for fine gentlemen was silk, which could be seen when the man was seated and the leg was partially exposed.

Today, men wear socks in place of formal hosiery. They are available in various lengths, materials, patterns, and styles to complement every type of apparel.

Today's men's and women's hosiery industry has significantly expanded. The product is so important as a fashion accent that the industry, once dominated by "less-than-household-names," now includes offerings by designers who have made their reputations on fashion apparel. Primarily through licensing agreements, names like Donna Karan, Calvin Klein, and Liz Claiborne grace the products. The market has become so popular that department and specialty stores, as well as off-site merchants, have expanded their inventories to merchandise all varieties of hosiery.

Hosiery Construction

All types of hosiery are knitted. Only the fibers and methods of knitting differ from one type to another. Although modern technology has enabled hosiery to be produced faster and better than ever before, the methods of construction are much like those produced in the early years.

Stockings that use the **full-fashioned** construction are produced in flat form, in the desired size and shape. A back seam is then stitched to finish the assemblage. The product is dyed, placed on a form, and heat set for retention. *Seamless* hosiery uses a one-piece construction that forms the hosiery by use of circular knitting machines. The product is made according to the desired size and shape. Like the full-fashioned type, it is dyed and heat set.

Pantyhose is constructed in two ways. One may use individual stockings and a panty, which are ultimately stitched together to form the product. Some manufacturers create pantyhose as one-piece constructions on special machines. In both cases, the items are dyed and heat set.

Socks construction follows the same stages as stockings and pantyhose. They are knitted on circular machines, either in a natural color that must be bleached to better accept later dyeing or, if a pattern is desired, different colored yarns are knitted together, eliminating later coloring.

Materials

The majority of dress hosiery is produced in some form of nylon. The fiber has been regularly enhanced through various techniques that add elasticity, texturing, less shine, and other visible and functional characteristics. Sometimes it bears more exotic names, but it is still nylon.

Nylon hosiery also takes on different appearances depending on the weight of the yarn and the number of loops knitted per inch. **Denier** is a term that applies to the fineness of the yarn, and **gauge,** to the closeness of the knit.

Socks are made of a variety of fibers such as cotton, wool, cashmere, acrylic, polyester, and nylon. To prevent slippage, an elastic band might be inserted at the top of the sock or a "ribbed" construction might be used above the ankle. To give the appearance of a luxury product and provide function and comfort to the wearer, two or more yarns may be used in the construction.

One of the most important features of hosiery is color. The industry takes its cue from the apparel markets and produces varieties of hues that enhance and coordinate with the wearer's garments. Thus, even the colors that are considered to be neutral have subtle differences that change from season to season.

Sizes

Men's hosiery generally comes in a standard size that fits all from 10 to 13. These sizes correspond to shoe sizes that range from 8 ½ to 12. With the significant stretch in men's hosiery fibers, there is little need for other sizes. In some cases, producers will manufacture smaller and larger sizes.

Women's socks also use a single size, because most women can be accommodated with the one-size-fits-all concept. In the case of pantyhose, size is generally determined by the wearer's height and weight (Figure 13.11). They usually range from size A for women whose heights are from 4 feet 11 inches to 5 feet 3 inches and whose weights range from ninety-five pounds, to size F for the heaviest and tallest figures that include heights of 5′1″ to 5′7″ and go to weights beginning at 155 and end at 170 pounds. Sizes B, C, D, and E fall somewhere between the measurements of A and F. Most companies include a size chart on the package to ensure proper size selection. In cases of inexpensive pantyhose, a one-size-fits-all measurement is used.

For the tiniest figures, some manufacturers tailor their pantyhose in petite sizes, whereas larger-sized women are treated to queen sizes.

Children's hosiery comes in a variety of sizes. Newborns to age one usually wear sizes that range from 4 to 5 1/2; older children wear sizes that run up to 8 1/2. Preteen and young

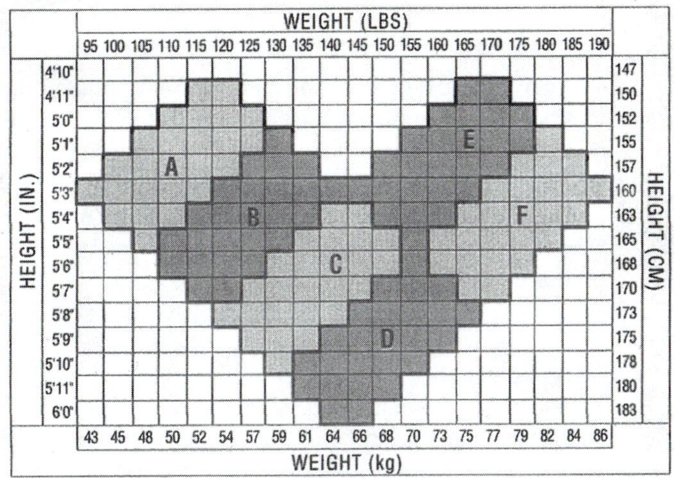

Figure 13.11 This chart aids in the selection of the appropriate hosiery size.

teenage girls wear a range that begins at 9 and concludes at 11. Preteen boys and young teenage boys usually wear from 9 1/2 to 13. Some children's manufacturers are using S, M, and L for their hosiery.

Styles

Today's hosiery manufacturers offer many styles for both dressy and casual attire.

Pantyhose. Hosiery that combines stockings and a panty and covers the body from the toes to the waist. They come in seamed or seamless styles.

Stockings. Hosiery that comes in pairs and reaches from the toes to the thigh. To prevent sagging, they are worn with garters or garter belts.

Tights. The same as the pantyhose concept, except that the product is produced of an opaque material.

Anklets. Socks that reach just above the ankle and may be ribbed, plain, or cuffed.

Crew socks. Socks that use heavy ribbing in the design and reach about four or five inches above the ankle.

Tennis socks. A style that covers the foot and ends beneath the ankle. It usually has elastic around the body, and an ornamental pom-pom that peeks over the sneaker with which it is worn.

Knee-highs. A type of hosiery that reaches above the calf. Men wear finer types for dresswear, whereas women use them primarily under pants.

Tube socks. Shapeless socks that conform to the foot and are worn for athletics.

Many hosiery manufacturers produce pantyhose in different variations for purposes that might be decorative or functional. Table 13.1 features terms used to describe certain styles of pantyhose.

TABLE 13.1 Pantyhose Styles

Control top	A pantyhose that features a yarn such as Spandex in the panty portion of the design.
Sandalfoot	A model that eliminates heel or toe reinforcement. It is worn with sandals and avoids the unsightly portion of hosiery that is present in regular styles.
Textures	Styles that use fancy patterns in their design.
Demitoe	A pantyhose with an abbreviated reinforcement at the toe.
Support	A term used to describe hosiery that uses Spandex along with another fiber, usually nylon, for better control.
Mesh	Hosiery that uses knitted fabric resembling mesh.

SCARVES

Many countries have had scarves as part of their dress for centuries. Spain, for example, introduced the **mantilla,** a lace version worn over the head. It was popularized in America during the Kennedy reign in the White House when it was the choice of the president's wife Jackie as a head covering worn to church. The British, French, and Chinese each had their own versions that have remained popular within their own borders as well as in other places. These large scarves were not the only styles favored by the people. Smaller versions, oblong shapes, and others were favorites.

Scarves, as we use them today, are both functional and decorative. On a stormy winter day, there is nothing quite as warming as the woolen muffler that prevents the wind from making the body feel colder. At the other extreme, the large silk square is ever present, often displaying the name of a famous designer and telling the world that it is as treasured as the apparel it augments.

American fashion emporiums began to feature silk squares of all sizes in the 1950s (Figure 13.12). Some were at modest price points that featured creative motifs, and others, imported from the world's fashion capitals, were silk treasures that were signed by such marquee designers as Gucci and Hermes. Since that period, others have joined the bandwagon either by producing their own collections or lending their names, via licensing agreements, to accessories manufacturers.

The industry continues to grow, as demonstrated by the size of the merchandise assortments in fashion operations.

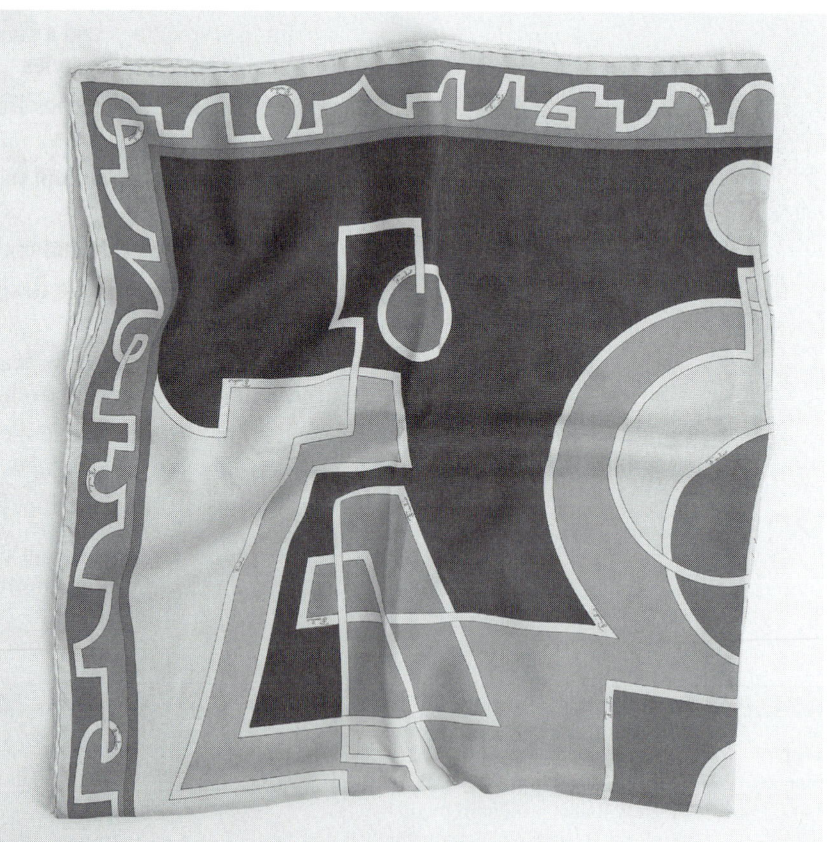

Figure 13.12 This Pucci scarf was fashionable in the 1950s.
(Courtesy of Dorling Kindersley Media Library.)

Scarves Construction

Unlike shoes, handbags, and other more intricately produced accessories, scarves are simple to make. Natural fibers such as silk, wool, and cotton and a host of man-mades serve as the basis of the scarf. Some are individually silk-screened to create a design that parallels a painting or work of art, whereas others are cut from rolls of fabric that have been printed, or dyed solid colors before being cut and sewn. Others are knitted versions that are constructed to the desired sizes.

The motifs range from typical paisleys and flowered prints to geometrics. The edges of the costly varieties are hand rolled, whereas the mass-produced, inexpensive types have their edges finished by machine.

They may be made into squares, rectangles, oblongs, and triangles, depending on their final use. Sequins, beads, fringe, and other trimmings are used to enhance some of the designs.

Styles

As do other accessories, scarves come in a variety of styles.

Ascot. A piece of material that comes to two points and is worn one over the other around the neck. Often, it is held in place with a decorative stickpin.

Shawl. A large piece of cloth in a rectangular or triangular shape that covers the neck and shoulders and is worn over a dress, suit, or coat. It is sometimes accentuated with fringe.

Mantilla. Taken from the head covering of Spanish ladies, it is a lace scarf that has either straight or scalloped edges.

Cowboy Scarf. A square that is folded into a triangular shape worn with the point to the front and knotted in the back.

Muffler. A knitter or woven oblong-shaped scarf that is worn around the neck to provide warmth (Figure 13.13).

Stole. An oversized rectangle that is worn over a suit or dress. It is made of wool or fur.

Care of Scarves

Like any other fabric accessory, care should be given according to the fibers used in the construction. Silk scarves that are costly should be professionally dry cleaned to ensure continuous pleasure, as should the woolen varieties. Those made of cotton, linen, or launderable man-made material may be washed according to the directions on the hangtags. Since many types are worn directly around the neck, the natural oils from the hair and body tend to soil them. In these cases, regular cleaning is recommended.

Stoles, oblong and oversized scarves, are often made of fur. They require the same care as any fur garment, including cold storage during the summer months.

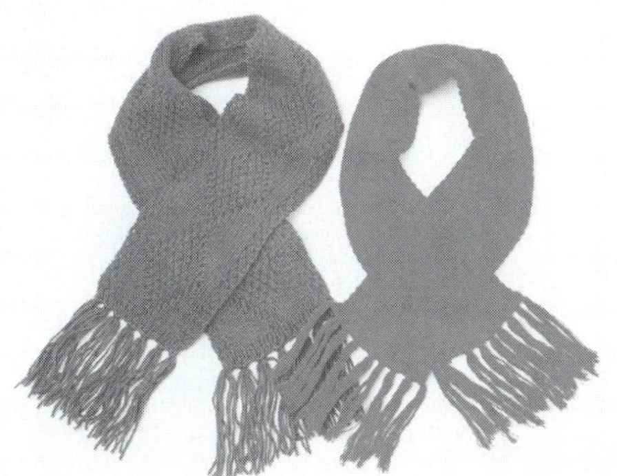

Figure 13.13 Mufflers provide warmth as well as style. *(Courtesy of Pearson Learning Photo Studio, John Paul Endress.)*

UMBRELLAS

When a rainy day is in the forecast, many people prepare themselves for the eventual downpour by carrying an umbrella with them. Some even use them on sunny days to shade themselves from the harmful effects of the sun's rays. Whatever the case, this accessory is both functional and fashionable.

The umbrella dates back more than 4,000 years, beginning with the civilizations of Assyria, Egypt, Greece, and China, where many citizens used them. Many centuries later, in the 1500s, the use of the umbrella spread to Europe. In England, only women used them until Jonas Hanway popularized their use in the 1700s after discovering them on a trip to Portugal. Another Londoner, John MacDonald, began to use one made of silk in 1778. The "Hanways" were carried by English gentlemen of that period. Today, of course, everyone grabs an umbrella to stay dry. All types ranging from the traditional *sticks* to the *automatic* and *folding* varieties are commonplace throughout the world.

Styles

Several umbrella styles are popular. They vary by shape, size, function, and fabrics. Each has a number of similar parts: the *frame*, the metal form on which it is built; *ribs*, metal supports that are used to hold the cover of the umbrella, known as the *canopy*, and that number from 8 to 16; the *shaft*, or pole, which may be stationary or collapsible; *spreaders*, the rods that move up and down when the umbrella is opened; and the *finial*, or the decorative design at the umbrella's top. Most of today's umbrella canopies are made of nylon because of its durability, with the frames generally made of steel or fiberglass. In terms of styles, the following list features some of those that are in use today:

- *Stick* a long, narrow umbrella that either fits into a case or tube and is fitted with a band with snaps, making it less cumbersome when carried. Sometimes the tube is omitted to make the umbrella's fabric or trim visible.
- *Automatic* used either on a stick or collapsible umbrella, with a shaft that extends to full height with the release of button found somewhere on the handle.
- *Bubble* a dome-shaped canopy usually made with a vinyl cover.
- *Ballerina* the bell shape often used for children's umbrellas, with a ruffle at the edge of canopy (Figure 13.14).

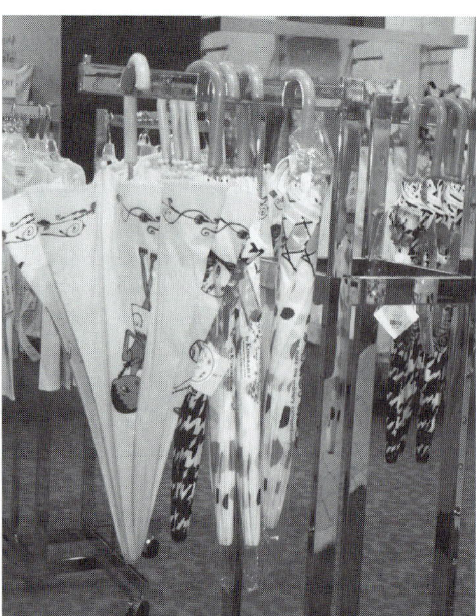

Figure 13.14 Children's umbrellas often use figurative images as design enhancements.
(Courtesy of Ellen Diamond.)

- *Collapsible* a type that is reduced in size, when not in use, by one-half; the flick of the button in the handle brings it to full size.
- *Golf* oversized umbrella that is not only used on the golf course, but also for times when extra coverage is needed; may feature special logos that serve as promotional devices.

Merchandising the Umbrella

Like other products, umbrellas are available from the typical outlets such as brick-and-mortar merchants, catalogs, and Web sites. Two other places where umbrellas are typically sold include:

- *Museum Shops.* Whenever a museum features a "blockbuster" exhibit such as paintings by Monet or Van Gogh, the gift shop is generally stocked with umbrellas that have been designed to feature the artist's work. They are excellent promotional pieces that carry the name of the museum for significant periods of time.
- *"Opportunistic" Street Vendors.* As soon the rain starts to fall, many street vendors are ready to accommodate pedestrians with umbrellas. They are usually bargain-priced and generally are the collapsible type.

EYEWEAR

Initially used primarily as functional devices, eyewear has taken on a fashion-oriented persona. Like clothing and accessories, eyewear helps people achieve individualized looks that oftentimes become their "signatures." Jackie Kennedy Onassis, for example, made oversized eyewear the rage, and it soon became the choice of women everywhere.

First introduced by the Chinese around 10 A.D., as a means of protecting their eyes from evil spirits, the first glasses that were used to help the elderly correct their reading problems were introduced in Italy in the 1260s. While eyesight improved, the problem with the early models was the inability to keep them from slipping down the nose. The Spaniards tried to improve the slippage problem by attaching ribbons to them and tying them around the ears. This solution wasn't terribly successful and didn't please the wearers. In 1730, an English optician, Edward Scarlett, added rigid sidepieces to sit on top of the ears. This was the beginning of the eyewear that combine function and fashion today.

Benjamin Franklin, often credited with the invention of eyeglasses, in fact, invented the bifocal lens in 1780. Tired of changing reading glasses to distance glasses, he developed a lens that would enable him to manage his "seeing" needs with one pair.

In addition to the traditional glasses, other types were used, including the *monocle*, a single round glass that fits over the eye, and the *lorgnette*, a long-handled, handheld style.

In addition to the standard glasses, 1827 saw the beginning of a new concept, a lens that would be placed on the eye's surface to improve sight. The English astronomer Sir John Herschel first developed the idea, and glassblower F. E. Muller produced the first eye covering in 1887. By 1929, the *contact lens* had been perfected and began to gain acceptance.

Sunglasses made their initial entry in 1929 when Sam Foster convinced Woolworth to sell his "Foster Grants" in its Atlantic City, New Jersey, store. Their popularity soared when the Hollywood stars started to use them (Figure 13.15).

Today, eyewear is a major segment of the fashion industry. Designers who first made their marks in the apparel field have crossed over into eyewear. Most have entered into licensing agreements with major companies to have their styles produced and marketed. Ralph Lauren, Yves St. Laurent, Armani, Gucci, Prada, Hilfiger, Boss, and Versace are just some of the names that grace the frames.

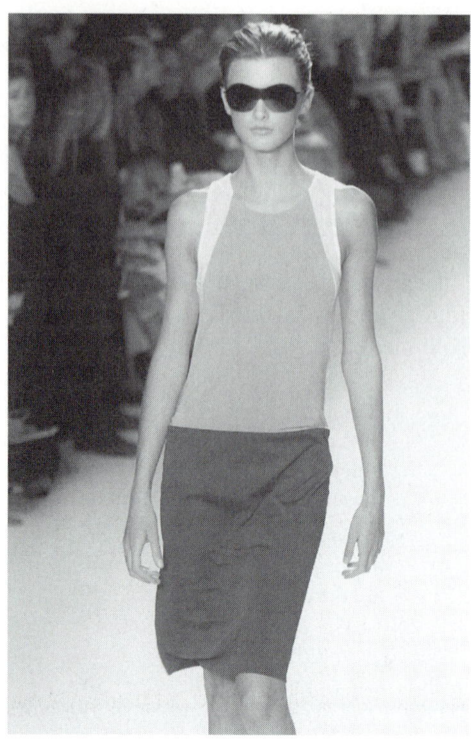

Figure 13.15 Sunglasses add glamour to any outfit. *(Courtesy of Corbis/Bettmann, Reuters/Mike Segar.)*

Frame Styles

A variety of different styles is available, with the choice dependent upon personal preference, vision, and the fashion of the times. The popularity of frames changes from time to time. Some are:

Granny glasses. Small circular glass frames that sit at the edge of the nose and are used primarily for reading.

Aviators. Oversized glasses that were popularized by pilots in World War II (Figure 13.16).

Rimless or three-piece. A style that eliminates the need for a frame to hold the lens in place.

Semirimless. A style that uses a rim at the top, with the rest being rimless.

Goggles. Tight-fitting style used underwater to protect the eyes and for sporting activities.

Panto or preppy. Small frames with a wire frame that houses round or oval lenses.

Mask or shield. Glasses that wrap around the face, usually worn for sporting events.

Frame Materials

Numerous materials are used to hold the lenses. These include:

Plastics. A wealth of plastic frames is available in fashion colors as well as black, a big seller. Others come in a variety of patterns, with the most popular being tortoise.

Steel and iron. These strong materials are mostly produced in gold and silver, but are also available in black, white, and fashion colors.

Titanium. This lightweight metal is extremely flexible, giving the wearer a durable frame (Figure 13.17).

Base metals. These are generally used under other metals to provide durability. One of the more popular choices is nickel silver.

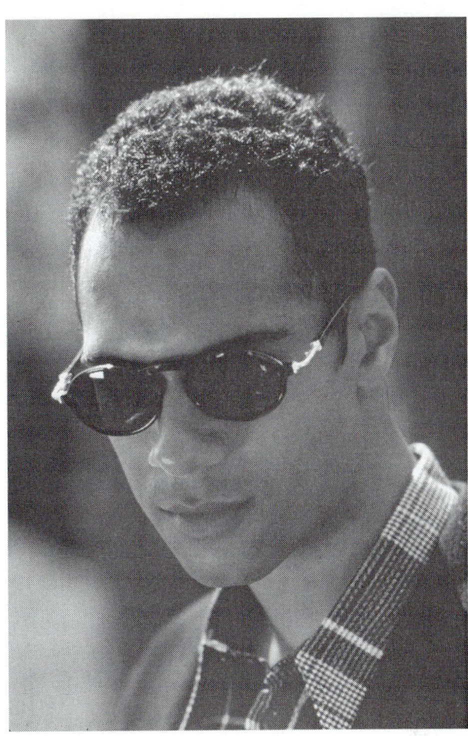

Figure 13.16 These frames are a variation on the aviator style.
(Courtesy of Ellen Diamond.)

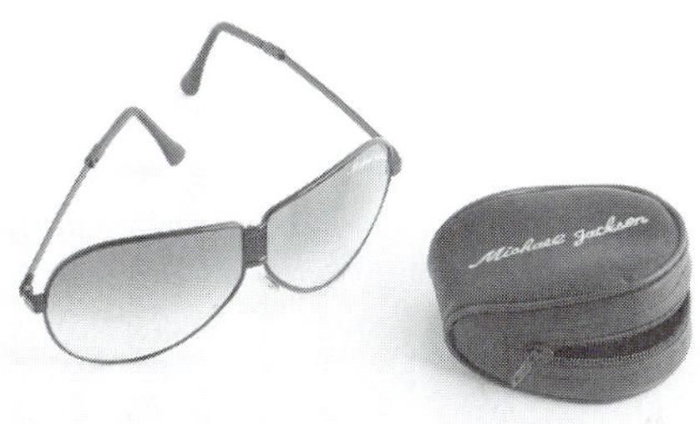

Figure 13.17 Titanium frames are lightweight and durable.
(Courtesy of Dorling Kindersley Media Library.)

Wood. High-fashion frames are produced with a number of different types of woods.

Buffalo horn. One of the by-products of slaughtered buffalos is their horns. Many designers are using them to give the frame an ivory appearance.

Lens Types

Several lens types may be fitted into a variety of frames to help improve eyesight:

- *Single vision.* designed for one purpose, to improve reading or correct distance problems, for example.
- *Bifocals.* a multipurpose lens with one section for reading and another for distance.
- *Trifocals.* three distinct areas available for reading, mid-range purposes such as computer use, and distance correction.
- *Progressive.* A type of lens used to improve reading, mid-range, and distance problems without the noticeable "lines" on bifocals and trifocals.
- *Tinted.* coloring applied to the lenses.

Lens Materials

The vast majority of lenses produced today are either made of plastic or mineral. The use of plastic gives the wearer a lightweight product. Some products feature a polarizing lens that involves the insertion of a filter between two layers. A coating may also be applied to provide scratch-resistance and reduce glare.

Marketing Eyewear

In addition to traditional marketing techniques, designer logos add appeal to frames. Famous designers who have captured a vast audience in the fashion industry are affixing their signatures via the logo route, to the *templepieces* of frames. With so many consumers motivated to buy designer labels, this type of marketing has captured a large segment of the glass-wearing market. Some designers have developed more than one logo, such as Dior, for use on frames.

Merchandising Eyewear

The industry merchandises its products in several different ways, including selling them in stores, optical outlets, catalogs, and the Internet, even on street corners. The choice generally depends on the price of the product and its use.

- *Stores.* Department stores, specialty shops, pharmacies, supermarkets, mass merchandisers, and warehouse outlets each have successfully merchandised eyewear. Some department stores and warehouse outlets such as Costco have on-premises optical departments that produce eyewear to the specifics of the customer's prescriptions. The upscale department and specialty stores are home to a wealth of different sunglasses that are either the prescription types or "ready-mades" in a wide range of styles and prices. Supermarkets and pharmacies also feature *readers*, which are inexpensive, nonprescription eyewear.
- *Optical Outlets.* Both chains and independently owned stores are the major outlets for prescription products. They generally carry the more expensive glasses, many of which feature designer frames, and offer such services as optometrist evaluation and tinting.
- *Catalogs.* Both independent catalogs and those of department stores feature a wide range of nonprescription eyewear. They are either private brands or those that carry the logos and signatures of marquee designers.
- *Web Sites.* The number of Internet outlets featuring glasses continues to increase every year. Eyewear is available in just about any designer name and usually offered at prices below those charged in optical outlets and traditional stores.
- *Street Corners.* In most shopping districts around the world, street vendors sell a wide variety of designer eyewear. Most often, they are counterfeits and sell for a fraction of the cost of the authentic eyewear.

Internet Resources for Additional Research

www.familyforest.info/gloves.htm features the history of gloves.
www.thehatsite.com/historyofhats.html examines the history of hats beginning with primitive man.
www.nahm.com/hosieryterms.html offers a complete glossary of hosiery terms.

Merchandise Information Terminology

Signature scarf
Trank
Fourchettes
Quirks
Bolton thumb
Quirk thumb
Skeleton lining
Taxing
Table cutting
Pull-down cutting
Inseam
Outseam
Overseam
Pique seam
Half-pique
Pointing
Button lengths
Mitten
Shorty
Driving glove
Gauntlet
Mousquetaire
Slip-on
Cones
Crown
Brim
Blocks
Buckram
Plaiting
Baseball cap

Beanie
Beret
Cowboy hat
Sherlock Holmes
Derby
Fedora
Panama
Bonnet
Cloche
Gaucho
Alpine
Turban
Top hat
Tam O'Shanter
Breton
Cartwheel
Sailor
Nehru
Garden party
Ski cap
Picture hat
Slouch
Toque
Hood
Profile
Fez
Pantyhose
Knee-high stockings
Bobby socks
Leg warmer
Full-fashioned
Denier
Gauge
Crew socks
Tube socks
Control top
Sandalfoot
Textured pantyhose
Demitoe
Support hose
Mesh pantyhose
Mantilla
Ascot
Shawl
Cowboy scarf
Muffler
Stole

EXERCISES

1. Take an old glove that is ready to be discarded and separate its component parts. Affix each part to a foam board and label the technical names, along with the purposes each serves.
2. Visit a fashion retailer's hosiery department and take note of the different size classifications used on the packages. From the knowledge gained, prepare a graph that explains the proper size for each wearer.
3. Prepare a report on the types of women's hats offered for sale in a store, catalog, or Web site. Take pictures of the hats, with the store manager's permission, or make copies of the styles featured online. The style of each hat should be labeled.

Review Questions

1. What phenomenon gave a boost to glove sales in the 1980s?
2. What is a *trank*?
3. Define the term *fourchette* and tell the benefit it serves in glove construction.
4. Name and differentiate between the two major types of thumbs used in making leather or fabric gloves.
5. Distinguish between full and skeleton linings in gloves.
6. Why are the more expensive leather gloves *table cut*?
7. Describe the method used in pique seaming.
8. Through what system are women's gloves measured?
9. How does a mitten differ from traditional gloves?
10. Over what type of form is the felt hat shaped?
11. Describe the process of plaiting used in the construction of straw millinery.
12. At what size intervals do men's hats progress?
13. What is a *pillbox*, and who popularized it in America?
14. What is the distinguishing feature of a bonnet?
15. How did DuPont help to revolutionize the hosiery industry?
16. Explain the style *pantyhose*.
17. In what way has Spandex helped in the sale of pantyhose?
18. How is seamless hosiery constructed?
19. Differentiate between the terms *denier* and *gauge*.
20. What is a mantilla?

CHAPTER 14

Cosmetics and Fragrances

After reading this chapter, you should be able to:

- Trace the history of cosmetics from ancient times to today.
- List and describe the different product categories that comprise cosmetics.
- Discuss a three-pronged approach for the application of makeup.
- Define common terms related to cosmetics.
- Explain the need for proper skin care before makeup application is considered.
- Describe the various types of sun protection products.
- List and explain the four fragrance categories.

When historians trace Egyptian history, they discover that beauty was an integral part of the culture as far back as 4000 B.C. Through numerous archeological digs, researchers discovered jars of salves from this epoch. Highly developed cosmetics were used as early as 1550 B.C. and included products to reduce stretch marks, minimize wrinkles, eliminate scars, and even encourage new hair growth. The use of eye makeup has also been attributed to Egyptian women. Not only was it used for aesthetic reasons, but also to "avert the evil eye."

Also around 1500 B.C., Chinese and Japanese women used rice powder to paint their faces pasty white. Eyebrows were shaved and plucked, and teeth were painted gold or black. Henna dyes were used to stain the hair.

As time progressed and cultures merged, cosmetics took on an even more important place. The Greeks' use of cosmetics significantly increased, as did the Romans' centuries later. Around 1000 B.C., upper-class Greeks wore wigs to hide the fact that they seldom bathed. Upper-class women, as did their Asian counterparts, used white face powder. When some wanted a little color, they chose ochre clays laced with red iron for lipstick.

In 100 A.D. Platus wrote, "A woman without paint is like food without salt." This is an indication that cosmetics were soon to become commonplace among the people.

As the centuries moved forward, cosmetics became more and more acceptable and evident. In the fourteenth century, Elizabethan England was the place for fashionably dyed red hair, and egg white was the choice for well-to-do women to use on their faces. The fifteenth and sixteenth centuries were popular for a wealth of cosmetics, with France and Italy taking the lead as the chief centers of cosmetics manufacturing. Red rouge and lipstick were prominent among the cosmetics worn by all except the very poorest class in the seventeenth and eighteenth centuries. In the nineteenth century the French developed chemical processes to replace the natural fragrances used in cosmetics. During the 1920s, America took the lead and began to mass-market cosmetics.

The key in cosmetics in recent decades is diversity. With $20 billion in annual sales, it is one of the most important of the fashion-oriented industries. Products are available through many channels, including department and specialty stores, boutiques, catalogs, and the Internet.

Fragrances also date back for centuries. For thousands of years, man has practiced making fragrances not only for beauty, but also to enhance spiritual states. The burning of essence was used in religious rites in ancient China and Egypt and ultimately led to the use of perfumes as we know them today. The Greeks developed flower ingredients that enabled

EXERCISES

1. Using fashion magazines as your resource, examine the cosmetics advertisements for different types of products. Select five ads that concentrate on one product such as lipsticks or mascara, and mount them on a foam board. Adjacent to each ad, list the product benefits that each delivers to the consumer.
2. Prepare a visual rendering of a female's face, including the characteristics of which it is comprised. Using this template, visit a local cosmetics store for the purpose of examining a specific line and selecting the different makeup products that should be used for each of the face's components. Each area of the drawing should feature the name of the product that will enhance its appearance and the benefit it delivers.

Review Questions

1. Briefly describe where cosmetics were first used and what types of products were popular during those times.
2. What were some of the cosmetic uses in Elizabethan England in the fourteenth century?
3. What are the major color cosmetics available to today's users?
4. What is mascara? What purpose does it serve the wearer?
5. Differentiate between prefoundation and foundation products.
6. In what way does an eye pencil differ from an eye liner?
7. List and describe the three major lip enhancers available in cosmetics.
8. What is the purpose of dermatological testing in the cosmetics industry?
9. Differentiate between opaque and translucent makeup finishes.
10. What is the difference between a skin cleanser and a toner?
11. Why are moisturizers used as a daily regimen?
12. How does an SPF of twenty-five differ from one that is fifty?
13. What care must be exercised in the application of sun tanning cream?
14. How does perfume differ from cologne?
15. What is the major purpose for the use of eau de parfum?

SECTION FIVE

Home Accessories and Decorative Enhancements

CHAPTER 15

Tableware: Dinnerware, Flatware, Glassware, Holloware, Tabletops, and Candle Holders

After reading this chapter, you should be able to:

- Explain the manner in which dinnerware may be purchased.
- Discuss how dinnerware should be cared for to increase its usefulness in dining.
- Make the case for the importance of "open stock" flatware.
- Differentiate between the different patterns available in glassware.
- Describe the typical glassware styles and purposes they serve.
- List the different sizes in which tablecloths are available and the seating allocation each serves.
- Explain the importance of the tabletop when runners are used in place of tablecloths.
- Discuss the importance of candle holders to table settings and other interior and exterior environments.

One of the largest segments of the home furnishing arena is tableware. As we examine interior design photographs from the past decades, we are often made aware of the extravagant table settings that graced the homes of the upper class. Grand dinnerware, glassware, silverware, candelabras, and table accessories, each perfectly coordinated with the others, resulted in breathtaking presentations. While the privileged class was fortunate enough to enjoy these fabulously designed table components, the masses were generally relegated to more functionally oriented tableware. Instead of the grandeur of sterling silver, elegantly embellished bone china, crystal stemware, antique candlesticks, and hand-crafted brocade table linens, serviceable substitutes were the order of the day. Of course, many middle-class households tucked away "the good china" for special occasions.

If we fast-forward to the late twentieth century, we find significant changes in the home furnishings arena. Much of the credit is due to the creative talents and marketing skills of Martha Stewart. She almost single-handedly made consumers aware of the ways in which they could dress their tables at modest expense and deliver a finished setting that could rival the most expensive and elaborate installations. Imparting her knowledge of "good taste" to the masses, Stewart helped transform lackluster tableware departments into exciting arenas that others soon emulated.

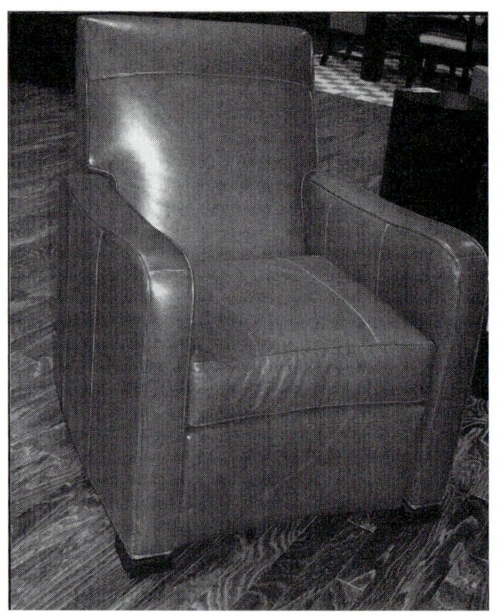

Figure 16.1 Upholstered leather furniture offers comfort with class.
(Courtesy of Ellen Diamond.)

Other accessories are equally important to the overall impression that the room or office setting will immediately convey to the viewer. These include lighting, sculpture, pottery, candles, plants, basketry, and other decorative and functional pieces. Rounding out the needs to provide both beauty and practicality in any room are floor coverings, a topic that will be fully explored in Chapter 18.

FURNITURE

When interior designers and other industry professionals interface with their clients in terms of furniture selection and acquisition, they generally begin their discussions with periods and/or country and regional classifications. Each features particular styles from which choices may be made. The decision may be to stay within one general classification or to opt for an eclectic approach that combines the elements of two or more periods.

While volumes have been written about furniture styles, we offer here a brief overview of popular period and country classifications.

Period Classifications

Each period has a focus of its own and is represented with specific styles. While the popularity of each often peaks and wanes from time to time, they are always available to satisfy the consumers' needs.

COLONIAL

When America was in its infancy, its inhabitants for the most part came from England. Many brought furniture with them to begin their new lives. Known as **colonial,** or early American, the pieces bore classical lines. Case goods were primarily manufactured from mahogany, and upholstered pieces were generally made of silk and cotton that featured checks, plaids, and floral patterns.

Those who prefer this period of furniture generally select items that have been carefully copied from the original offerings. Of course, the originals are comparatively expensive, thus making the reproductions more likely to be found in the typical interior setting.

REGENCY

Also originating in England was the **regency** period, often referred to as the *Federal* style. Unlike the colonial category that typically followed simple lines, regency furnishings are more formal. Mahogany and a wealth of black lacquered woods were case goods mainstays with brocades, moirés, and damasks used for upholstered pieces and draperies.

BIEDERMEIER

A departure from the English influence, **Biedermeier** originated in Germany in a neoclassical period. The lines are simple and are often used as accents with other furniture periods. Original pieces are extremely costly, making reproductions more popular.

VICTORIAN

Just before the turn of the twentieth century, **Victorian furniture** became the rage. Unlike the simple lines of the colonial period, a more massive appearance was emphasized. Chairs with curved backs, oversized sofas, fringe embellishments, chintz, damasks, velvet, and brocade fabrics are typical of this home furnishings classification.

ARTS AND CRAFTS

While the Victorian era was reigning, a less elaborate style was introduced to the furniture world. Clean lines and fine materials exemplified the **arts and craft** movement and gave the consumer an elegant, yet simple choice. Incorporated into many of the designs are stone, brick, copper, oak woods, and fabrics that bore small, geometric patterns.

MODERN

Early in the twentieth century, several different influences appeared on the furnishings scene. As a group they are known as the *modern* style, but individually they are identified as art nouveau, art deco, and Danish modern.

Curved lines and patterns replete with birds and curved lines are typical of **art nouveau.** Lilies and irises are abundantly used along with stylized birds. Also prevalent are peacocks and snakes in the fabrics. Glass pieces are used as adornments as are stained glass windows.

Modernism and clarity are the elements that comprise **art deco** designs. Popularized in the 1920s, it was used in many of America's great buildings and theaters such as the Chrysler building and Radio City Music Hall in New York City. Merging functionality with decorative elements such as curved contours, highly polished surfaces, and ancient pyramids, it was seen in a host of different furnishings such as the coffee table, which it introduced; in satin, leather, and velvet fabrics; and in many different unique accessories such as tortoise shells and animal skins.

Following the introduction of art deco was **Danish modern.** Asymmetrical shapes and clean lines were typical of this period that originated in Scandinavia. It is still popular in contemporary homes and offices.

Country and Regional Classifications

In addition to the traditional periods that make up furniture offerings, other styles epitomize country and regional collections. Each features a wealth of different characteristics that are found in furniture designs and accessories for the home. Most popular are those that are classified as English, French, Mediterranean, American, and Scandinavian.

ENGLISH

English country case goods are primarily constructed of old pine that has been previously used in floorboards and walls, or newly constructed woods that replicate the used pieces. The upholstered counterparts are dominantly covered in floral chintz fabrics that feature strong reds, greens, and blues. Needlepoint and tapestry pillows are often used as accents or enhancements. Making the room setting typically English is the use of wooden floors and oriental rugs on top of them.

FRENCH

Originating in the small towns of the Provence region in France such as Avignon, Arles, St. Remy, and Aix-en-Provence, this class of furniture has become a staple in the United States. The case goods and accent pieces are usually constructed of fruitwoods and are either stained or hand painted. Upholstered chairs and sofas are generally covered in polished cottons and *toiles* that depict scenes of the region. Primarily colored with red, blue, green, and yellow fabrics, except for the toiles, which feature more subtle pinks and blues, they give a distinct look to the furniture. With a multitude of enhancements such as throw pillows and other accents, country French designs impart a distinctive, homey impression.

MEDITERRANEAN

The countries that border the Mediterranean Sea, such as Italy and Greece, are responsible for the furnishings that have come to be known as *Mediterranean*. Painted case goods and frames for chairs dominate this classification of furniture. Simple white linen and cotton fabrics are typical. Flooring is often terra-cotta tiles that provide functionality. For added pizzazz to this simple style, painted ceramics are often the choice as accents.

AMERICAN

When the early settlers arrived in America, many brought with them furniture from their native England. Those who did not, embraced a simpler design that was primitively constructed. In addition to the case goods that were primarily functional, small calico prints and gingham checks adorned the upholstered pieces, with wooden planks covered with braided rugs for flooring. Four-poster beds also typify the furniture and are covered in patchwork quilts.

In addition to settlers from England, others came from Spain. Dominant were rough-hewn wooden pieces with colorful rugs and pottery used as accents. Native Americans also produced styles similar to the Spanish.

LIGHTING

When a professional interior designer addresses lighting requirements, he or she must consider the period of the furnishings that make up the space, the light sources that will be employed to illuminate the areas, and the types of fixtures that will most appropriately complement the furniture and accessories that have been purchased.

Light Sources

Today's offerings are more extensive than at any other time. Different types of light serve different purposes. One may be used merely for overall illumination purposes, while others might be used to accent and highlight the room's accessories.

Typically, the choices are fluorescents, incandescents, and halogen lamps. Each offers the user a different result.

INCANDESCENTS

Most often the choice for overall lighting is the **incandescent bulb.** They come in the standard bulbs that are used in lamps or as floodlights that are generally used in recessed installations or in tracks. They are also available as spotlights used to define certain areas.

Today's choices have been expanded through the availability of low-voltage lamps. Unlike the older variety of incandescents that had a limited lifetime and ultimately cost more,

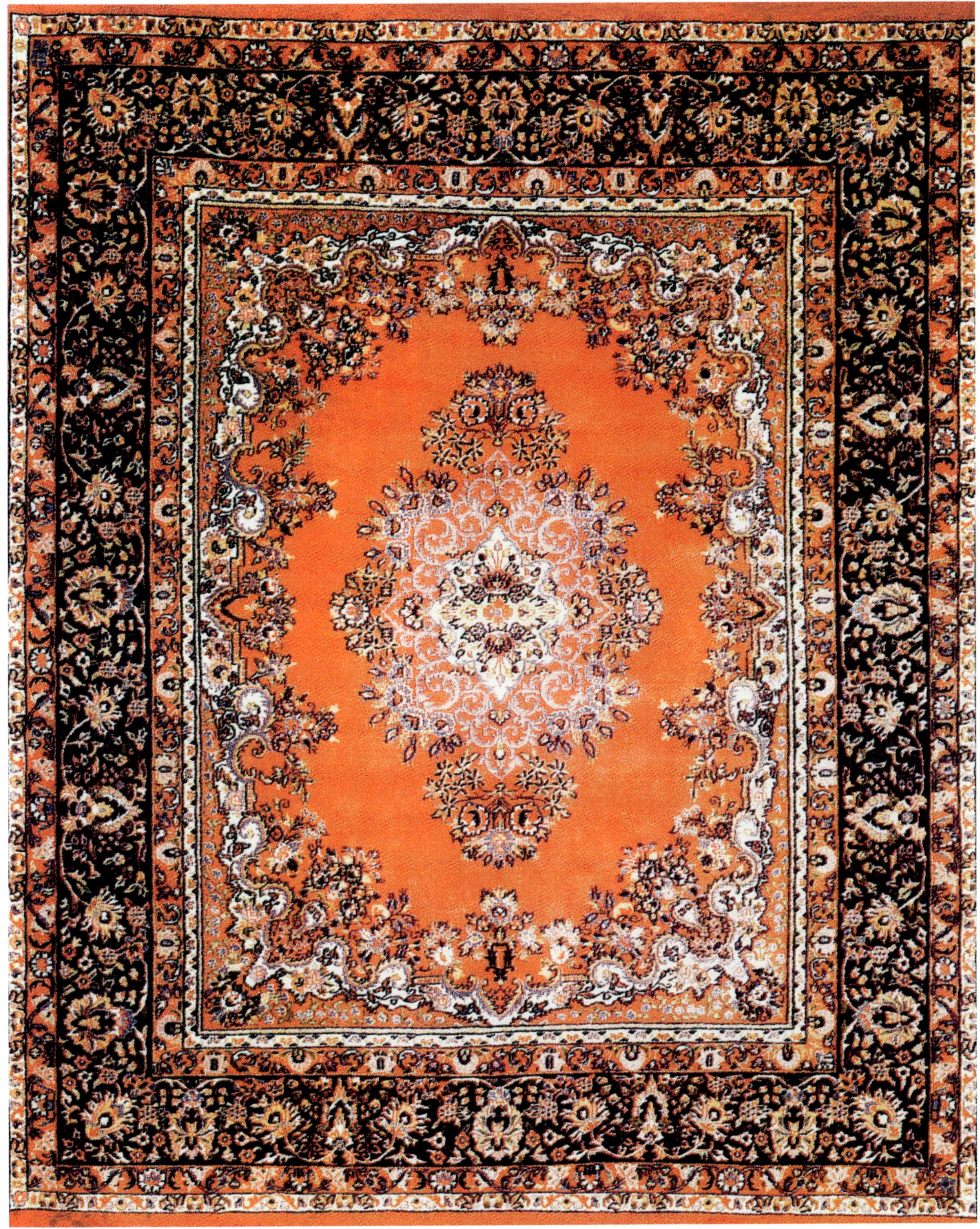

This "sirouk" design is typical of rugs made in India.
(Courtesy of Ellen Diamond.)

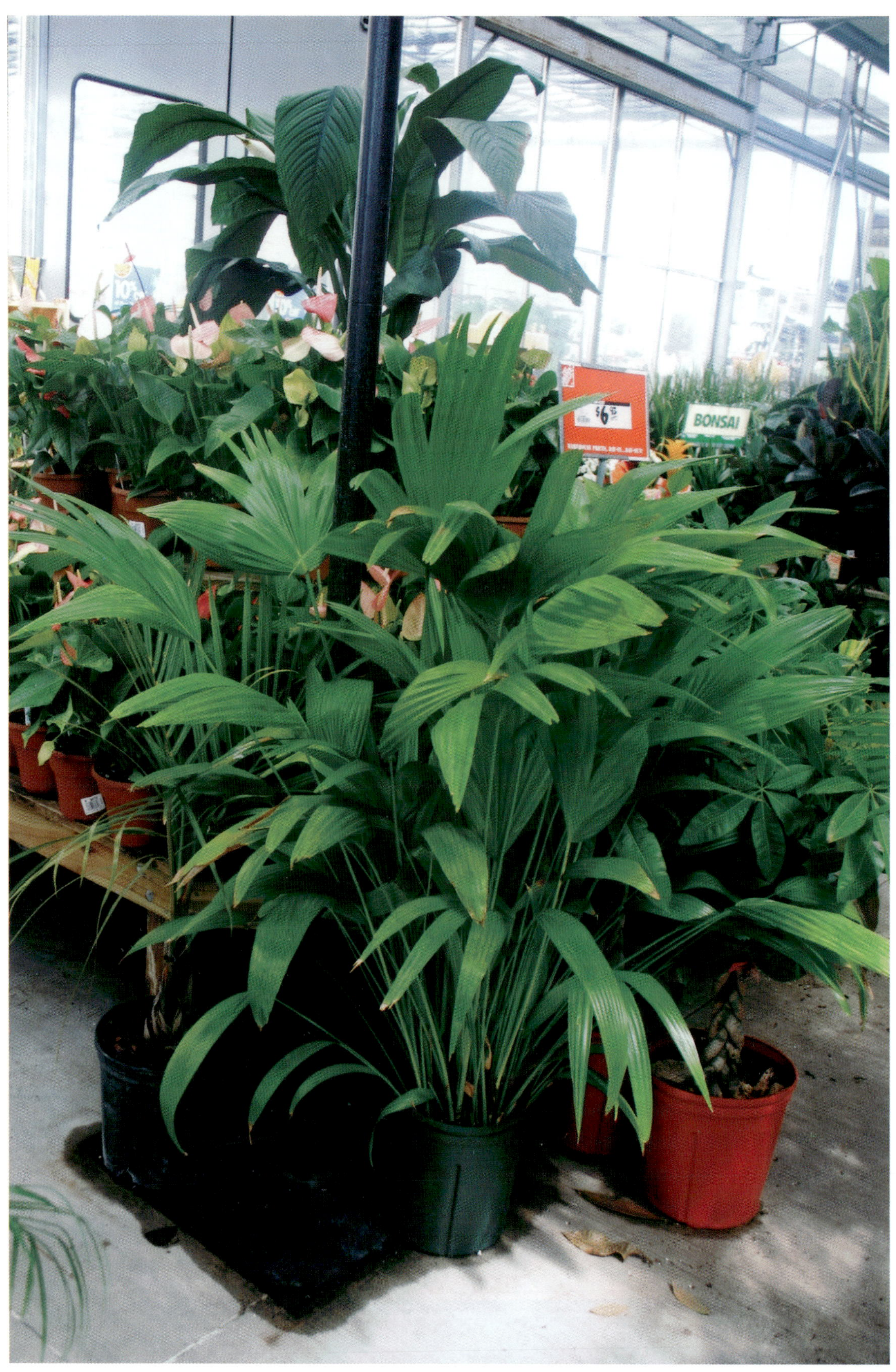

Live plants have turned ordinary rooms into exciting places.
(Courtesy of Ellen Diamond.)

the new types are longer lasting and easier to maintain. They also throw two-thirds less heat than the traditional bulb.

FLUORESCENTS

For cost efficiency and long-lasting results, some areas of the home call for the use of **fluorescent lighting.** In kitchens, for example, a recessed fluorescent fixture might be appropriate for overall lighting. It also might be used in valances that conceal these bulbs, yet generate sufficient light to illuminate particular areas.

While their popularity has waned in recent years, they are still used when the requirement is low-cost maintenance and effective, cool lighting.

HALOGEN LAMPS

When dramatic highlighting is the intention, no other lightbulb gives the same effect as does the **halogen lamp.** It is a whiter, brighter bulb that measures about one-quarter of the size of a standard incandescent. It may be used to enhance a specific part of a room or wash an entire wall. In addition to these attributes, it has about double the life of an incandescent bulb.

Lighting Fixtures and Systems

The options for light fixtures and systems are numerous. They range from the sleek recessed lighting systems to the ornate chandeliers and many types in between.

RECESSED LIGHTING

When a more modern approach to lighting is the aim, the use of **recessed lighting** is often the choice. The fixtures are recessed into the ceiling, and may be used to house incandescent floodlights for overall coverage and spotlights to pinpoint certain objects or areas of a room. In addition to the stationary fixtures, many can swivel to provide greater flexibility.

TRACK LIGHTING

While recessed lighting is generally stationary and some may turn a little, the need may be to use a more flexible system of lighting. The answer is to use **track lighting.** Tracks come in two-foot, four-foot, six-foot, eight-foot, and twelve-foot lengths and can be arranged in many ways with the use of flexible connecters.

For the best lighting, whether it is to "wash a wall" with lights or accent particular objects, the track should be placed three feet from a wall that is eight or nine feet high, and four feet from walls that are ten or twelve feet high.

Once the track has been selected, the next step is select from the hundreds of different styles of containers or "cans" that are available. They range from the simplest contemporary cans to those that fit any design décor.

DECORATIVE LIGHTING

The chandelier has been a mainstay in interior design for hundreds of years. Period films have long featured these extravagant lighting fixtures to depict elegance and opulence.

Today's homes continue to feature chandeliers of every type, ranging from gilded, ornate styles embellished with crystal to more contemporary models that are often constructed from steel. In between are the carved, wooden lighting fixtures, wrought irons, glass, metallic, and other types. Some styles feature "cup" shades that conceal the bulbs and provide a decorative accent to the chandeliers, while others feature ornamental exposed bulbs.

Whether they are placed in hallway entrances or over dining tables, they are considered to be an integral part of interior design, often as the focal points in environmental settings.

TABLE LAMPS

Used more as decorative accents than for overall illumination, table lamps have remained popular ever since the lightbulb was invented (Figure 16.2). Designers and those who prefer

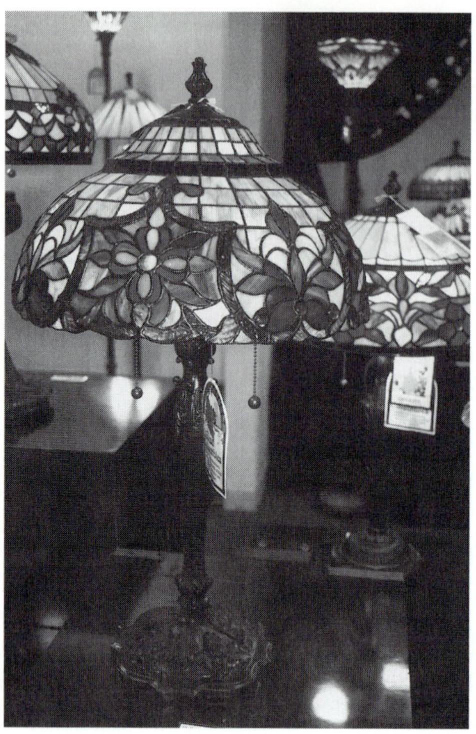

Figure 16.2 This Tiffany-inspired lamp provides a unique style and warm lighting.
(Courtesy of Ellen Diamond.)

to tackle their own decorating problems have hundreds of different styles from which to make their selections. Most often, the choice of lamps comes after the furniture is purchased so that they can be chosen to enhance interior design.

Every price point includes a vast assortment of table lamps. Ranging from antique to contemporary styles with a host of models in between, they include massive creations that might serve as a room's focal point and the smallest styles that might merely serve the reader who is enjoying a good book in bed.

WALL SCONCES

Decorative receptacles known as **sconces** are also found in many different materials and styles. They are used as wall accents, generally in pairs, to give some light, but more often, as a means of extending the room's design concept. Often used in period settings, antiques are made of bronze, wood, brass, and glass, with chrome and steel the choice for more modern settings.

WALL ART

Today, more than ever before, art is available in many different formats. These include original works, numerous limited edition prints, and posters. Each classification serves a different purpose and is generally chosen with cost in mind.

Original Art

Just as this classification implies, each work of art is created one at a time by an artist who wishes to deliver his or her "canvas" to a limited audience. When individuality and exclusivity is the aim of the designer or the consumer, **original art** is the choice.

The cost of these artistic works range from the exorbitant to the more modest (Figure 16.3). Museum quality works, such as those created by old masters or highly recognized artists, are extremely limited and are only within the reach of a few. Some people or companies have collections of these works and use them as the focal points of their environments. At the other

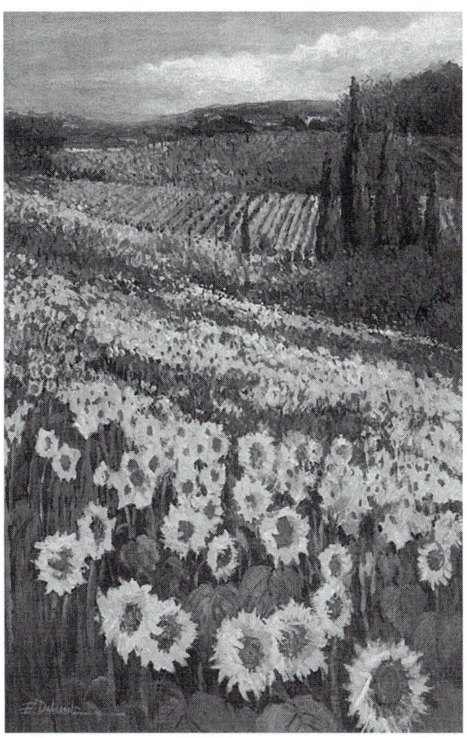

Figure 16.3 Original painting prices run the gamut from "priceless" to affordable.
(Courtesy of Ellen Diamond.)

end of the price scale are more modestly priced originals. They might be found in art fairs, galleries, catalogs, or online. These, too, give the collector a sense of individuality and serve to enhance any interior.

Original paintings are available in numerous media, including oils, acrylics, and watercolors. Subject matter ranges from the traditional landscapes and still lifes to the more contemporary abstracts. Selection of these artistic works usually is based on the furnishings they are intended to complement.

Limited Edition Prints

When price is a factor, and the intent is merely decorative in nature, **limited edition prints** are generally the choice. They are produced by the artist and his or her production team using a variety of techniques. Most common are lithographs, serigraphs, woodcuts, etchings, monprints, and giclees, a relatively new process that has been enthusiastically received by the interior design world. The term *limited edition* indicates that only a certain number of pieces are sold to the public. The number of the piece in the edition is indicated as is the total number that has been produced. For example, if there is an edition of 100 and the individual piece being purchased is the fifteenth to be run, the numbering will appear as 15/100. Extra pieces, known as **artist proofs,** are samples used by the artist to determine if the print meets his or her standards; they are also available for purchase. They are clearly marked with the letters *A.P.* on the face of the work.

Limited edition prints should be accompanied by documentation that indicates the method of production, where and when the piece was produced, and how many prints are in the edition. This gives the purchaser a history of the piece and helps to determine its worth.

LITHOGRAPHS

One of the oldest forms of print production is called **lithography.** Most lithographs that are considered to be quality pieces involve the artist's hand. These are called *original stone lithographs* and are the most expensive. Less costly lithographs include *original plate lithographs* and *mylar plate lithographs*.

- *Original stone lithographic* production begins with the artist hand drawing the image on limestone or marble. The entire edition is hand printed, then signed and numbered individually by the artist. A mark or *chop* is also embossed on each piece, indicating its authenticity.
- *Original plate lithography* is created by the artist who draws his or her composition on an aluminum plate. The plates are less expensive than their stone counterparts and easier to transport. Like the stone pieces, they are individually produced, signed, and numbered. They are a popular alternative to the stone prints since their costs are considerably lower.
- *Mylar plate lithography* requires the drawing to be accomplished on a mylar sheet. The rendering is then transferred to a photosensitive lithographic plate and then printed. Numbering and the artist's signature is the same as in the other two techniques.

SERIGRAPHS

Another popular method of producing prints is called **serigraphy** or silk-screening. For fine art products, the artist creates an original image, then transfers it onto a number of different screens made of mylar for each color. Then, each is mounted on a wooden or metal frame. A film that adheres to each screen is cut away wherever color penetration is to take place. Colored inks that match the original image are then applied, one at a time, by forcing them through the image areas that are not protected until all of the colors have been used to complete the work. The number of screens used depends upon the number of colors in the work. Each screen must "fit" perfectly so that the final piece will be rendered flawless.

WOODCUTS

A type of *relief print*, a **woodcut** involves the use of a raised printing surface. The artist prepares his or her drawing on a block of wood, and carves away the surfaces that are not to be printed. The raised areas, those that are left intact on the wooden surface, are inked and pressed onto the paper to produce the image.

ETCHINGS

The process involves the scratching of a composition into a coated metal plate that is ink resistant. The image is then given an acid bath to "etch" the scratched areas. **Etchings** enable the artist to produce artworks that are fine lined.

MONOPRINTS

Unlike the other types of limited edition prints that are used to produce a relatively large number of pieces, the **monoprint** is used to produce only one. The image is painted onto the surface of plexiglass, then uses a hand-turned press to print it. On occasion, a second print is made using the residual ink. It is called a *ghost*.

GICLEES

The newest form of limited edition prints is called the **giclee.** Taken from the French word for "to spray," the production is based upon the artist's original work that has been reproduced by computer. The term *giclee* is often used interchangeably with the word *iris*, because that is the name of the original computer printer that was used in giclee production.

The process begins with a digital photo or a high-quality transparency of the artwork. The image is then downloaded onto a computer. The artist and the printmaker then make adjustments to the computer-produced image, refining the elements to carefully match the original work of art. These adjustments include color balance, contrast, and density. Once the artist approves the computer image, a digital file is printed out on the giclee printer.

The printing process involves the wrapping of a high-quality archival paper, or canvas, onto a large drum in the printer. The drum rotates while nozzles spray the inks across the wrapped drum. The process takes about forty-five minutes to complete.

Once the piece has dried and is sprayed with a protective coating, it is ready for sale or to be further enhanced by the artist. **Print embellishment** has become a popular option to

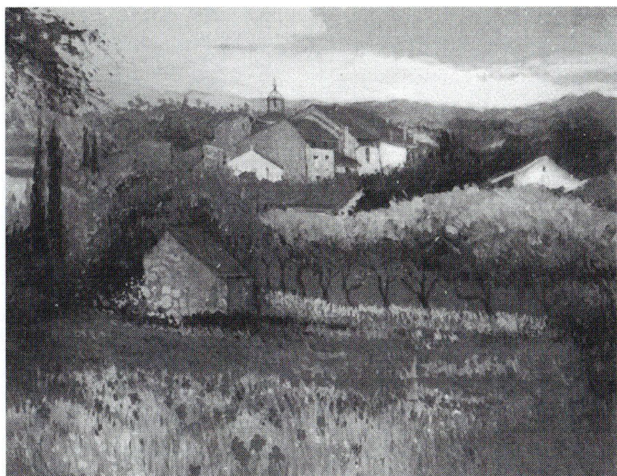

Figure 16.4 Giclee prints are high-quality alternatives to an original.
(Courtesy of Ellen Diamond.)

give each print an individualized appearance. While embellishing is done on paper prints, the vast majority is used on canvas. The result is a more textured and highlighted piece of art that is often mistaken as the original piece of work (Figure 16.4).

Open Editions

Rather than limiting print production to a set number of pieces, many artist works are reproduced as an **open edition**. If the market calls for thousands of pieces, as in the case of prints of works created by well-known artists and sold in museum shops, the images are run over and over again, sometimes for many years.

Any of the processes used for limited editions may also be used for open editions. The difference is that these are not hand signed by the artist, nor are they numbered. The artist's signature is in the plate. Since there are often a countless number of pieces in the open editions, they are modestly priced.

DECORATIVE FRAMES

The selection of the appropriate frame can make a work of art even more exciting. This is also true in the case of mirrors. Today's frame manufacturers produce the widest selection possible for consumers. The offerings may be those that are custom constructed from moldings and made to fit any size or shape; **standardized frames,** or ready-made types available over the counter; and antique frames often chosen to enhance paintings that hang in homes that feature antique furnishings.

Custom-Made Frames

Art galleries often feature a wealth of framing materials to fit any décor. Walls and walls of moldings ranging from the most ornate to the simplest are ready to be transformed into frames. The materials are most often woods that have been stained, gilded with gold or silver leaf, bleached, or painted. Hand carved or machine crafted, they feature styles that range from the heavily carved baroque types to the more simple contemporary (Figure 16.5).

For simple tastes, metallic frames are often the choice. They come in a variety of finishes that include gold, silver, copper, and a variety of colored paints. They are generally narrow moldings that are used to merely outline the artwork rather than add dimension. It should be noted that while most of the metallic frames are simple presentations, some simulate the carvings found in ornate wooden frames.

Lucite is still another material widely used for modern works of art. In addition to the typical frame mountings, "boxes" are created in which the art may be mounted. To give these

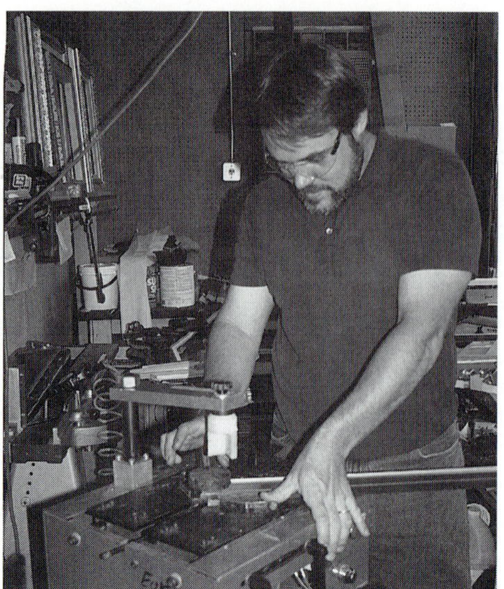

Figure 16.5 Custom-made frames are constructed in any size and style to perfectly enhance artwork. *(Courtesy of Ellen Diamond.)*

settings a more luxurious visual effect, the back wall of the box is often lined with an elegant silk or other fabric that complements the colors in the painting or print.

FRAME ENHANCEMENTS

After the framing material has been selected, the next step is to add one or more accents to the finished product. Oil and acrylic paintings and giclees on canvas are often framed with the addition of a linen liner that is attached to the frame and gives additional dimension to it (Figure 16.6). The liner usually measures a minimum of $^{1}/_{2}$ inch and a maximum of $1^{1}/_{2}$ inches, and it is typically a neutral color such as cream or white and its many variations.

For works of art that are painted with watercolors or prints such as lithographs, serigraphs, woodcuts, and etchings, which are printed on paper, **mats** are generally used. They come in a wide variety of widths ranging from a minimum of one inch to six inches or more.

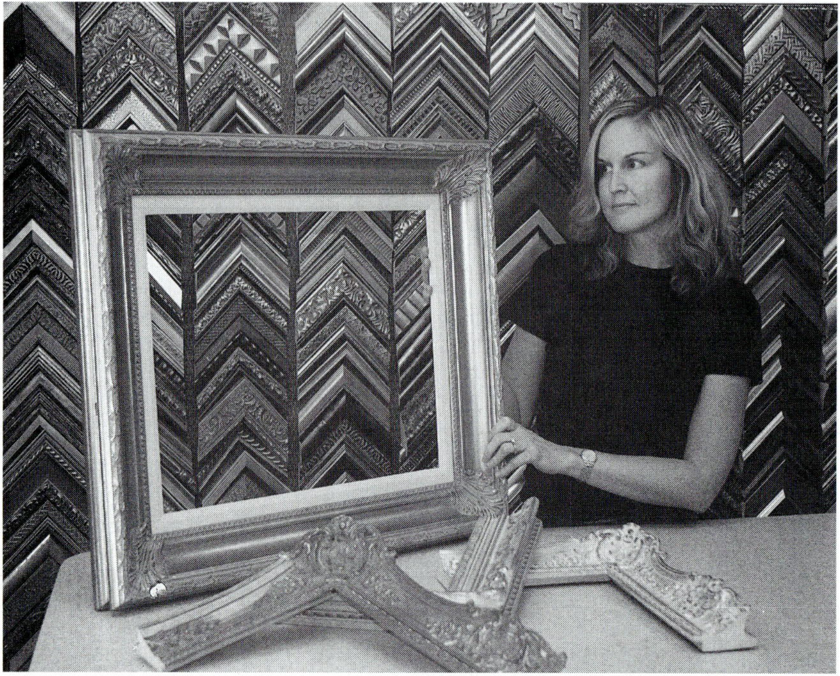

Figure 16.6 A completed custom-made frame features a liner to provide dimension. *(Courtesy of Ellen Diamond.)*

They are sometimes used in multiples of two or three to give more pizzazz to the piece. Color selections are numerous, ranging from a variety of whites to most any color. Common color choices are either a neutral or a color taken from the piece of art. It is essential that the mat be **acid free** so that it will be considered *archival*, or able to endure adverse atmospheric conditions. For the best visual presentations, the mats should be **bevel cut**.

Another accent that makes the frame even more attractive is the use of **filets**. These small metallic strips are attached to the mats to add even more dimension to the art.

Ready-Made Frames

When economy is the primary consideration or immediate acquisition is necessary, the choice of a ready-made frame is the answer. A variety of frames may be purchased in frame shops, hobby shops, and art galleries for immediate use. The only requirement for use of these frames is that the artwork is standard-sized. Typically the standard sizes are 5″ × 7″, 8″× 10″, 12″ × 16″, 16″ × 20″, 20″ × 24″, 24″ × 30″, 24″ × 36″, 30″ × 40″, and 36″ × 48.″ Occasionally, some manufacturers make other sizes available.

They are available in a variety of materials and styles and cost considerably less than their custom-made counterparts.

Antique Frames

In some cases, the frames that have been around for years are becoming more valuable than the paintings they hold. Serious collectors and museum curators are paying a great deal of attention to the frames that encase their works of art. The periods in which old paintings were created are increasingly being shown with frames from those eras. With the popularity ever increasing, the cost of these antique frames is reaching new heights. In fact, some frames are selling for $75,000 or more.

So popular are these frames that museums like New York City's Metropolitan Museum of Art have been putting on exhibitions to show frames without any paintings inserted in them. Many of the frames were created by famous artists such as Thomas Eakins, Charles and Maurice Prendergast, Milton Avery, Edward Hopper, and Andrew Wyeth, giving them even more distinction.

Protective Insertions

In order to protect art that is produced on paper, it is essential that a protective shield be used. Typically, the shield is glass or in some cases, plexiglass.

Glass is available in two formats, regular plate glass and **nonglare glass**. The former is clear and tends to present the most realistic image of the art. The latter is sometimes less clear and tends to dull the image. It is used, however, where the sunlight or intense daylight affects the viewing of the piece.

Plexiglass is an alternative that offers a nonbreakage advantage. This is often essential when the piece is to be shipped via commercial carrier.

Caring for Prints

While there is no guarantee as to the lifetime of any print, certain precautions should be taken to ensure their longevity:

1. Handle them carefully to make certain they are not damaged in shipping or through carelessness.
2. Protect them from extreme exposure to sunlight. Often, when exposed to extreme light for extensive periods, fading will take place.
3. Make certain that high-quality glass is placed over the print, especially if it is a limited edition, signed piece.

4. Repair "weakened paper," if this occurs, by attaching a high-quality paper that may be adhered to the work of art with an archival adhesive.
5. Remove wrinkles that may have occurred by applying moisture to the area. When this has been finished, the next step is to apply gentle pressure with blotters and weights.

Valuable works on paper sometimes need restoring. It is best to take these art pieces to a professional. These individuals may be found on the Internet through any search engine.

WALL COVERINGS

The interior designer's first challenge is to decide upon a style or period that will suit his or her client's needs and then follow with furniture selections, lighting, and perhaps wall art. The next step is often the selection of a wall covering that will enhance those choices. These include the use of paint, fabrics, papers, mirror, and novelty materials such as raffia that will perfectly complement the elements in the setting.

Today's designers and consumers have a wealth of materials from which to choose that will help bring all of the room's "ingredients" together.

Paint

Once merely a covering to bring some color to a room, paint has come a long way in terms of its choices and application. Even some high-fashion clothing designers, such as Ralph Lauren, and home furnishing gurus like Martha Stewart have created lines of paints that feature different textural surfaces. With modest expense and relatively quick application, rooms may be transformed into venues with special visual appeal.

Paint comes in two basic formulas, oil-based and latex. Each has its own characteristics that make one more suitable than the other for specific purposes.

Characteristically, oil paint thins out with the addition of mineral spirits or turpentine. Its drying time is much slower than that of latex paint, delaying the addition of a second coat often from eight to twenty-four hours. Odor is one of the negatives of oil paint during its application and drying periods, often making it unpleasant for the painter as well as the inhabitants of the home being painted.

Latex paint is the alternative to oil paint, with many characteristics that are different and advantageous to oil paint. It thins with water and thus cleans up easily. Spills, brushes, spatter marks, and rollers clean up quickly with the use of soapy water. It dries extremely fast, often from one to six hours, thus enabling a second coat to be applied in much less time than when oil paints are used. With practically no odor, it has become the choice of most painters.

Table 16.1 presents a performance comparison chart for top-quality paints, which was constructed by Bob Vila, perhaps the best known of today's home improvement gurus.

APPEARANCE CHARACTERISTICS

Within each of the classifications several different appearances are available. They range from the shiniest to the dullest.

- *Flat* is the word used for lusterless, shine-free appearances.
- *Low luster* paints are often referred to as those with *satin* finishes. They are resistant to marking and therefore are excellent choices for kitchens and bathrooms.
- *Semigloss* is somewhere between the flat and high gloss paints. It is easy to clean, therefore making it practical for use on doors and trim.
- *High gloss* paint renders a shiny surface. It is excellent for areas such as doors that get a great deal of use.

TABLE 16.1 Paint Comparison Chart

Category	*Oil-Based*	*Latex*
Durability	Excellent adhesion; better than latex on heavily chalked surfaces	Excellent adhesion; better elasticity than oil
Color retention	Not as good as latex, more likely to chalk and fade in sunny exposure	Superior resistance to color-fading, especially when in bright sun
Ease of application	More difficult to apply due to greater "drag," but goes on heavier for better one-coat hiding and coverage	Goes on smoothly and easily with less brush drag
Mildew resistance	Vegetable-oil base can provide nutrients for mildew growth; most products contain mildewcide to minimize growth	Less likely to grow mildew
Versatility	Can be used on most materials, but for new stucco or other masonry, a sealer or pretreatment is required	Can be used on wood, plaster, stucco, and brick surfaces
Odor	Stronger odor than latex	Very little odor
Cleanup	Turpentine, paint thinner, or other solvent	Simple water cleanup
Drying time	Eight to twenty-four hours	One to six hours

PAINTING TOOLS

Basically, the painter has three types of tools from which to choose: brushes, rollers, and painting pads. Other tools are used to create faux effects. Each offers a different advantage to the user.

- *Brushes* four inches come in a variety of natural and synthetic fibers, sizes, and shapes. For large areas, flat brushes that measure from three to four inches are most popular since they cover large areas in less time. Moldings and window sashes are best painted with angular or round brushes that measure from one to three inches. They also are available in different length handles, with the choice dependent upon the comfort and needs of the painter.
- *Rollers* are excellent choices for covering large areas. They come in a variety of types to cover smooth, semismooth, semirough, and extra-rough surfaces.
- *Painting pads* are primarily used for edging. The pads come on short-handled devices that may be lengthened with poles if the area is difficult to reach.
- *Faux painting* effects such as marbling, striping, and graining may be achieved with some common household products. For example, if a marbled effect is the goal, it is easily achieved with the use of a plastic bag to remove the wet glaze and reveal the initial color. A dry artist's brush may be used to give the surface a lined effect, and a comb may be used to achieve fine lines. A piece of screening mesh may be used on which paint is poured and a "toothbrush"-like implement is brushed to force the paint through the holes forming a spattered effect.

SURFACE PREPARATION

For the best results, paint surfaces must be carefully prepared before the paint is applied. The following are some steps professional painters address before they apply a coat of paint.

1. The correct tools must be carefully selected before the process begins.
2. Once the job is to begin, attention should be paid to proper ventilation, including opening doors and windows and using ceiling fans.
3. The surfaces must be completely cleaned, including the removal of dust, mildew, grease, and chipped paint.
4. If new plaster has been applied, it must be left to dry completely.
5. If there are cracks or open seams in the surface, they must be filled with a patching or spackling compound and left to dry before sanding takes place.

6. If a wooden surface is to be painted, and it has a shiny or glossy surface, it must broken into with sandpaper and primed with an undercoat.
7. Nails that protrude from the surface must be "countersunk" and evened with a fine-grade putty.
8. If the wall surface is not perfectly smooth, it is best to use flat paint since shiny types tend to emphasize the imperfections.
9. If the surface has never been painted, or the new color is much lighter than the original, it is best to use a prime coat before the regular paint is applied.
10. When wood with "knots" is being painted, a coat of a product such as Kilz should be used to conceal the imperfections.

EXERCISING CARE WHILE TACKLING THE JOB

Do-it-yourselfers face some hazards in taking on a job like this. Consider these precautions:

- Hands should be protected from solvents and other chemicals by wearing chemical-resistant gloves.
- When spraying paint, the eyes should be protected by the use of safety glasses with side shields.
- Contact lenses should be avoided since there could be the possibility of trapping vapors between the lens and eyeball, causing some irritation.

Wallpaper

The word *wallpaper* in the home furnishings industry has come to mean more than just the paper product. It is generally used by design professionals and consumers alike to include vinyl.

Each of these products is used to bring aesthetic qualities to the walls of homes and offices. Unlike paint, which comes in solid colors, wallpaper products are available in every conceivable period and color combination that enhance and augment the room's furnishings. In addition to the beauty it brings to the eye, it also often serves a functional purpose, in that many of today's paper and vinyl surfaces are durable and easy to clean.

With a wide variety of patterns, textures, and designs, wallpaper introduces light, mood, and personality to any environment. It also has the ability to cover imperfect walls, often a problem in older structures.

CLASSIFICATIONS

The following are the major classifications of wallpaper:

- *Vinyl-coated paper* is comprised of a paper **substrate** that has been sprayed with vinyl or acrylic. These styles are easy to care for and are scrubbable and strippable. Unlike plain paper that has not been coated, they are grease resistant and somewhat moisture proof.
- Instead of using paper as its substrate, *coated fabric*, commonly referred to as *wallpaper*, uses fabric that has been sprayed with vinyl. It is considered more breathable than regular wallpaper.
- *Paper-backed vinyl* involves laminating a paper substrate to a solid, decorative, vinyl surface. It is durable, scrubbable, and peelable. Since it resists moisture, stains, and grease, it is practical for most any room in a home.
- *Fabric-backed vinyl* is either a vinyl film that has been laminated to a fabric or paper substrate, or one that is a combination of a paper substrate/ground combination.
- *Stringed wallpaper* has fine threads laminated to a paper substrate. The strings are usually cotton, linen, or silk. Extreme care should be exercised when cleaning this surface.
- *Flocked wallpaper* is a classification that features a three-dimensional effect. The process involves the imparting of cotton, rayon, silk, or nylon fibers from a "hopper" onto a pattern that has been printed with an adhesive material such as varnish. The varnish "catches" the fibers and, when dried, results in velvetlike surfaces.

- *Natural fiber laminates* use such materials as jute, wool, cork, sisal, and grass that have been dyed or bleached and are constructed by laminating them to a paper backing. After the lamination process, the product is then printed to achieve the ultimate pattern.
- *Foils* are produced by laminating a thin sheet of aluminum foil or mylar onto paper. After the lamination process, designs are then printed on the surface.

MEASURING FOR THE JOB

Once the choice has been made, it is essential that the right amount of paper be ordered for the job. This is extremely important, because often vendors do not accept wallpaper returns. If a professional wallpaper hanger is employed, then he or she will do the measuring. Do-it-yourselfers can use a basic formula to determine the proper amounts.

The area of the room is measured, along with its height. Once this has been accomplished, the next step is to measure the windows and door openings so that they can be subtracted from the walls that will be covered.

Let's say the room measures fifteen by twenty feet with an eight foot ceiling, with two windows of three by four feet and one door that measures three by eight feet.

$$15' + 15' + 20' + 20' = 70' \text{ (walls)}$$
$$70' \times 8' \text{ (ceiling)} = 560 \text{ square feet}$$
$$3' \times 4' \times 2' \text{ (windows)} = 24'$$
$$3' \times 8' \text{ (1 door)} = 24'$$
$$560 - 48 = 512 \text{ square feet (walls + ceiling)} - \text{(windows + door)}$$

The number achieved from these calculations is then divided by 25 (the number of square feet in a single roll).

$$512/25 = 20.48\text{, rounded up to } 21$$

Other considerations must include the **repeat** of the wallpaper pattern and an extra allowance if the room is odd-shaped. A wallpaper supplier, once given these figures, will be able to determine the proper amount of paper to complete the job.

WALLPAPER CONSIDERATIONS

In addition to examining the different wallpaper categories and measuring to determine the amounts needed for the job, here are some other considerations to address:

- *Preparation of surfaces other than drywall and plaster.* When the underneath surfaces are paneled or bricked, they may be covered with wallpaper if they are carefully prepared. Lining paper is the best way to conceal the irregularities of these surfaces.
- *Hanging wallpaper.* When one opts to hang his or her own wallpaper, the challenge is not as difficult as one might think. The best results are accomplished when the manufacturer's instructions, available from the place of purchase, are carefully followed. Step-by-step instructions include the application of the wallpaper paste (unless the paper is prepasted), the matching of patterns, and the cutting of the rolls into strips.
- *Choosing the right wallpaper type for particular rooms.* If the project is for a kitchen, for example, the choice should be a scrubbale, stain-resistant paper; for a sunny area, one that is colorfast should be considered. These will give greater life to the paper.
- *Preparing the right equipment for the installation.* The tools and equipment should be selected before the installation takes place. Such items as scissors, utility knife, putty knife, level, ladder, sponges, drop cloths, paste brush, paint brushes and rollers, and paste adhesives satisfy minimum needs. If in doubt, paint retailers will help determine the actual needs for the job.

It should be noted that many retailers such as Home Depot and Lowes conduct clinics for do-it-yourself enthusiasts. These seminars take all of the guesswork out of paper installation and make the task a simple one to master.

WALLPAPER CARE

The proper care will ensure long-lasting use. The first step is to determine whether or not the paper is washable. If this is the case, then certain rules should be followed. These include careful sponging with a mild detergent in warm water, beginning at the bottom of the wall and working upwards toward the ceiling, making certain that the soapy solution is fully rinsed after it has been washed, and drying the paper with a soft, lint-free cloth. Abrasive cleaners such as scouring powder should be avoided since they will harm the paper.

For papers that are not washable, it is best to use a dry-cleaning sponge, a variety of which are available at wallpaper outlets. For the best results on these papers, follow the manufacturer's instructions.

DECORATIVE ACCESSORIES

Very often, when one enters a room, his or her attention is drawn to one or more of the accessories in it. The furniture that has been chosen sets the mood of the room, but the artistic pieces often give it a personality. The accessories available in today's marketplace can cost anywhere from thousands of dollars for a one-of-a-kind antique or contemporary work to many that sell for a few dollars. Those that demand the highest prices are generally found in galleries that specialize in rare and unusual creations while those that retail at the lower price points are often found in brick-and-mortar operations, in catalogs, and on the Web sites of such companies as Pier 1, Bed, Bath & Beyond, and Crate & Barrel. Even flea markets and swap meets sell accessories for the home, usually at bargain prices. Whatever the artistic level of this group of home furnishings, they are meant as environmental enhancements.

Within the general decorative accessories are many different types found in the home or business.

Categories of Home Accessories

Countless types of accent pieces, or accessories, fill households and businesses. Included are statuaries, urns, live and artificial plants, baskets, clocks, vases, and mirrors. In addition to their aesthetic appeal, some are also functional, in that they serve useful needs. Baskets, for example, may be used to hold magazines, and clocks, of course, are timekeepers.

STATUARIES

Striking statues are sometimes used as focal points in a room. They come in a variety of sizes and run the gamut from ceramic to wood. All around the globe, statues dating back hundreds of years, along with products that have just come off the assembly' line, fill stores, open-air markets, galleries, and designer showrooms. In Xian, in the People's Republic of China, for example, life-size replicas of thousands of warrior statues found underground are available for sale. Produced with the use of molds, taken from the originals, they are cast in plaster, and then finished in natural tones. Homes all over the world use these statues as focal points, especially when the setting is Asian oriented. In Greece, replicas of the Cyclades are also used in the home. They are available in white plaster or marble and are used in many contemporary settings. That region also produces a great number of different statues that represent the times of ancient Greece.

Wooden statuaries are also available. They are mass-produced with the use of lathes that can create the most intricate designs. Of course, hand-carved pieces are also found in homes, with many coming from Haiti, Jamaica, St. Thomas, and other Caribbean islands.

Marble figures are another decorative home accessory. Those that intrinsically valuable are hand carved with the use of hand and power tools. They too come from all parts of the world and fill every type of environment.

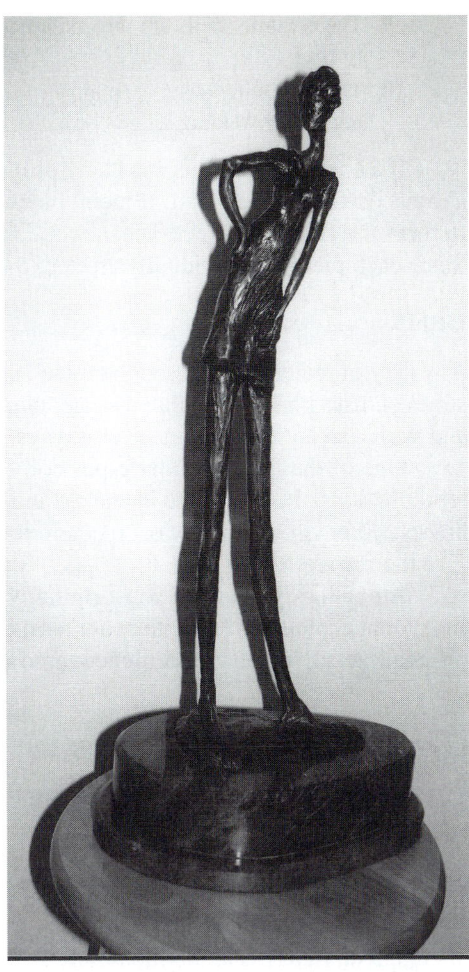

Figure 16.7 This bronze statue was produced with the lost wax method.
(Courtesy of Ellen Diamond.)

Bronze statuaries are is popular in today's homes. Since the production process is time-consuming and tedious, they are comparatively costly. The process that is used when several pieces are to be reproduced is called the **lost wax method** (Figure 16.7) and involves several steps:

1. The artist creates a design out of one of several materials. It might be a wire armature that has been covered with clay or a claylike substance, a wooden construction, or a metal base, each of which is also covered in clay.
2. The piece is examined to determine how it will be laid out or "sectioned" for the molding process.
3. The original sculpture is first sealed, then a mold release agent is applied to allow the mold, which is constructed with silicone, latex, or polyurethane, to be removed without damaging it.
4. The original is then covered with a coat of rubber and then subsequent coats of the same material until the desired thickness is achieved. When the rubber is completely set, a backup shell, made of plaster or fiberglass, is applied to support the rubber for the wax poring process.
5. The backup shell is then removed and the rubber gently pulled back so that the original sculpture can be removed.
6. The mold then receives the first coat of wax, then additional coats as deemed necessary. When sufficient drying has taken place, and it is completely cooled, the backup shell and mold are removed, leaving a wax casting.
7. The wax is then cleaned to remove any unwanted lines that may have occurred during the wax pouring process.
8. A secondary mold is then made by dipping the wax casting into a liquid binder material and covering it with a fine ceramic shell, or "slurry." This process is repeated as many as ten times so that it will be strong enough to hold the molten bronze.

9. The ceramic shells are then placed in the kiln, at which time the wax melts, and then left to cool.
10. The remaining piece is an unfinished bronze casting, which is finished by means of sanding and/or welding.

If a one-of-a-kind piece is being produced, a building-up method may be used in which various parts are assembled. If metal pieces are used, they are welded and soldered together to form the finished object. When wooden pieces are assembled, glues and nails are used. Since each piece is individually crafted, the cost is considerable.

URNS

A variety of materials are used to create urns, with ceramics leading the way. Other urn construction uses plaster, simulated stone, metals, and woods. They come in a variety of shapes and sizes and are finished in several ways.

One of the more popular types comes from the Provencal region of France. They are reproductions of those found in ancient times and have been faithfully reproduced for today's household environments. Most of them are glazed in a variety of colors and "antiqued" to give them a worn look.

A popular type of urn was originally used to hold and ship olives from Greece. Once functional containers, today they are used as focal points in many settings. Some of them are original pieces that have been uncovered in archeological digs, while others are reproductions cast in concrete.

LIVE AND ARTIFICIAL PLANTS

More and more designers are incorporating plants in their room settings. They provide a texture that is different from the rigidity of case furniture, the fabrics that cover upholstered pieces, and accessories that often employ ceramic, wood, and metallics in their structures.

The choice is either live plants or artificial replicas. Palms of all types, rising to heights of eight feet, ficus trees, spathiphylum, and numerous others are commonplace in interior environments. For purists, live plants are the choice (Figure 16.8). Of course they are sometimes difficult to maintain, requiring attention be paid to light and heat conditions. Their artificial counterparts are trouble-free and serve the same general purpose as the real thing.

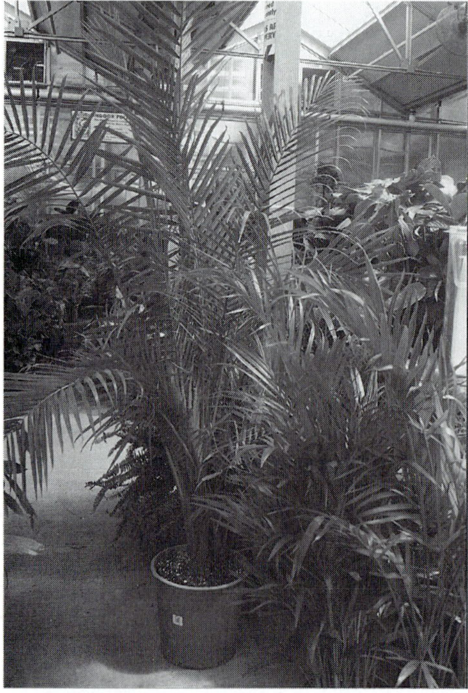

Figure 16.8 Live plants are used extensively in room settings.
(Courtesy of Ellen Diamond.)

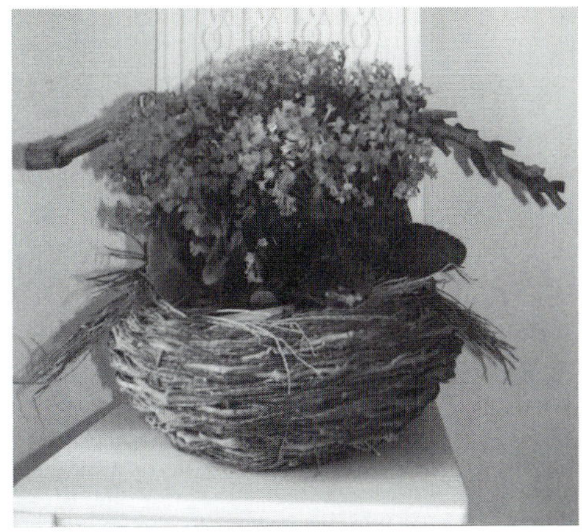

Figure 16.9 Baskets filled with plants are excellent accessories for the home
(Courtesy of Ellen Diamond.)

Orchids are particularly popular, where color is desired. Many varieties are available, ranging from the rarest to the most common. They require careful attention to thrive. Here, too, artificial types are often used in place of live plants.

A visit to any nursery will immediately reveal the wealth of plants suited to any design scheme or environmental conditions. These include bromeliads, ferns, cacti, geraniums, bonsai, African violets, and kalanchoes.

BASKETS

Wicker, reed, and other types of materials are woven into baskets that stand alone or are used to hold a variety of objects such as magazines, plants, and other items (Figure 16.9). They are plentiful in a variety of shapes and sizes, with the vast majority being modestly priced. More costly baskets are produced as works of art and may be obtained in galleries that specialize in these products. In cities like Taos and Santa Fe, New Mexico, artisans painstakingly produce intricate designs that cost several hundred dollars. Similarly, many of the regions of the world produce their own specialties that represent particular patterns.

CLOCKS

Although they are primarily considered to be functional products, many are used for their decorative appeal and grace the environments of homes. Majestic grandfather clocks, antique and contemporary, serve as focal points in entranceways and in corners of a room with spotlights to highlight them (Figure 16.10). Others are the table variety that sit on mantles and shelves, on walls, or in groupings with other decorative accessories. Some consumers are clock enthusiasts who collect clocks and display them as they would fine art.

VASES

Used as containers for fresh flowers, vases come in a variety of materials that include glass, ceramics, brass, silver, bronze, and Lucite. Retailers such as Crate & Barrel and Pier 1 merchandise large selections of the modestly priced pieces, while galleries feature the collectors' items. They are available in many different sizes, shapes, and styles and used with every type of décor.

MIRRORS

Although their primary purpose is functional, mirrors are used as decorative enhancements in just about every room in the house. They may either be framed to enhance the décor, or used as "wall-to-wall" installations in which they immediately give the impression of a larger space.

The variety of shapes and frames enable the user to select the perfect one that fits the specific room. Shapes include square, rectangle, round, oval, and others that are designed to mimic gothic arches or unusual architectural features. The materials that frame mirrors are wood, iron, metallics, inlaid and "veined" mirror, and plastics.

The mirrors themselves are either plain edged or bevel edged and are available in clear panes or somewhat antiqued finishes.

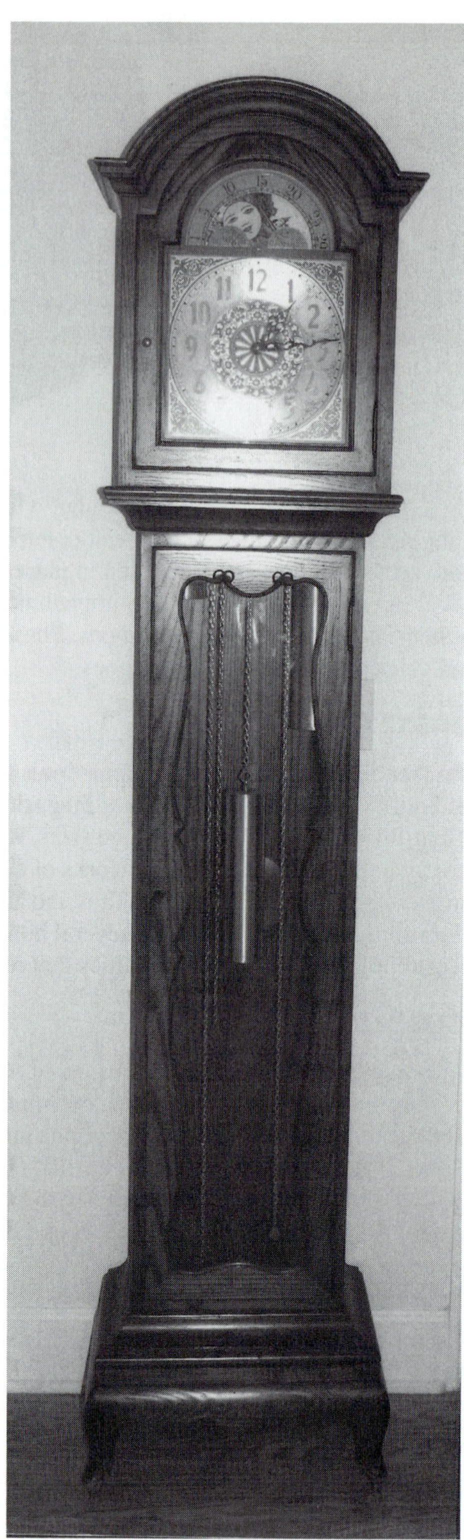

Figure 16.10 The grandfather clock provides a focal point in a room.
(Courtesy of Ellen Diamond.)

Internet Resources for Additional Research

www.collectorsguide.com/fa/fa010.shtml offers recommendations for preserving works of art on paper.
www.bobvila.com is master craftsman Bob Villa's how-to site.
www.interiordec.about./com/od/furniturestyles/ offers information on furniture styles.
www.answers.com/lighting for technical information on lighting and light sources.
www.wallpaperinstaller.com/anatomy.html explores different types of wallpaper.

Merchandise Information Terminology

Case goods
Upholstered furniture
Colonial furniture
Regency furniture
Biedermeier
Victorian furniture
Arts and crafts period
Art nouveau
Art deco
Danish modern
Incandescent bulb
Fluorescent lighting
Halogen lamp
Recessed lighting
Track lighting
Sconces
Original art
Limited edition prints
Artist proof
Lithography
Serigraphy
Woodcut
Etching
Monoprint
Giclee
Print embellishment
Open edition
Standardized framing
Mats
Acid-free mats
Bevel cut
Filets
Nonglare glass
Substrate
Pattern repeat
Lost wax method

EXERCISES

1. Prepare a research report on antique furniture, beginning with its origins and following it until the present time. An abundance of information may be obtained on the Internet by using your favorite search engine. In addition to the written portion of the paper, assemble pictures of different antiques and label their periods and styles.
2. Lighting continues to play an ever-important part of exciting home illumination. Contact a lighting company, many of whose addresses are on the Internet, for the purpose of gaining a telephone, personal, or e-mail interview with a company representative to learn about the latest trends in lighting. Try to obtain pictures of some of the lighting systems the company sells, and mount them on foam board for presentation to the class.
3. Visit a fine art gallery in your area to learn about how to properly choose art for the home. Write a paper on the gallery representative's suggestions and accompany them with photographs of ten pieces of artwork, their styles, and prices.

Review Questions

1. What is the difference between case goods and upholstered furniture?
2. What is another name used interchangeably with colonial furniture, and what are some distinguishing features of this period?
3. Differentiate between art deco and art nouveau.
4. How has the lighting industry improved the incandescent bulbs used to illuminate homes and business spaces?
5. Why may a track lighting system be more advantageous than a recessed system?
6. What does the term limited edition mean in the world of art?
7. Explain the three major types of lithographic reproduction.
8. Name the most recent form of printmaking and the basic steps involved in its making.
9. How can one be certain if there will be a ready-made frame to fit a finished piece of wall art?
10. Why is paint generally the wall covering of choice for most household areas?
11. Compare the color retention and odor characteristics of oil-based and latex paints.
12. What is the primary use of a painting pad?

13. How is vinyl-coated paper produced?
14. In addition to the wall's measurements, what other consideration must be addressed when ordering the proper amount of rolls of wallpaper?
15. What are some of the pieces of equipment and supplies that are necessary to install wallpaper?
16. Discuss some of the materials used in the creation of statuaries.
17. What is one of the most popular methods of producing statuaries when several of the same pieces are needed?
18. Why are plants so important as elements in a room setting?

CHAPTER 17

Bedding and Bed Linens

After reading this chapter, you should be able to:

- Compare and contrast the different types of mattresses available for consumer use.
- Explain the construction techniques used for innerspring mattresses.
- Describe the difference between *latex foam* and *memory foam* mattresses.
- List the various sizes of mattresses and the purposes that each serves.
- Explain the different types of bed pillow fillings and the advantages of each.
- List and explain the different types of convertible bedding available for consumer use.
- Describe the construction factors in sheets, pillowcases, and shams.
- Evaluate the different types of down used in comforters.

Where consumers once had a limited number of **foundations** on which to sleep, today's choices are numerous. They range from traditional beds and mattresses to those that convert from sofas and are primarily used when space is a problem and temporary sleeping accommodations are required. For example, in major cities like New York, where "apartment sharing" is the norm, a sofa bed is often the answer. Seating by day, with easy conversion to a sleeping space at night, this alternative is becoming popular.

Whether the bed is of the conventional type or any of the convertible possibilities, the selections are vast and are based on size, mattress types, and price.

The enhancement of the bedding is accomplished by the choice of **bed linens** that one selects. Once relegated to relatively unknown designers, today's linens arena has become a major segment of the fashion industry with marquee designer names lending their talents to produce exciting products. Names like Ralph Lauren grace the multitude of elements that dress up bedding.

BEDDING

The furniture and accessories on which we sleep are collectively known as **bedding.** Mattresses, foundations, and convertible beds make up the classification (Figure 17.1). The choices are more numerous than ever before, making it imperative for the consumer to be able to assess them before making a purchase.

Mattresses

Choosing the right mattress requires careful study and evaluation. The need might be for one that is merely a basic foundation that serves general requirements or one designed to deliver special contours and characteristics.

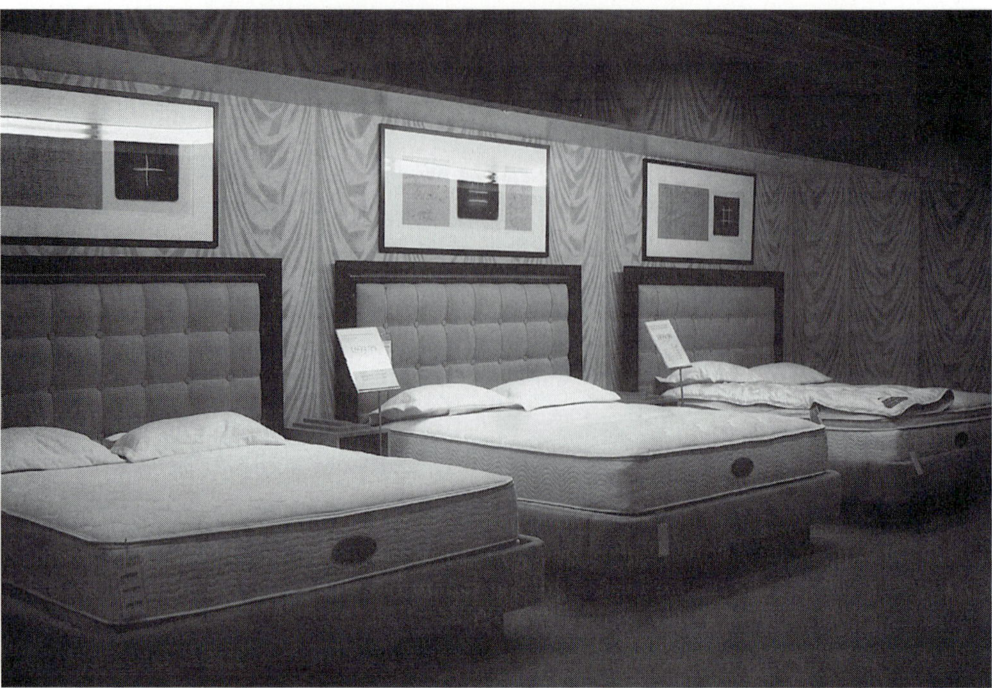

Figure 17.1 Mattresses are sometimes set on decorative upholstered platforms to add a fashion flair. *(Courtesy of Ellen Diamond.)*

When shopping for a mattress, different factors should be addressed to make certain it will fulfill the specific needs of the consumer and deliver the best available product. Some questions that should be addressed include the following:

1. *Is there sufficient support to properly handle sleeping requirements?* The entire body must be supported at all points, with the spine being kept in the same position as if the individual were standing. The body's natural curve should be considered and made to relax on the chosen mattress so that, upon rising, stiffness and soreness will not be present.
2. *Does the mattress deliver the required degree of comfort?* "Extremely firm" or "overly soft" are some of the words that one hears from consumers in their selection process. While these are personal preferences, the key is to obtain one that delivers comfort as well as proper support. Even the firmest mattresses are replete with cushioning materials to deliver comfort as well as a superior foundation. The core of the mattress makes the difference. One should test the product before making a decision.
3. *How long will the mattress continue to supply durability?* No matter how superior the product is when new, it will eventually lose the characteristics it had when first purchased. Therefore, it is important to evaluate the warranty that comes with the mattress and determine if it will adequately serve the user for an extended period of time. Warranties generally do not guarantee that support and comfort will be delivered for specified periods of time, but rather that defects will be covered. A careful reading of this document will tell the purchaser exactly what will be covered.
4. *Is the mattress the right size to fit the space requirements and needs of the occupants?* A room should be carefully measured and evaluated to determine exactly what size mattress will be appropriate. If a single individual is the sole user of the mattress, then a single or double mattress will be sufficient. However, if two people share the bed, then a queen- or king-sized product is more appropriate. Of course, space is a factor that must be considered along with preference. Today, mattresses that are six inches longer than standard sizes are available to accommodate taller people. The key is that there must be sufficient comfort for those occupying the bed.
5. *Should the mattress and foundation be a matched set?* It is imperative that a set be purchased to ensure comfort and the deliverance of satisfaction for as long as possible. Mattresses and the foundations upon which they lie are carefully designed and engineered to

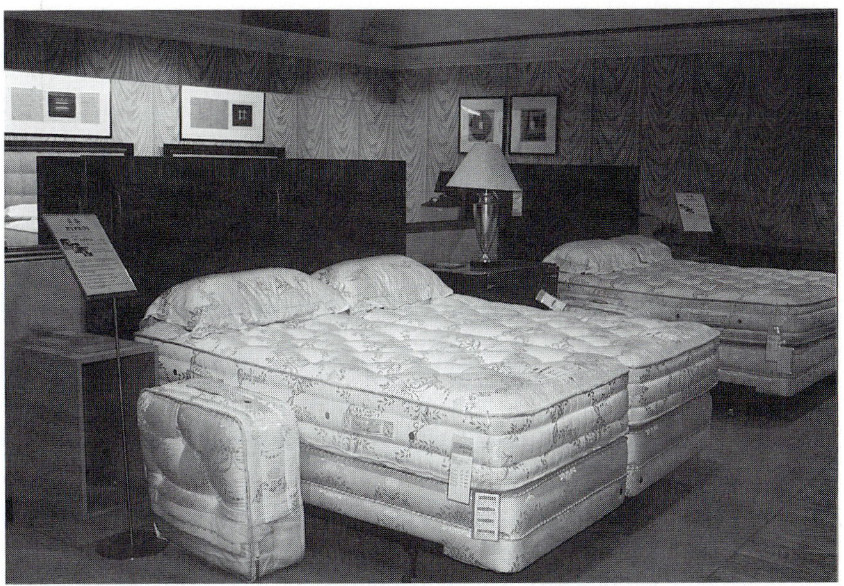

Figure 17.2 A mattress and matching foundation deliver the best possible sleep. *(Courtesy of Ellen Diamond.)*

deliver the best possible sleep (Figure 17.2). Using a new mattress on an old foundation might impede comfort and durability.

MATTRESS CONSTRUCTION

After carefully studying these questions, it is advisable to learn about mattress construction and determine if it meets individual requirements. The elements that comprise a mattress are as follows:

Foundation. The purpose of the foundation is to act as a buffer between the individual's body and the product. It acts as a shock absorber and is designed to support the body while fending off the wear and tear that comes from nightly use. It also offers support, flexibility, and durability.

Mattress Core. The middle of the mattress, or its **core**, may be constructed of different elements. Traditionally, the core is comprised of springs, but many products are foam-based. Others are either air or water mattresses.

Upholstery Layers. Usually the layers that encompass the mattress core are comprised of fabrics and cushioning elements. The fabrics are generally jacquard patterns and the under layers are often foam or other cushioning agents.

MATTRESS TYPES

The most widely manufactured mattresses are the innerspring and foam varieties. Other types include those that are air-filled and water-filled. The selection of a particular type depends upon the personal preferences of the users.

Innerspring Mattresses. The most popular choice is the **innerspring.** These types of mattresses are available in a wide range of products and include those that are extra firm, firm, or cushiony soft. The choice depends on personal comfort level and the support required.

The spring systems are comprised of steel coils. The thickness of these coils, the number of them in the construction, and the manner in which they work together contribute to the support of the body and their durability. Coil count alone, however, while important, is not the only consideration in the selection of an innerspring mattress. All too often manufacturers use a significant number of coils, but use low-quality coils in their production.

Since it is difficult for the layman to properly investigate the coil construction, it is advisable to make the purchase from a reliable resource where different mattress cross-sections may be examined.

The major coil systems are the **pocket-coil** type in which the individual coils are wrapped in muslin and are found in the high end of the market; **coil-on-coil** in which finer coils rest on top of the innerspring and provide more bounce; and **open-coil,** which uses many rows of hourglass-shaped coils, generally found in lower-priced mattresses.

Covering the springs is padding. Generally constructed of two layers, the padding provides comfort for the user. Each is made of foam. The top padding is often polyurethane, and the layer beneath is foam or cotton cushioning. Some of the higher-end mattresses provide a third layer for extra softness.

The outer layer of the mattress is covered with **ticking,** a term used to describe the fabric coverings for mattresses and box springs. These striped cotton materials are extremely durable. For more aesthetic appearances, more and more manufacturers are using sateen, jacquards, and damasks.

Foam Mattresses. Foams mattresses have become the preference for many household users. One of the major reasons for their success is that they are hypoallergenic and serve the purposes to those individuals who are sensitive to some of the materials that may be used in the construction of innerspring mattresses.

They are available in two formats, latex foam and memory foam. **Latex foam** is derived from the rubber tree and has natural qualities that conform to every contour of the body. It is considered to be the perfect sleeping material. It provides superior back support and relieves pressure. Allergy sufferers readily embrace foam because it is dust mite resistant and inherently antimicrobial. Rounding out its benefits, it is breathable and warmer in the winter and cooler in the summer. It retains its firmness level, maintains independent supports even when shared by two people, and improves body circulation.

Memory foam is made of **Visco elastic.** It is heat and pressure-sensitive material that gently supports the body. The material responds to body temperature and conforms to pressure, weight distribution, and support. Initially introduced in hospitals in 1989 to increase comfort and prevent bed ulcers, it is now widely used in the home.

Air Mattresses. One of the advantages of this type of mattress is that it may be adjusted to deliver the individual's desired firmness. Within a matter of seconds, different firmness levels may be reached by filling the mattress with different amounts of air. The mattress is constructed from heavy-duty vinyl that is encased in a foam shell. The outside covering is made of ticking, the same material used to cover the more conventional types of mattresses.

Water Mattresses. Once considered revolutionary, the **water mattress** was popularized in the late sixties and early seventies and is still used today, but in declining degrees. While it is said to be comfortable to the user and prevent bedsores, it has several disadvantages. The bed's weight can reach as much as 1,000 pounds, and the gurgling sounds and "waves" that may come from movement can rob users of sleep.

The water mattress is placed on a pedestal base that houses a decorative frame. Imperative to its use is the addition of a heater that will eliminate the cold surface it is prone to emitting.

MATTRESS SIZES

Several different standard mattress sizes are readily available. Others, such as round mattresses, may be custom-made. The standard sizes are:

- ***Twin*** the smallest of the mattresses, made to sleep one person. It measures 39 × 76 inches.
- ***Twin extra long*** as wide as a standard twin but four inches longer. It is 39 × 80 inches.
- ***Full or double*** meant to sleep two people, but is often used as a spacious size for one. It measures 54 × 75 inches.

- ***Queen*** sleeps two and is both wider and longer than the double-sized mattress. It measures 60 × 80 inches.
- ***King*** the largest of the mattresses, measuring 78 × 80 inches.
- ***Cal-king*** narrower and longer than the king mattress, measuring 72 × 84 inches. Like its name, it is found most often in California.

MATTRESS DEPTHS

In the last few years, the depth of mattresses has come to surpass the traditional measurements. Since mattresses are offered in these different thicknesses, consumers are alerted to make certain they have selected the appropriate sheets to fit them. The three classifications are:

- *Standard.* Seven to nine inches.
- *Deep.* Ten to fifteen inches.
- *Extra Deep.* Fifteen to twenty-two inches.

MATTRESS FOUNDATIONS

The most popular of the mattress foundations is the box spring. The best type uses helical coils throughout. The construction uses a wooden frame that encases springs that are tied together. The more springs and the better quality wire of which they are made, the better the box spring.

The springs are covered with padding insulation that is constructed from foam, felt, or cotton batting and then topped with the same ticking as the mattress. In better-quality box springs, corner guards are fitted so that the friction of the mattress on the spring will not damage the ticking.

Open coil springs are flat constructions that are left uncovered. The main problem with these springs is that they are prone to damage the fabric of the mattresses because of the friction caused by body movement.

Wooden platforms are sometimes the choice on which to place mattresses. They are usually made of solid, heavy plywood bases and are encased with decorative frames. During the 1970s they gained popularity as a decorating device in modern décors.

PROTECTIVE LEGISLATION

Congress and state legislatures have passed many laws to protect the health and safety of their constituents, even as they sleep. Thirty-one states and the federal government require manufacturers to identify mattresses constructed with new materials. Nineteen states mandate that mattresses constructed from used materials be identified.

CARE OF MATTRESSES

1. Spring mattresses should be regularly rotated at least every three months to ensure uniformity of wear.
2. Mattress pads should be used to protect them from soiling.
3. The mattress should be used on a proper base, such as a matching box spring, to ensure proper ventilation.

BED PILLOWS

Optimizing the sleep experience generally depends on the selection of the proper pillow. Unlike yesteryear, when pillow choices were extremely limited, today's offerings include different fillings and different shapes.

FILLINGS

Each of the materials that fill bed pillows provides different experiences and comfort levels. They range from the finest *down* to *latex.*

- **Down** is the most expensive of the materials used in pillows. It comes from the undercoat of the waterfowl and is extremely soft and lightweight. The best variety is *goose down.*

- **Feathers** for pillows come from a variety of fowl. Unlike down, which only uses the soft filaments, feather construction uses the entire quill making it less expensive, but not nearly as soft. Duck, chicken, goose, and turkey are some of the fowl feathers used in pillows. Goose feathers are considered to be the best, with chicken the poorest and least expensive.
- **Feather and down** combinations are often found in pillows. The purpose is to reduce cost but still provide some of the comforts of down.
- **Foam** is a popular pillow choice especially for those with sensitive skin. Its hypoallergenic characteristic eliminates the potential for adverse allergic reactions. The construction includes the solid molded variety and the shredded product. The former is likely to provide longer-lasting service. Foam pillows are available in different grades ranging from soft to firm.
- **Fiberfill** pillows are also hypoallergenic and are generally made of polyester materials. They are lightweight and comfortable alternatives to foam and offer another allergy-free material.

SIZES

Numerous pillow sizes are available to fit the sizes of the beds on which they are used. Table 17.1 indicates common sizes, dimensions, and uses.

Convertible Bedding

In crowded living quarters, a substitute for a traditional bed can save space and serve dual purposes. The mattresses and pillows used for these **convertible beds** are generally the same as those used in the more conventional types, but the bed types themselves are different and might be considered as alternates to typical bedding.

CONVERTIBLE SOFA BEDS

As the name implies, these beds are hidden in sofas and chairs and convert to beds. They come in a variety of sizes with queen- and double-sized mattresses generally featured. Once the cushions are removed, a quick pull of a fabric handle opens the sofa to a bed. They are equipped with many different types of mattresses in terms of construction and thickness. They are covered in every possible fabric or leather, and come in a variety of styles that can easily fit any décor.

STUDIO COUCHES

Usually measuring thirty-nine inches wide, the **studio couch** is actually two sets of mattresses and springs. By day it appears to be a couch, and by night, the bottom spring and mattress pull out to become a bed.

FUTONS

A mattress that is either rolled up and stored or used in conjunction with a frame is called a **futon**. Many of today's contemporary homes use futons on frames where space is extremely limited. The futon mattress is generally covered with a decorative fabric and draped over a wood or metal frame to be used as a sofa.

TABLE 17.1 Pillow Size Characteristics

Size	*Dimensions*	*Uses*
Standard	20 × 26 inches	Used with a standard size pillowcase; one for a single bed and two for a double bed.
Queen	20 × 30 inches	Two on a queen-sized bed; used on standard-sized pillows.
King	20 × 36 inches	Two on a king-sized bed.
Euro	26 × 26 inches	Used to house euro pillowcases; good for propping up while reading or as decorative accents.
Travel	12 × 16 inches	For extra comfort on long trips.

BUNK BEDS

Bunk beds are stacked one on top of the other and are generally used in children's bedrooms. The upper bed is reached by a ladder. They come in a variety of styles ranging from early American to contemporary.

TRUNDLE BEDS

The **trundle bed** is by all appearances a traditional sleeper. The difference is that it might have storage space underneath, or a separate mattress on which another person may sleep. In either case, the under piece is pulled out by means of a handle or "pull."

MURPHY BEDS

The ultimate space-saving bed is called a **Murphy bed.** It looks like a cabinet or "breakfront" against the wall. The façade may be lined with shelves or other decorative embellishments. When retrieved from the wall, a bed, ranging in size from twin to king, is revealed.

BED LINENS

Bed linens, which are both functional and decorative, include sheets, pillowcases, shams, blankets, comforters, bed spreads, bed skirts or dust ruffles, duvets, and throw pillows (Figure 17.3). Each is available in a variety of fabrics, designs, and styles.

Sheets

Mattresses are covered in sheets that are either fitted or flat. Generally, fitted sheets fit snuggly over the mattress with the flat sheet used between the fitted sheet and the blanket or comforter. They are available in matching or contrasting pairs, but are also sold individually to enable consumers to design their sleeping environment.

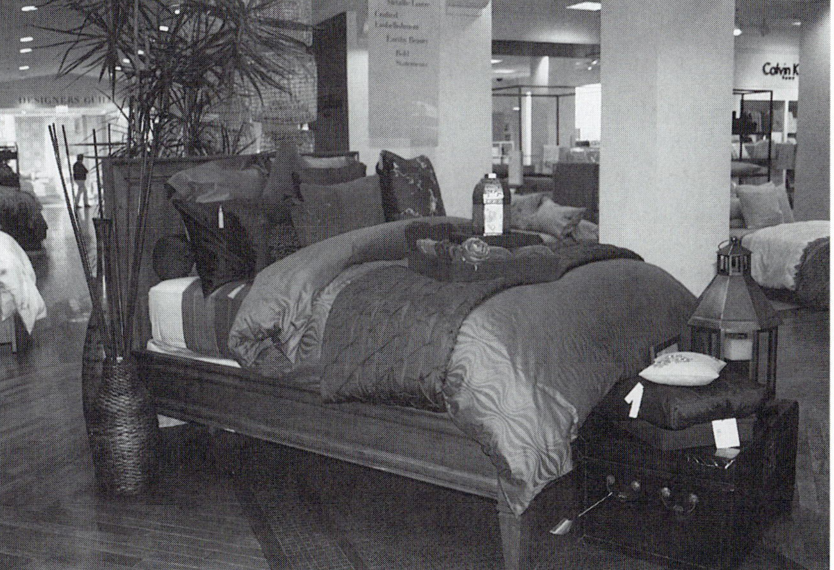

Figure 17.3 Decorative throw pillows add fashionable accents to beds.
(Courtesy of Ellen Diamond.)

FITTED SHEETS

Fitted sheets are made to snuggly cover the mattress. They are available in the following standard sizes:

Twin	39 × 76 inches
Twin X-long	39 × 80 inches
Full (Double)	54 × 75 inches
Queen	60 × 80 inches
King	78 × 80 inches
Cal-king	72 × 84 inches

FLAT (TOP SHEETS)

The **top sheet** is a flat construction that is larger than its fitted counterpart. Its sides fall several inches below the top of the mattress. The following standard sizes are available:

Twin	66 × 104 inches
Twin X-long	66 × 114 inches
Full (Double)	81 × 104 inches
Queen	90 × 110 inches
King	108 × 110 inches
Cal-king	108 × 119 inches

Pillowcases

The changeable coverings of pillows, or pillowcases, come in three basic sizes:

Standard	21 × 35 inches
Queen	21 × 39 inches
King	21 × 44 inches

The standard and queen sizes are sold in pairs, while the king size is sold individually. They are available as parts of sets, matching the sheets, or in individual patterns that coordinate with the sheets.

Oftentimes, a manufacturer will offer a *bed-in-a-bag* ensemble that includes a top and fitted sheet, two pillowcases, and a comforter, the latter of which will be discussed later in the chapter. This type of ensemble generally is geared to the cost-conscious consumer and offers a package that usually sells for less than the sum of the individual pieces purchased separately.

Shams

In addition to pillowcases, **shams,** or decorative coverings are used on pillows. These casings feature ruffles, eyelet embellishments, and other decorative touches that are used more as enhancements in a bedroom than for functional purposes (Figure 17.4). They are not intended to be slept upon, as are regular pillowcases, but are used to deliver eye appeal.

Shams are available as matching elements to sheets and pillowcases, or as contrasting pieces that give the consumer the flexibility to create more exciting environments. They come in the same sizes as regular pillowcases but generally feature "extensions" or contrasting trim that makes them aesthetically more pleasing.

SHEET, PILLOW CASE, AND SHAM CONSTRUCTION

The construction of sheets, pillowcases, and shams varies considerably. Woven fabrics are by far the most popular. The major difference from one to another is the **thread count** of the material (Figure 17.5). The thread count is determined by the number of horizontal and

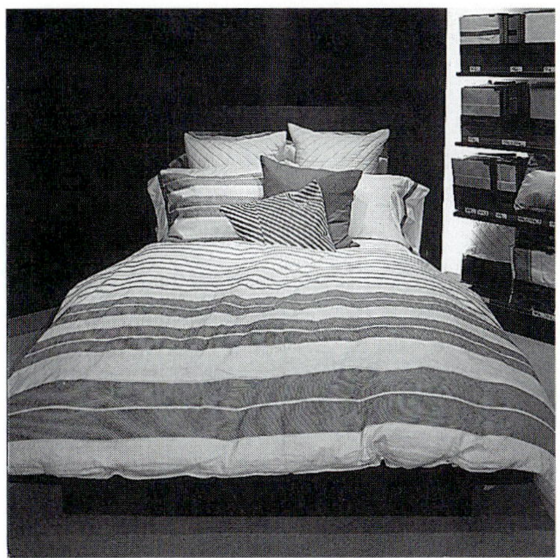

Figure 17.4 Contrasting shams make for a decorative touch.
(Courtesy of Ellen Diamond.)

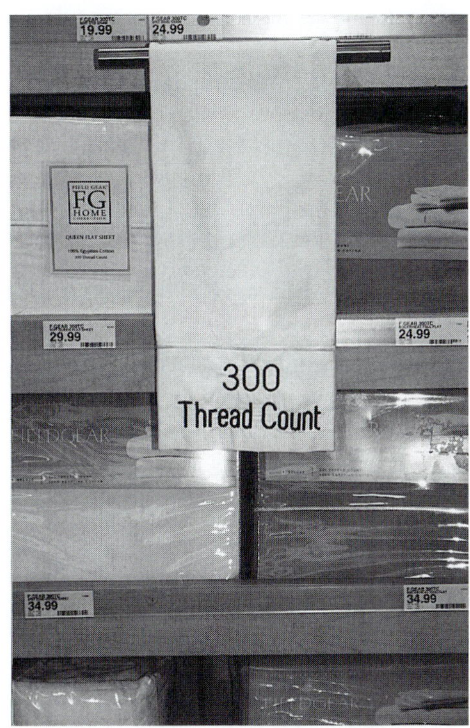

Figure 17.5 Bed linen construction is based on thread count.
(Courtesy of Ellen Diamond.)

vertical threads per square inch of the cloth. The poorer quality, known as **muslin,** has thread counts of 160 or less. The better-quality bed linens are classified as **percale** and features thread counts of at least 180. The former is a coarse type of construction and sells for considerably less than percale.

Today's quality bed linens continue to improve with some constructions featuring thread counts of 600. These luxury products not only feature high counts, but also finer-quality yarns such as *Egyptian cotton,* which contribute to their comfort levels.

In addition to the typical all-cotton goods found in most bed linens, a variety of blends such as cotton and polyester are available to provide consumers with products that resist wrinkling. Textures include the smooth types, typical of most linens; extra smooth, which resemble satins; and brushed flannels, which offer comfort and extra warmth.

In addition to the basic cloth used in their construction, embellishments such as embroidery, unique dyeing and printing such as silk screening, and unusual hemming such as scalloping are available, with each contributing significantly to the selling price.

A small percentage of the product offerings are knitted. These are generally cotton or cotton-blend materials that feature perfect fit because of their elasticity.

Comforters

These bed coverings are used both as decorative enhancements and to provide warmth. **Comforters** are not fitted pieces, but loose-fitting "covers" that extend several inches over the edges of the bed (Figure 17.6). They are available in the following standard sizes:

Twin	68 × 86 inches
Double	80 × 90 inches
Full/Queen	88 × 88 inches
Queen	86 × 94 inches
King	110 × 96 inches

Some vendors suggest using one size larger than the standard bed size to provide more coverage.

Comforters are available as matching elements in a bedding ensemble or as individual coverings that coordinate or contrast with the sheets, pillowcases, and shams. A large percentage of comforters are down-filled. They are covered in basic white cloth and are meant to be used with duvets, a covering that will be discussed later in the chapter.

TYPES OF DOWN COMFORTERS

The word *down* is meant to describe the soft, undercoat of fowl without the quills. Several types of down are available in comforters:

- *White goose down* is considered the best and longest lasting. It is white and extremely durable and has more fill power than duck down. It is a luxury product.

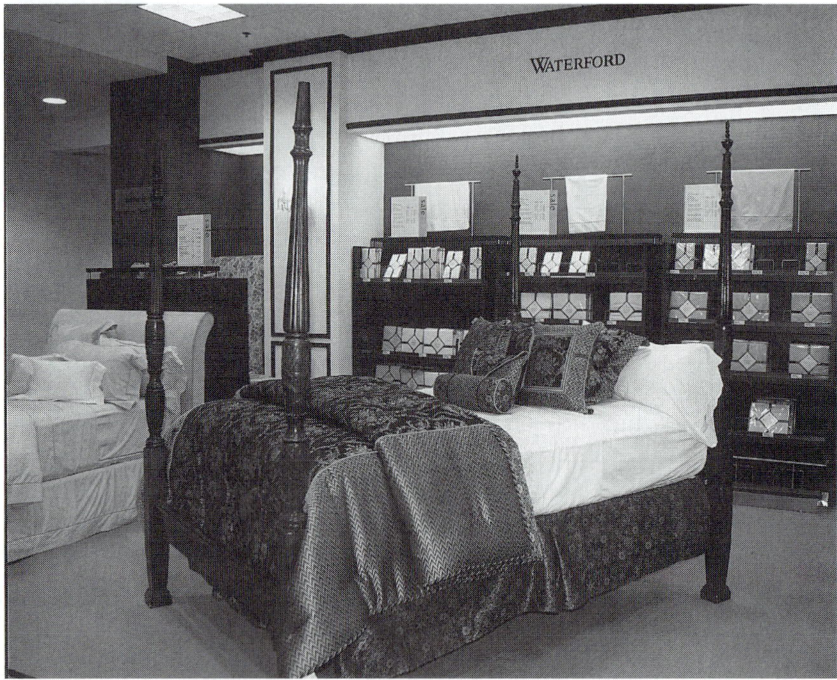

Figure 17.6 Comforters are loose-fitting "covers" that extend over the edges of a bed to provide warmth and decorative enhancement.
(Courtesy of Ellen Diamond.)

- *Eider down* is a brown product. It is considered to be the finest of the down products and is affordable only to the wealthy.
- *Hungarian goose down* is a fine product that has strong clusters. It is moderately priced.

Bed Skirts

The decorative edging used to cover the box spring is called a **bed skirt** or **dust ruffle.** It comes in a variety of designs, ranging from the shirred or gathered variety to the more contemporary box-pleated type. The cloth used for bed skirts may be the same as the sheets and pillowcase used on the bed, or contrasting types that aesthetically coordinate and enhance them. Eyelet, jacquard, brocade, ticking, velvet, satin, and embroidery are found on bed skirts.

Duvets

A cover that closely fits over a plain comforter, usually one that is down-filled, is called a **duvet**. It is slightly larger than the comforter it is to cover, and is generally fastened with Velcro, buttons, zippers, or snaps. The benefit of a duvet is that it can be easily changed to bring different looks to the bed (Figure 17.7). During the warmer weather months, the cover might be lightweight, while the winter months might call for a heavier cover to provide extra warmth.

Bedspreads

The formal covering for a bed is the **bedspread.** It generally comes in two lengths, either to the floor and completely covering the mattress, boxpring, and bed frame or to the edge of the mattress. The latter is known as a **coverlet.** In either case, this decorative enhancement may be manufactured in the same materials as the rest of the bed linens, in coordinating patterns, or in totally different designs and materials that give the bed a degree of individuality.

Bedspreads are either fitted constructions that carefully frame the top of the bed or loose-fitting types that are called *throws.*

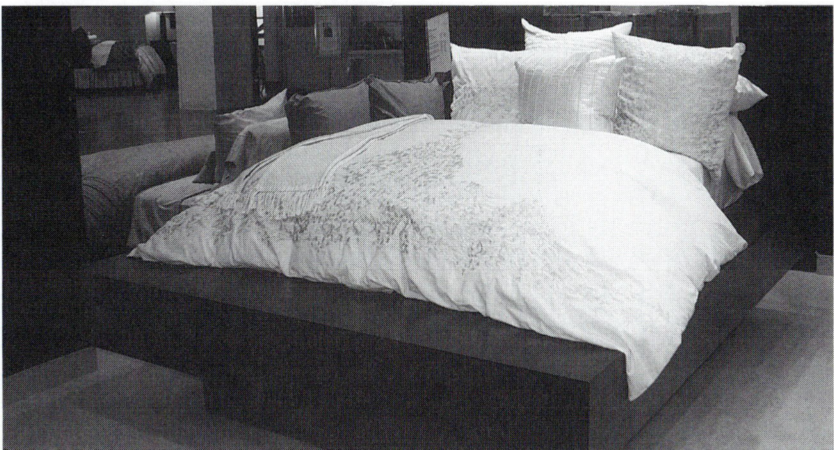

Figure 17.7 A duvet fits over the down comforter and may be changed to produce different looks.
(Courtesy of Ellen Diamond.)

Blankets

Being both decorative and functional, blankets provide color and comfort for the user. They are available in sizes that are the same as flat sheets and in a wide range of fibers and fabrics. Blankets are generally knitted and come in a variety of weights, with lighter ones for summer use and heavier ones for winter. Wool is the primary fiber used in blanket construction, although blends are available for those who want to be able to wash them without having to worry about shrinkage. For greater dramatic effects and more warmth, specialty fibers such as cashmere are available.

Electric blankets were the rage during the 1970s and are still sold today. However, many people are fearful of the long-term adverse affects that have been known to be associated with electric blankets, making them less desirable in many households.

Most blankets are woven, with some using a napped finish to provide extra warmth. Some are knitted by machine or hand, with intricate patterns adorning their surfaces.

Throw Pillows

The use of decorative **throw pillows** has enabled consumers to add pizzazz to the bed (Figure 17.8). They are used at the head of the bed as adjuncts to pillowcases, shams, and bolsters. They come in numerous fabrics that may be embroidered, quilted, ruffled, and even hand painted. The fabrics in throw pillows are satin, sateen, velvet, velveteen, brocade, jacquards, plaids, prints, and anything that will enhance the bed linen ensemble.

They range in size from the standard 16 × 16 inches to 24 × 24 inches and also come in oval, oblong, and rectangular shapes.

Bed Linen Marketing

One look at the prices charged for bed linens immediately reveals a wide range. As in the case of apparel, the quality of the material and the construction of the finished product contribute to the cost. Another factor in the pricing of bed linens is the signature of the product. There are basically four approaches to their marketing:

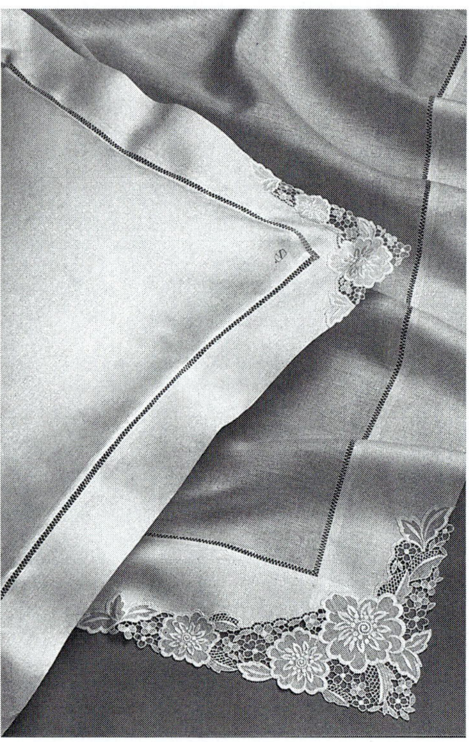

Figure 17.8 Throw pillows give extra pizzazz to the bed.
(Courtesy of Ellen Diamond.)

1. *National brands* such as Cannon and WestPoint Pepperell are the most prevalent offerings. Companies like these have been in business for many years and have established themselves as the marquee labels consumers often look for to satisfy their needs.
2. *Designer labels* have made enormous inroads in the bed linen industry. Names that grace apparel such as Ralph Lauren have entered this field via licensing agreements with linens manufacturers and have captured an ever-growing segment of the market. These brands tend to be more costly than the typical national brands.
3. *Private labels* have become an integral part of the marketing of bed linens. Major retailers have entered into contracts with national brand producers who design and manufacture linens that bear their own labels. In this way retailers eliminate the price competition of well-known brands and designer labels.
4. *Generic labels* are those that have little name recognition, but still deliver a wide range of products. They tend to cost less than the other entries since they are not heavily advertised or promoted, thus lowering marketing expenses.

Internet Resources for Additional Research

www.interiordec.about.com/od/allaboutbedlinens presents articles about upscale bed linens and product resources.

www.mattresstraditions.com offers information on mattresses.

Merchandise Information Terminology

Foundations
Bed linens
Bedding
Mattress core
Coils
Innerspring mattresses
Pocket-coil
Coil-on-coil
Open-coil
Ticking
Latex foam
Memory foam
Visco elastic
Water mattress
Twin size
Twin extra long
Full or double size
Queen size
King size
Cal-king size
Down
Feathers
Feather and down
Foam
Fiberfill
Convertible beds
Studio couch
Futon
Bunk beds
Trundle bed
Murphy bed
Fitted sheet
Top sheet
Shams
Thread count
Muslin
Percale
Comforter
Bed skirt/dust ruffle
Duvet
Bedspread
Coverlet
Throw pillow

EXERCISES

1. Visit a merchant that specializes in bed linens for the purpose of comparing the different product qualities. The following chart should be completed for five sheets and pillowcases that are featured in the retailer's collection.

COMPARISON CHART			
Brand	*Thread Count*	*Ornamentation*	*Price*

2. Visit a bedding store for the purpose of comparing the mattress offerings. Select five different mattresses and answer the following questions for each:
   a. What type of inner foundation is used in the product?
   b. Which element is used in its "core" construction?
   c. Are coils used in the construction, and if so, which type is used?
   d. In your opinion, is the price appropriate for the mattress?
   e. On what type of foundation is the mattress most likely to provide the most comfort?
3. Log onto any search engine to locate merchants who specialize in down comforters. By using the key words "down comforters," you should find several different vendors. Select a vendor that offers a wide variety of these comforters and compare the offerings. A chart should be constructed that features the different types of down, the prices of each, and their characteristics.

Review Questions

1. Define the term *bedding* and list the various products that make up this classification.
2. What are some of the considerations that should be addressed when considering a mattress purchase?
3. What types of mattresses are available to the household user?
4. Which coil system is found in high-end products?
5. Differentiate between latex foam and memory foam mattresses.
6. What addition is necessary to the waterbed to make it a viable sleeping surface?
7. What is the difference between a king and Cal-king mattress?
8. What is the best variety of down?
9. What are the dimensions of Euro pillows, and what purpose do they serve?
10. How does a futon differ from the traditional convertible sofa bed?
11. Does the trundle bed serve any other purpose than storage?
12. Do flat sheets and fitted sheets serve different purposes? If so, what are they?
13. Define the term *thread count*.
14. What is the purpose of a duvet?
15. What is the difference between a traditional bedspread and a coverlet?

CHAPTER **18**

Flooring: Rugs, Carpet, and Hard Surface Materials

After reading this chapter, you should be able to:

- Discuss the different types of floor coverings available for in-home and commercial use.
- Describe the many carpet classifications, their production techniques, and advantages and disadvantages.
- Discuss the regions of the world that produce oriental rugs and the different characteristics of each.
- Avoid the pitfalls often associated with the purchase of oriental rugs.
- Describe the vast assortment of rugs available in addition to the orientals.
- List the advantages and disadvantages of hardwood floors.
- Explain the popularity of ceramic tiles.
- Discuss the use of poured floors in home and commercial environments.

Today's home and commercial environments feature more types of flooring than at any other time in history. A wealth of products—rugs, carpet, wood, ceramic, vinyl, linoleum, and poured flooring—are available in a wide range of styles and prices. Not only do these floor coverings provide the user with aesthetic advantages, but also are functionally sound to fit most any requirement.

Rugs come from practically every part of the globe, with each offering designs and motifs that immediately enhance the surroundings in which they are placed. They may be hand or machine crafted, new or antique, and composed of different types of fibers and yarns. They range in price from under $100 to more than several thousand dollars. Some with unique designs and construction techniques are considered to be priceless.

Carpet, unlike rugs that come in specific sizes, are sold by the yard and housed in rolls. They are also produced at various price points and styles. Carpet is available for household use and heavily trafficked areas that necessitate commercial grades. The typical rolls of carpet are produced in a wide range of standard and fashion colors that will fit most any designer's needs or in custom colors and patterns for more unique settings (Figure 18.1).

Hardwood flooring is another surface that features both decorative and functional advantages. Used either alone or as under surfaces for area rugs, the choices are significant. Different natural wood and engineered patterns are simply installed or intricately placed to form artistic patterns.

Ceramic tiles are yet another type of flooring found in both homes and industrial settings. Available in a wide range of sizes, patterns, and colors, they are considered to be one of the most functional flooring materials available.

The characteristics of ceramic and wood were discussed in Chapter 6. In this chapter, we explore the styles used for flooring.

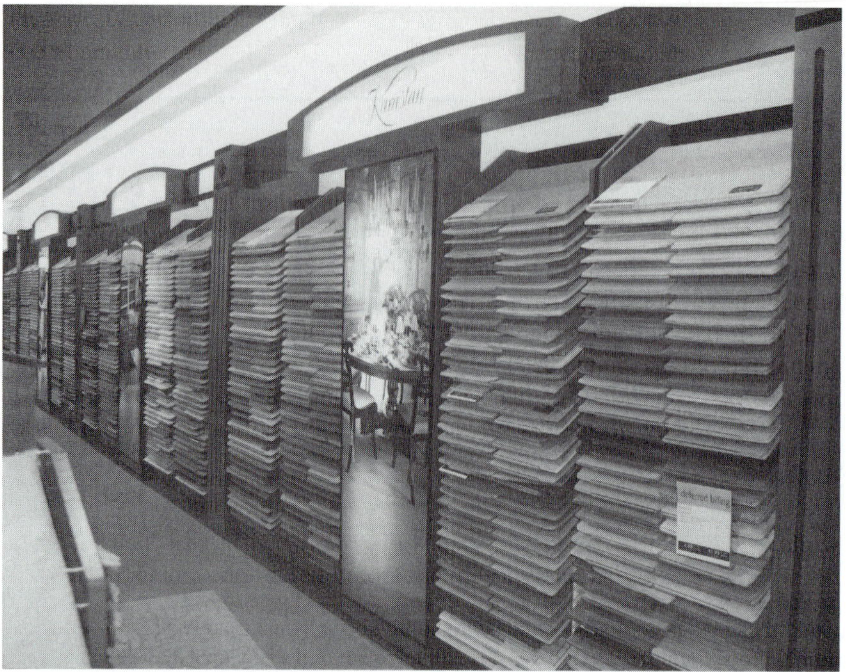

Figure 18.1 Carpet samples show the wealth of available options. *(Courtesy of Ellen Diamond.)*

Vinyl is yet another flooring product that serves the needs of consumers and professional interior designers alike. They come in a wide range of patterns and tile sizes that fit any décor. As an alternative, vinyl in rolls is less costly and appropriate for certain needs.

Linoleum is a hard surface material that comes in rolls and is generally chosen where price is the primary consideration.

Poured floors such as terrazzo and concrete are yet other surfaces used where durability is the key requirement. Although they are available in a variety of patterns and colors, their main feature is functionality.

CARPET

When carpet is initially chosen for home or commercial use, it is generally selected on the basis of appearance. Of course, price and durability are also important factors in their ultimate selection. Before the final decision is made, several factors should be considered.

Construction

Carpet is constructed in many ways, including tufting, weaving, needle punching, flocking, and knitting.

TUFTING

The vast majority of carpet made today is made by the **tufting** process. The procedure involves the sewing or punching of face pile yarns into a backing by a special machine that is equipped with numerous needles. The tufts are inserted lengthwise into a primary backing. In finer carpet the tufts are close together, giving the finished product a denser quality and appearance. The tufts are then set in place with the use of a latex compound that is laminated to the secondary backing. This final backing or layer gives the carpet additional strength.

The primary backing used in tufted carpet is usually made of polypropylene. For fine-gauge carpet, polyester is sometimes used in place of polypropylene. The secondary backing for tufted carpet is also mostly made of polypropylene, with jute or foam used to a lesser extent.

WEAVING

Woven carpet has been available for many centuries. Before the invention of machines, the products were hand woven. The process for both is virtually the same, with different types of weaves used for specific appearances and qualities. For more detailed information on weaving, refer to Chapter 2.

Basically, to produce a woven carpet, two sets of yarns are intertwined. These are the pile yarns, commonly referred to as *face yarns*, and backing yarns that result in a single "fabric." The three most common types of woven carpets are velvet, Wilton, and Axminster (Figure 18.2).

- **Axminster** is a machine-woven carpet that features an enormous number of colors and colorful patterns.
- **Wilton** is woven carpet made in variety of patterns and textures but with a limited number of colors in the patterns.
- **Velvet** carpet features a level surface or cut pile and is made of yarns that have very little twist.

NEEDLE PUNCHED

Needle-punched construction requires the assembly of *fiber webs* that are compacted and interlocked by means of barbed felting needles. The advantage of this type of construction is that the carpet can be printed, flocked, and embossed, the latter giving it textural effects. The angling of the needles and the mixing of fiber deniers (weight) produce textures such as corduroy. After the carpet has been woven, weather-resistant latex is applied to the back. The process is relatively low cost and is used primarily for indoor/outdoor carpet.

FLOCKING

Few carpets are made with the **flocking** process. The appearance resembles velour and offers a product that is resilient and crush resistant. The "fabrics" are usually backed with a secondary backing material to add body and dimensional stability. The carpet is sometimes used for bathrooms.

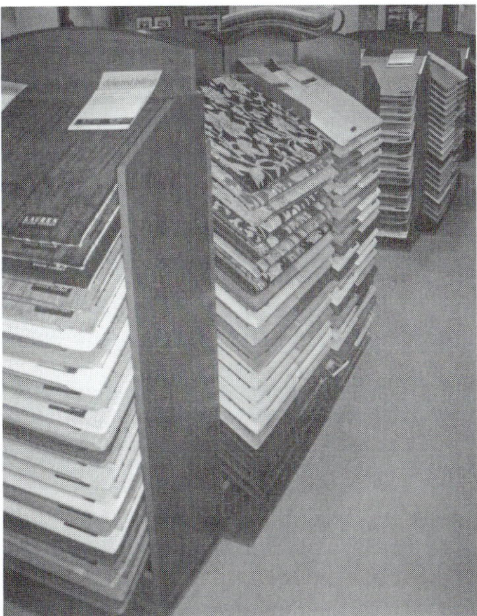

Figure 18.2 Woven carpet samples feature a variety of patterns from which the consumer may choose. *(Courtesy of Ellen Diamond.)*

KNITTING

The process is done on a **knitting** machine, and when finished, is backed with a coat of latex and a secondary backing material to provide stability and strength. It is used in a small percentage of carpet production.

SCULPTURING

A variation of the weaving technique, **sculpturing** produces a multilevel loop carpet. Two sets of loops are woven into the carpet; the taller ones are sheared and the shorter ones remain uncut to produce a sculptured pattern. This textured carpet, often with variegated coloring, has the added advantage of camouflaging soil.

Textures

A choice of textures is available to suit one's personal preference, décor, and durability requirement. They range from the smooth, plush surfaces to those that are rough textured. The variations depend upon size and twist of the yarns. The following are some popular textures.

LEVEL LOOP PILE

Loops all of the same height are produced to give the surface a pebbly appearance. For commercial purposes, the close loops make cleaning easier and improve durability.

MULTILEVEL LOOP

Instead of the uniformity of the level loop texture, **multilevel loops** are produced in a variety of different heights. This texture hides soiling extremely well.

CUT PILE

Unlike level loop and multilevel *loop* carpet, the loops in **cut pile** offerings are cut away. Velvet or Saxony carpets have a level surface, but differ in yarn twist. The former is constructed with yarns that have been slightly twisted, producing a smooth surface; the latter are more tightly twisted. It should be noted that one of the characteristics of cut pile velvet is the appearance of footprints when someone walks on it. It is considered to be the "beauty" of the construction, but should be avoided if that type of surface is not desired (Figure 18.3).

FRIEZE

A rough, nubby appearance is characteristic of **frieze** carpet. The yarns are tightly twisted and may either be replete with loops or cut for an even appearance. The advantage of this type of carpet is durability.

RANDOM SHEARED

In the **random sheared** process, only the higher loops are sheared, producing a high/low loop carpet. The sheared areas are less reflective than the unsheared and appear to be brighter and lighter in color.

CARVED

Distinctive patterns may be achieved by cutting away some of the surface. **Carved carpets** cover soil and require less maintenance.

Carpet Classifications

Numerous types of carpet are produced. Some take their name from their construction techniques, while others are named for their point of origin or intended purpose. In addition to those already discussed, the list includes Berber, Saxony, indoor/outdoor, and sisal.

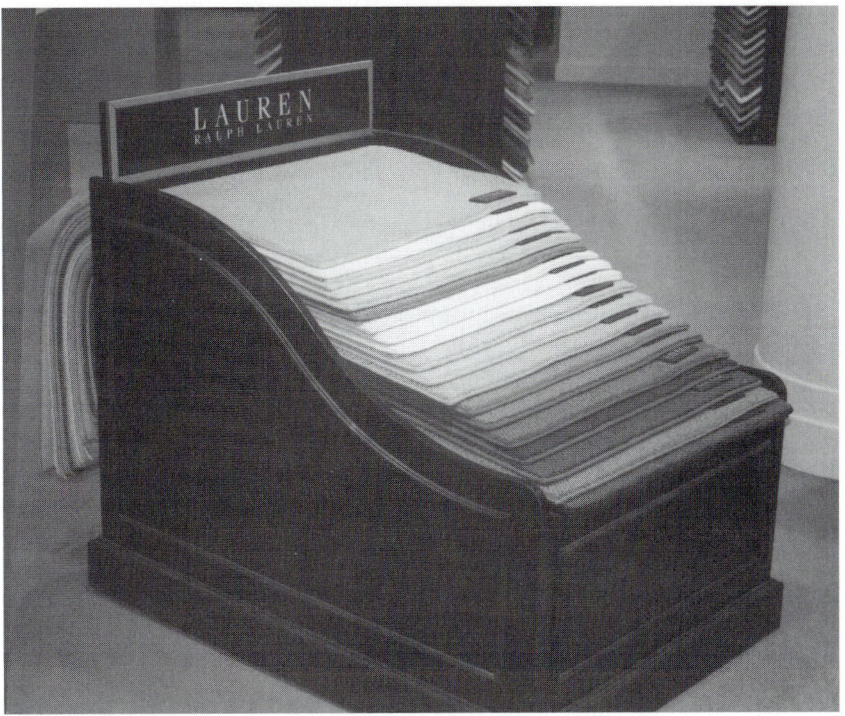

Figure 18.3 Cut pile, such as these offered by Ralph Lauren, are mainstay carpets. *(Courtesy of Ellen Diamond.)*

BERBER

Initially produced in off-white, **Berber carpet** appears to have the leathered looks of the garments worn by the Berber tribes of North Africa. The construction involves the use of flecked, looped yarns. The end result might be an even surface or one that is multileveled. Berbers are available in a wide range of colors. Generally, their use is in less formal settings.

SAXONY

Carpets that are extremely dense and have well-defined tufts are called **Saxony.** Those that feature the smoothest, densest piles are also known as *plushes*. Because they impart a feeling of elegance, they are generally used in more formal environments.

INDOOR/OUTDOOR

As its name conveys, **indoor/outdoor carpet** is made for both interior and exterior use. It is extremely durable and can withstand the adverse elements of the outdoors, and can also meet the demands of kitchens and other high-traffic areas. Generally, a rubber or latex backing is used on the product.

SISAL

Made from a natural plant, **sisal** is usually woven and comes in many colors. It is a frequent choice for less formal environments.

RUGS

The wealth of rugs produced today comes from virtually every part of the world. Each has a special personality that separates it from the rest. Ranging from the exotic patterning found in Oriental rugs to the more contemporary geometrics, the choice is based upon personal preference, décor, price, and aesthetic characteristics.

Hardwood floors are generally the undersurfaces on which rugs are placed. They may cover almost the entire floor or be used to distinguish certain areas from the rest of the floor.

Oriental Rugs

The true **oriental rug,** or **Persian** as it is often referred to because the first such rugs were first produced in Persia (today called Iran), is the mainstay of many interior designers' flooring components. The Oriental rug is a special product. As defined by the Oriental Rug Importers Association, Inc., "It is handmade of natural fibers (most commonly wool or silk), with a pile woven on a warp and weft, with individual character and design made in the Near East, Middle East, Far East, or the Balkans."

There are many quality variations in these rugs with the wool or silk, intricacy of design, and knot density playing the most important role. The degree of detail, the number of different colors in the pattern, and the number of knots per square inch, each of which makes the product significantly more labor-intensive, contributes to the price.

Although Oriental rug making is still practiced today, its early roots are in evidence in the Hermitage Museum in St Petersburg, Russia, where a rug that dates back to 400 B.C. is on display. Today these types of rugs are created in India, Pakistan, China, and Romania.

CONSTRUCTION

The initial stage is the design of the rug. Once that is completed, a loom is set up with the vertical threads, or **warps,** laid on the loom. Next, the horizontal thread, called the **wefts,** are ready to be applied. The interlacing of these yarns ultimately produces the rug. Of course, the design that has been laid out must be carefully followed so that the final product will be identical to the drawing. Such details as the size of the loom, materials, and variety of colors must be determined before any actual weaving takes place. The actual drawing, called the **cartoon,** is set on graph paper, with each square or box representing a single knot.

The weaving technique is very much like the procedure described in Chapter 2; refer to that discussion for a better understanding.

MAJOR PRODUCTION SOURCES

Many countries produce these rugs, with each offering something special. The more important Oriental rug producers are Iran, India, China, Pakistan, Romania, Turkey, Tibet/Nepal, and Afghanistan.

Iran. The first Persian rugs were produced in the 1500s. They became the best known of the rugs from this part of the world when the makers started to export them to Europe and, later, the New World. Starting in the 1850s, American, English, and German companies established factories in Meshed, Tabriz, Kerman, and Arak (formerly known as Sultanabad). These were royal factories where only the finest materials and procedures were used to manufacture the rugs.

The rugs from that region continue to be produced at very significant levels and are considered of the highest quality. In addition to the large factories, much of today's product's come from "cottage industries" found in the small towns and villages.

The finished rugs are available in an enormous range of designs, coloration, sizes, and weaves. They are generally named after the district in which they were made. Some of the better-known villages include Bakhtiari, Hamadan, Shiraz, Kurd, and Karaja. The most sophisticated, however, come from Tabriz, Kashan, Nain, and Kerman.

India. Influenced by the Persian culture of the time, rug weaving was introduced in India in the sixteenth century. They were primarily created in Jaipur, Kashmir, Agra, and Benares, where they are still produced. Their production not only rivals their Persian counterparts, but also is responsible for a unique creativity of their own (Figure 18.4).

India continues to be one of the major sources of pile and flat-woven rugs. They produce a wide range of qualities, designs, colorations, and sizes. One of the major reasons for

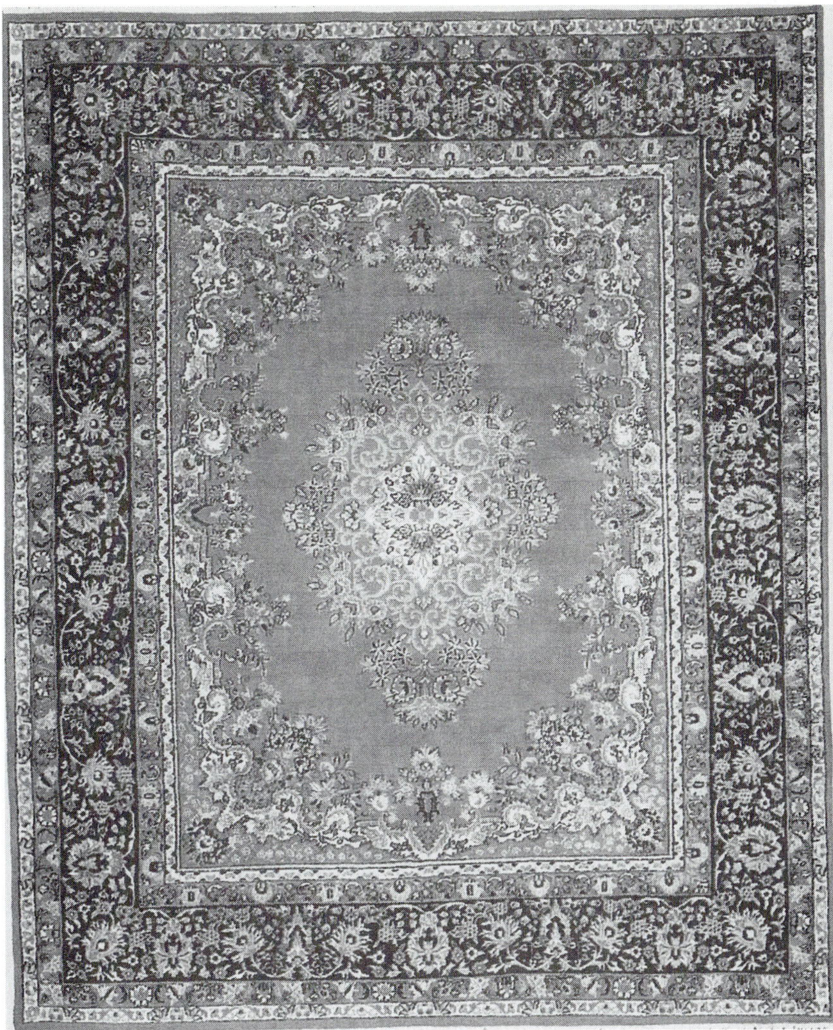

Figure 18.4 The Sardur design is typical of rugs produced in India. *(Courtesy of Ellen Diamond.)*

their success is their ability to quickly adapt to the ever-changing tastes of the Western world. Indian weaving is a cottage industry in villages throughout the Mirzapur/Bhadohi region.

In addition to the production of pile rugs, for which they are famous, Indian rug makers also create flat weaves, known as **dhurries,** and chain stitch rugs.

China. Chinese rugs were first produced in the mid-1600s, and continue to be sought after today. Through the late nineteenth century, production was exclusively for local consumption, with the noble and upper classes being the primary markets. The popularity of Chinese rugs occurred in other areas in 1900 during the Boxer Rebellion when the palaces were looted and the rugs were sent abroad. Rug making eventually became a major industry in the Beijing/Tianjin region. American importers made their requirements known and Chinese rugs became the rage.

While there are many small companies with just a few looms, major Chinese manufacturers now operate facilities with several hundred looms, weaving traditional patterns and many contemporary designs as well.

Pakistan. Carpet weaving originated in this region in the mid-1500s when several weavers were brought from Persia. When India was partitioned in 1947, Pakistan remained as its own rug-producing region. With the assistance of government subsidies in the 1960s,

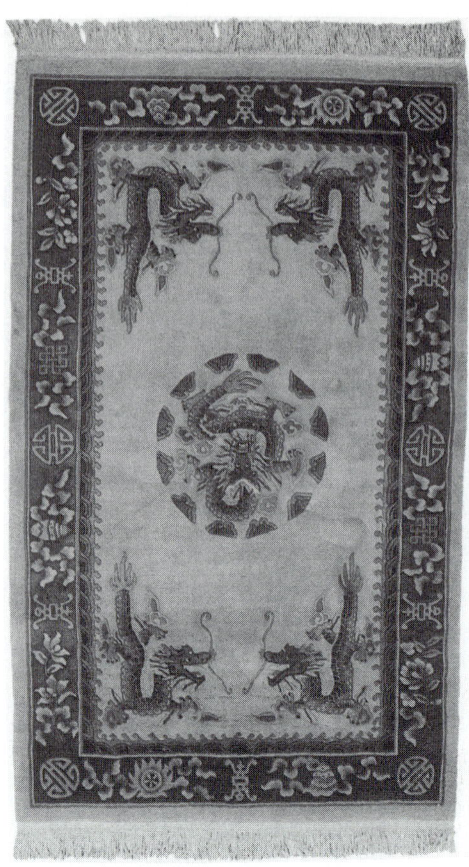

Figure 18.5 This is a traditional Chinese rug. *(Courtesy of Ellen Diamond.)*

it became one of the most important export businesses for the country. Unlike other rug-producing countries, rug weaving in Pakistan has remained primarily a cottage industry with only a couple of looms in each environment.

One of the reasons for their continued success is the willingness of Pakistani producers to create rugs that appeal to American decorative requirements.

Romania. Since the Middle Ages, Romania has exported its rugs. After World War II, government-sponsored weaving centers and cooperatives were established in which Persian designs were emphasized. Today, they continue to develop new qualities and designs that are required by their Western market.

Turkey. The rug-producing industry in this region dates back to the eleventh century. Today's production emphasizes the historic character of these antique offerings in contemporary colorations.

While Turkish rug manufacturers do export a great deal of their production, a significant number of rugs are made for both domestic and tourist interest. Tourists from all over the world come to Turkey, many of them intent on bringing home a "Turkey carpet."

These craftspeople have been credited with creative designs that bear unique handcrafted character. Experts in this industry predict they will become the "antiques of tomorrow."

Tibet/Nepal. In 1959, following China's suppression of Tibet, thousands of people fled to neighboring countries like Nepal. There, in the refugee camps, carpets were woven. By the 1970s, many of these carpets were exported to Europe. During the 1980s, the American market recognized these rugs as quality products and began to import them. These patterns emphasize "rustic charm," and feature a wide range of fashion colors.

Afghanistan. Unlike the more sophisticated Persian designs, the rugs produced in this region are more rustic. The vast majority of rugs are woven on small, portable looms, with

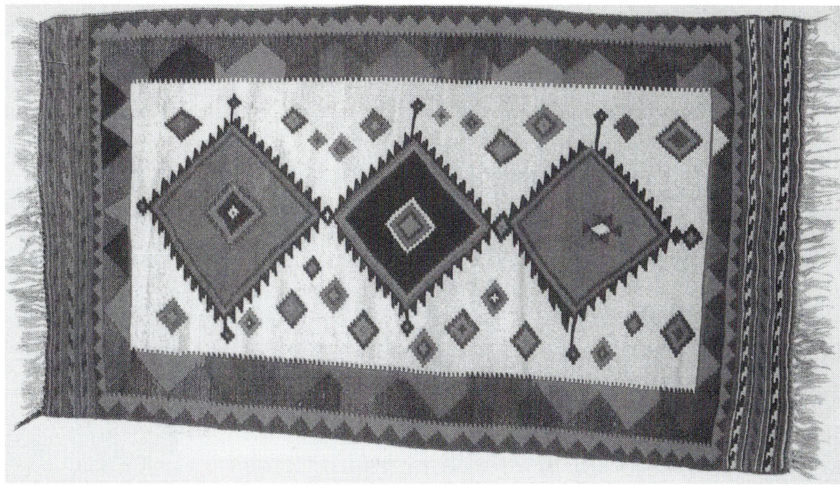

Figure 18.6 This is a typical Kilim rug.
(Courtesy of Ellen Diamond.)

much of the production earmarked for use in their homes. The number available is limited and the sizes are generally small.

TYPES OF RUGS

While the overall production coming from the aforementioned regions is classified as Orientals, they feature a variety of different styles. Included are *kilims* and *dhurries*, the major types, and others with lesser importance in terms of decorative use:

- **Kilims**—These flat-woven woolen rugs are produced mainly in Iran, India, China, Pakistan, Romania, Turkey, and Afghanistan. They are sometimes reversible (Figure 18.6).
- **Dhurries**—These flat-woven rugs are primarily produced in India, most often with yarns of cotton or silk.
- **Anatolians**—This generic name refers to rugs that come from the high plains of central Turkey.
- **Brailu**—Romanian rugs of the highest woven quality, with 105 knots per square inch, are collectively known by this term.
- **Drugget**—This pileless rug is from India or the Balkan countries.
- **Ghiordes**—This classic style of Turkish rug, often a prayer rug, typically features a narrow border and abstract flowers.

Table 18.1 represents the countries that are the main producers of rugs classified as Orientals and the dominant characteristics and colors of their production.

CARE OF ORIENTAL RUGS

Surprisingly, these rugs are designed to withstand harsh treatment. The skill involved in their creation helps them survive most normal use. With minimal care, they should last for many, many years.

These suggestions from industry professionals will extend the beauty of these rugs, and others, even further:

- *Vacuuming* should be done on a regular basis, at least every two weeks, to remove grit.
- *Professional cleaning* should be done every three to five years depending on the amount of evident soil. The process should be handled by an expert cleaner that specializes in Oriental rugs, and not the standard carpet cleaners that come to the home to clean wall-to-wall carpet.
- *Spills* should be attended to before the stain sets. Excess dirt should first be removed by scraping and then excess liquid should be blotted with a paper towel. A professional Oriental rug cleaner should be contacted for the exact type of cleaning agent to use.
- *Padding* should be used under the rug because it helps protect the rug from wear and also prevents slipping and wrinkling.

TABLE 18.1 Oriental Rug Characteristics

Country	*Characteristics*	*Colors*
Iran	Patterns, palettes, and weaves are linked to their indigenous culture; usually kilim constructed; geometric backgrounds with stylized flowers are dominant.	Reddish browns, blues, pastels, rose, greens
India	Flat- and pile-woven construction; wool and silk fibers used to produce rugs; dhurries, chain-stitch, and crewel-embroidered rugs are most dominant.	Dark reds, blues, contemporary colors that include jewel tones and pastels
China	Indigenous wool; floral patterns dominate, primarily in asymmetrical designs; some geometric patterning; products are either flat or pile woven; central medallion is often featured.	Dark reds, blues, contemporary colors
Pakistan	Indigenous and imported wools; repetitive octagonal motifs; gul (rose) motifs; geometric, contemporary designs.	Reds, rusts, ivories, pastels, peaches, corals, greys
Romania	Coarse, resilient wools; Persian-inspired designs; antique-style reproductions; kilims that feature folk art traditions; curvilinear floral designs.	Traditional and fashion colors
Turkey	Pile and flat weaves; wool and silk fibers; handspun and vegetable dyed fibers; recreation of Ottoman patterns; geometrics and curvilinear floral motifs.	Reds, blues, teals, greens, greys, peach, ivories
Tibet/Nepal	Primitive, hand-crafted looks; highly stylized patterns; Buddhist religion symbols; phoenix, dragon, and lotus symbols.	Reds, blues, lavenders, greys
Afghanistan	Vegetable-dyed hand-spun Afghan wool; coarse to medium waves; geometric patterns.	Dark reds, blues, blacks, ivories, greens

- *Carpet turning* 180 degrees every year will help even out the rug's exposure to traffic and sunlight.
- *Repairs* such as those needed to repair holes, tears, or worn surfaces, should be accomplished by professionals.

AVOIDING PURCHASING PITFALLS

With the significant cost attributed to the purchase of Oriental rugs, one must approach the transaction with considerable care. All too often, merchants use questionable tactics to entice potential purchasers to buy their products. Some of the suggestions made by professionals in the field include:

- Avoid places that offer prices that seem "too good to be true." Oftentimes, upon inspection of these advertised specials, the statement is absolutely true. When discounts are upwards of 60 percent or more, it is probable that the initial prices were inflated so that the deductions might be taken. Merchants are in business to make a profit, and any logical mathematics compels us to know that these exorbitant discounts do not leave any room for profit.
- Be wary of auctions sometimes advertised to take place in hotels and other temporary facilities. The quality of the merchandise and the prices are suspect. Since these are usually one-day events, the merchants will be off to another venue the next day and, if buyers are unhappy with their purchase, they cannot easily track down the seller.
- Be cautious about "going-out-of-business" sales often associated with rug merchants. These may be just marketing scams to entice people into thinking they are getting rock-bottom prices. Also if the company is going to suspend its business activities, it may add low-quality products to its inventory along with regular merchandise. Only a seasoned buyer can evaluate the actual worthiness of the rugs.

Other Rug Types

In addition to Orientals, numerous other rugs are used in both residential and commercial premises. They may be hand or machine made in many parts of the world. The range varies considerably in terms of styles, yarns, construction, patterning, and price. The following is a compilation of some of these rugs, along with the regions of the world in which they are produced. The list is by no means all-inclusive.

RYA RUGS

This deep pile rug was initially introduced in Scandinavia. **Rya rugs** were originally woven on a loom, but in later years they were produced on a canvas foundation where the yarns were knotted with a ratchet hook. They are rich in texture and are individually colored to meet the design requirements of the environments in which they will be placed.

FLOKATI RUGS

Flokati rugs are shag rugs that come in a wide range of colors. They are made in Greece of pure wool. They are used primarily as accents in any part of the home, with the bedroom as a primary location because of the warmth they provide.

SOUTHWESTERN RUGS

The vast majority of **Southwestern rugs** are produced in New Mexico and feature Navajo-inspired designs. They are primarily used as enhancements in rustic room settings.

ZAPOTEC RUGS

Hand loomed of 100 percent wool, **zapotec rugs** are produced in Oaxaca, Mexico. They are one-of-a-kind products that generally feature traditional Mexican and Mayan patterns. Each is fringed with two-inch borders.

NAVAJO RUGS

Taos, New Mexico, is one of the major areas in which **Navajo rugs** are created. They are handwoven by Navajo weavers and feature Native American designs.

RUGS INSPIRED BY FINE ART

Many renowned artists' motifs have been translated into rugs of all sizes. The artwork of Andy Warhol, for example, is used to produce a wealth of contemporary designed rugs, including abstracts and other subject matter.

Pablo Picasso is also a source of art-inspired rugs. They are primarily produced in Belgium of 100 percent New Zealand wool, considered to be the finest in the world.

BRAIDED RUGS

The yarns are braided in a manner similar to that used in hair braiding. The braids are then sewn adjacent to each other to form either an oval or round **braided rugs.**

HARD SURFACE FLOORS

Household and commercial environments feature a number of different types of hard surfaces, including wood, ceramics, marble, cork, linoleum, and poured materials. Each is selected to serve both aesthetic and functional needs.

Wood

The patterning obtained in wood installations ranges from simple planking to the most elaborate parquet designs. They are either used alone or as bases on which area rugs are featured. As we learned in Chapter 6, numerous types of wood are appropriate for flooring. The most widely used hardwood for flooring installations is oak, with maple, teak, and pine used less frequently.

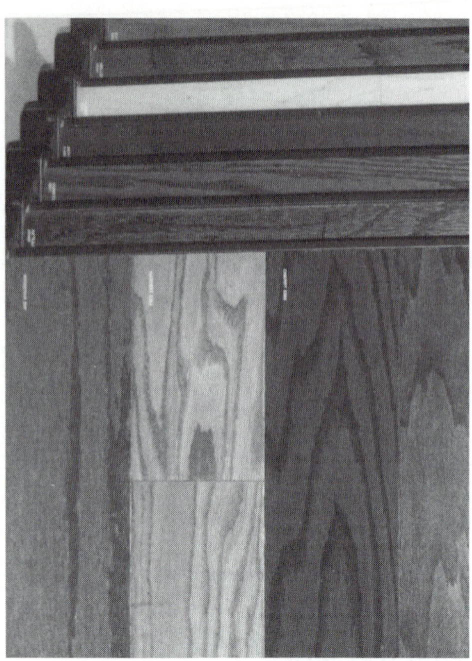

Figure 18.7 Plank flooring comes in many widths. *(Courtesy of Ellen Diamond.)*

TYPES OF WOOD FLOORS

Basically, three types of wood floors are used in every type of environment. Each offers a different feeling and is used to enhance the design of the room in which it will be installed. They are *plank, strip,* and *parquet.*

PLANK FLOORING

Planks of wood that have been used before and have been retrieved for new use come in widths that range from 2 to eight inches, with five and six inches the most typical (Figure 18.7). **Plank flooring** is most often used to provide a rustic look to interiors. Installations may either be uniform, using all of the same widths, or "random" with a variety of widths. Lengths may also be uniform or random to add interest to the design. Each plank generally features tongue and groove sides that interlock to provide a more secure foundation.

Strip Flooring. The strips are narrower than the pieces known as planking. **Strip flooring** measure 2¼, 1½, or 3¼ inches in width. It is also planked. Strip flooring may be installed diagonally for a more dramatic effect (Figure 18.8).

Parquet Flooring. The most detailed, artistic floors are created with the use of wood pieces that form geometric designs. In these pieces, different types of woods are generally used to give additional interest to the completed **parguet floor** design (Figure 18.9).

ADVANTAGES OF WOOD FLOORS

In addition to their aesthetic qualities, wood floors offer a host of different benefits to the user:

Resale Value. When used in home construction and design, professional sales agents report that the value of homes with wood floors will increase over the years. Wood floors generally help sell the property faster.

Minimum Maintenance. With no more than the use of regular vacuuming or sweeping with a broom, wood floors are easy to keep clean and in good condition. Occasionally, a professional wood cleaner should be used to bring the wood back to its original sheen and clarity.

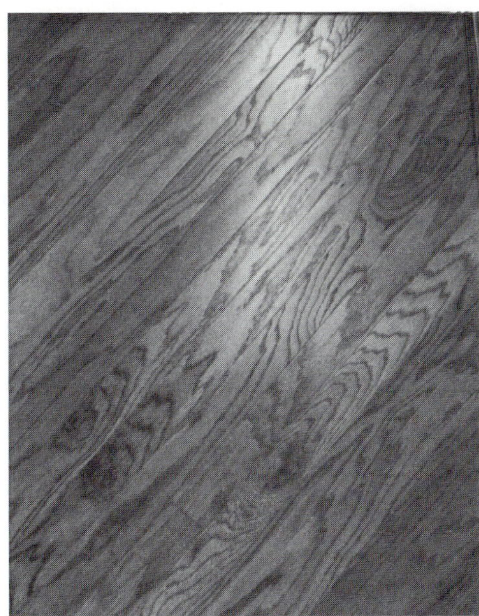

Figure 18.8 Strip flooring is often diagonally installed for greater design interest.
(Courtesy of Ellen Diamond.)

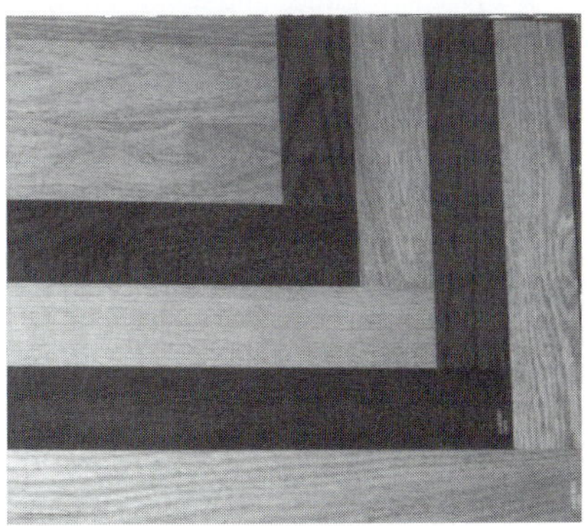

Figure 18.9 Contrasting colors and woods add interest to parquet floors.
(Courtesy of Ellen Diamond.)

Comparative Affordability. Unlike ceramic floors that have a tendency to crack and vinyl floors that eventually take on a "tired look," wood generally looks beautiful for long periods of time. If properly cared for, wood floors continue to serve the premises timelessly.

Significant Varieties. A walk through the showroom of any wood flooring merchant immediately reveals a host of different woods, finishes, patterns, and colorations. They range in style from the formal parquet squares to rustic planks. It is simple to fit any décor with the appropriate wood flooring.

FINISHES

Several different finishes may be applied to wood floors to protect them from harsh treatment. The vast majority are **urethanes** that remain on the floor's surface, along with varnishes and combination penetrating stains and waxes.

- *Oil-modified urethane* a solvent-based product that tends to eventually produce an amber glow; drying time is about eight hours.
- *Moisture-cured urethane* one of the most durable finishes, produced as a nonyellowing product with either a satin or glossy finish. While they are excellent surface protectors, these urethanes are difficult to apply. Another disadvantage is the strong odor released during application.
- *Conversion varnish* a durable finish that dries to a light amber color, but difficult to apply.
- *Water-based urethane* offers a nonyellowing clear finish that dries in a couple hours. It is comparatively easy to apply.

- *Penetrating stain and wax* a two-in-one product that provides color and sheen; when set, leaves a low-gloss satin finish.

CARE OF WOODEN FLOORS

The tremendous improvements that have been developed in terms of stains and finishes have made maintenance easier than ever. With the use of a soft broom or a soft vacuum cleaner attachment, cleaning is a simple task. Periodic cleaning with an appropriate wood floor product, which could be suggested by any floor-cleaning specialist, will help the floor maintain its freshness.

The National Wood Flooring Association also suggests several steps to minimize maintenance:

- Use only care products that are earmarked specifically for wood floors. Others might produce a slippery surface or dull finish.
- Use throw rugs inside and outside doorways to collect the grit, dirt, and other debris from being tracked into the house. These rugs prevent scratching.
- Avoid wet mopping. Standing water can dull and damage the finish.
- Wipe up spills immediately with a dampened, soft paper towel.
- Avoid the use of excessive waxing and try buffing instead.
- Place soft glides at the bottom of furniture legs to avoid scratching.
- Do not slide furniture from place to place as it will probably scratch the wood surface.
- Place an area rug in front of the sink if the kitchen has wood floors.
- Use a humidifier to prevent wood shrinkage during the winter months.

Ceramic Tile

Ceramic floor tiles are made from natural clay. **Bisque** is a term used to denote the body of the clay, with some having "white bodies" and others "red bodies." There is virtually no advantage to one over the other, except that they are chosen to produce a specific visual effect. Some tiles are *glazed porcelain,* which renders them stronger than the typical ceramic tile.

Quality is determined by a number of factors, including the clarity of the printed design, the artistry involved in the pattern, and the presence of undesirable spots in the design (Figure 18.10). Prices vary considerably and are based upon the originality of the artistry, the complexity of the manufacturing process, and the precision of the pieces.

TILE SELECTION

To make certain that the finished floor will satisfy one's desired needs, the following are some areas that should be considered before the tiles are purchased:

- The tiles should be consistently sized without any subtle variations in the batch. Since the firing in the **kiln,** the name given to the oven that is used, and the eventual cooling process may expand or shrink the tiles, slightly different sized tiles may be produced. This can cause difficulty in installation and an undesirable appearance.
- Since the areas to be tiled require several boxes of tiles, it is important to check the lot number and shade number to prevent product variation.
- The right sized tiles should be selected for the particular installation. Floors should use any sized tiles ranging from eight inch squares to fourteen inch squares. The choice depends on personal preference.
- Shiny surfaced tiles should be avoided since they are often slippery and have a poor abrasive resistance.
- Porcelain Enamel Institute (PEI) ratings should be considered before selecting tile. For floor use the PEI commends Class 2 for bathroom traffic; Class 3 for moderate to heavy foot traffic; Class 4 for residential, commercial, and light institutional traffic; and Class 5 for heavy to extra heavy traffic.

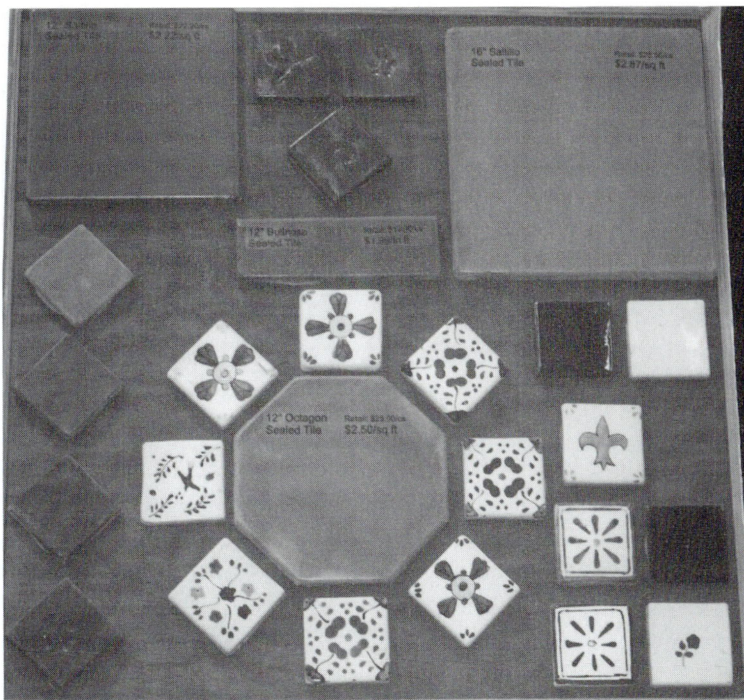

Figure 18.10 Different sizes and shapes are used to create unique ceramic floors. *(Courtesy of Ellen Diamond.)*

- The surface should be appropriate for the area to be tiled. For considerable traffic, unglazed tiles offer the advantage of exceptional durability. Glazed tiles offer a great deal of advantages such as resistance to staining and scratching, elimination of the potential for fading, and easy care.

TYPES OF CERAMIC FLOOR TILES

The following list describes the various ceramic tiles that are best suited to flooring needs.

- **Porcelain tiles** are dense, fine-grained, smooth tiles made by the dust-pressed method. They are available in mat, unglazed, or highly polished finishes.
- **Quarry tiles** are either glazed or unglazed and made from natural clay or shale. They most often come in a reddish color, but browns and grays are also produced, as are some fashion colors.
- **Terra-cotta** or **Mexican tiles** are handmade and vary in texture, color, and appearance (Figure 18.11). They come in a variety of shapes and are usually one inch thick. They are sometimes prefinished, but most often require the application of sealers after they have been installed. They are extremely durable and easy to maintain.
- **Terrazzo tiles** are produced by pouring marble or granite chips into a cement mixture. They are available in a variety of thicknesses and sizes.

Other Tile

Numerous other types of tile are available, some *hard surfaced* and others *resilient*. The most popular type is vinyl because of its considerable durability, availability in a wealth of colors and patterns, and ease of maintenance. Some of the different types include:

- **Solid vinyl** is the top-of-the-line choice, perfect for any room in the house or office. It is produced in patterns that are made to mimic marble, granite, and wood, and is long lasting and relatively easy to install.
- **Vinyl composition** is a mix of thermoplastic, fillers, and pigments. This tile is moderately priced, easy to install, and scuff-resistant, and it comes in numerous colors and patterns.

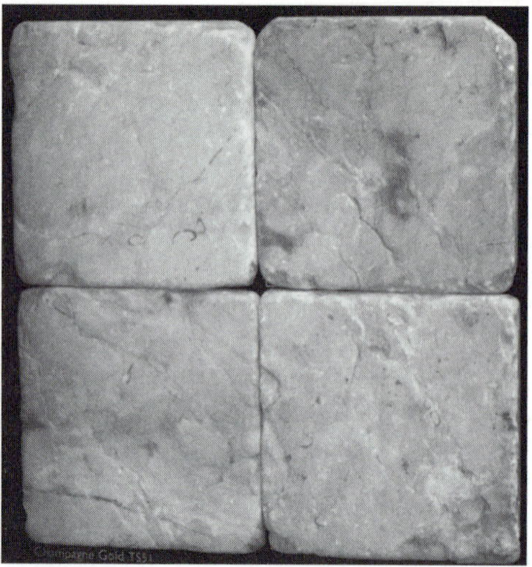

Figure 18.11 Terra-cotta tiles are handmade and feature unique markings.
(Courtesy of Ellen Diamond.)

- **Marble** is expensive in terms of the product itself and its installation costs. It is a hard, colorful, natural product that comes from many different parts of the world. Available in square tiles and slabs that measure as much as forty square feet, it is considered to be the most elegant of the flooring materials. Since it is a natural product, color variation is almost always present. One disadvantage is its potential for staining.
- **Granite** and **slate** are natural stones that offer great foundations both inside and outside of the home. They come in many patterns and colorations, with slight imperfections often visible. They are extremely durable.
- **Cork** is a resilient and versatile material. It is extremely durable and comfortable under foot. It produces a quiet sound when walked upon and is easy to maintain.
- **Metal** tiles, although the choice of many contemporary settings, are used sparingly. They are highly polished and emit a considerable amount of reflection. Although the thick tiles are durable, those made from finer-gauge materials are somewhat fragile.
- **Asphalt** is a resilient tile that is the most economical of all flooring tiles. It has color and pattern limitations and requires more maintenance than do many of the other tiles. It is also subject to cracking. This tile is primarily used in utility areas.

LINOLEUM

This type of flooring comes in sheets, is easy to install, and is extremely inexpensive. It is typically used in kitchens, hallways, and bathrooms where other flooring products are too costly and hard to maintain. It is installed over a wood subfloor, often with a layer of felt used between the floor and the linoleum.

Among the characteristics of linoleum:

- It has a resilient surface.
- It is composed of oxidized linseed oil, powdered cork, and wood flour and is pressed into sheets with jute backing.
- It is water resistant and heat and sound insulating.
- It is durable and flexible.
- It may be designed to imitate other flooring materials such as wood, slate, and even carpet.

While it does serve many purposes, linoleum has some inherent problems:

- Its chemical composition causes corrosion over time.
- It darkens over time due to its linseed oil content.
- Ultraviolet rays tend to darken linoleum.
- In heavy traffic areas it is subject to abrasion.
- Heavy furniture will leave marks.
- Exposure to alkalis found in many cleaning agents can cause pitting.

POURED FLOORING

One of the ways in which floors can be attractively covered and also provide completely durable surfaces is with the use of poured materials. The two major types are terrazzo and concrete.

Terrazzo

The material used is a composite that consists of marble, quartz, granite, glass, or other chips. It is paired with a binder and then poured to cover an entire floor or a mold that has been preformed. It then settles and is cured and polished to form the final surface.

Floors of this type are easy to maintain with regular washing, are extremely durable, and serve the needs of the user for many, many years.

Concrete

Used in homes, offices, retail settings, and other environments, it is easy to install and is cost-effective. It may be enhanced in a number of different ways. Typically, concrete may be stained, colored, painted, or left alone.

Its popularity is based upon several factors such as easy maintenance, ability to change its appearance, its use as an undersurface for carpet if a change in appearance is warranted, and its nonallergenic character.

TABLE 18.2 Floor Comparisons

Classification	*Advantages*	*Disadvantages*	*Care*
Rugs	Useful to define areas, may be moved from place to place, available in unlimited designs and colors, serve as design enhancement.	May move easily and cause slippage; possible fading of floor surface.	Easy to clean periodically with regular vacuuming, occasional professional cleaning to maintain appearance.
Carpet	Can be used to cover irregular surfaces, adds warmth and character to any room design, comfortable for feet, easy to install, comparatively cost-effective, available in both home and commercial grades.	If damaged it may be difficult to repair, colors may fade due to sunlight exposure, potential need for restretching, wear may be affected by heavy foot traffic.	Easily maintained with regular vacuuming, spots may be easily removed with the use of professional cleaning products, shampooing at regular intervals offer long-lasting beauty.
Hardwood	Durability, usable in simple or intricate designs, may be made scratch resistant with polyurethane finishes, serves as under surface for area rugs, available unfinished or prefinished.	May scratch if not properly treated, hard on feet, marks may be left when furniture is moved, hard to refinish blemished areas, periodic refinishing may be required to refresh surfaces.	Easily cleaned with special floor cleansers, professional cleaning to restore luster.
Ceramic tile	Extremely durable, comparatively inexpensive, available in a wealth of patterns, sizes, and thicknesses.	Hard on feet, potential for cracking and chipping, poor noise absorption.	Easy to damp mop; resealing when necessary.
Vinyl	Durable, easy to install, available in many patterns.	May crack, can leave marks on furniture.	Damp mopping.
Linoleum	Inexpensive, easy to install.	Cannot be installed over concrete, may crack or peel.	Damp mopping, periodic waxing.
Poured floors	Extremely durable, maintenance free, may be sealed, relatively inexpensive.	Difficult to repair chips and cracks, hard on feet, poor noise absorption.	Regular sweepings and damp mopping.

COMPARATIVE ANALYSIS OF FLOORING

As we have learned in this chapter, many different types of floors may be used in homes and commercial environments. Each offers the user different advantages and disadvantages. Table 18.2 features the primary characteristics and care requirements of each.

Internet Resources for Additional Research

http://www.addarug.com provides a wealth of information on contemporary, designer, Oriental, and Southwestern rugs.

http://www.floorbiz.com offers information on vinyl, marble, natural stone, slate, cork, and metal flooring.

http://www.armstrong.com features an overview of ceramic floor tiles in terms of function, quality, and price.

http://www.woodfloors.org offers information on wood floor surfaces and finishes.

http://www.concretenetwork.com provides an overview on the uses of concrete floors.

http://www.allfloors.com features a glossary of all carpet terminology.

http://www.jozan.net/rug-news features current news and articles on Oriental rugs.

Merchandise Information Terminology

Tufting
Axminster
Wilton
Velvet
Needle punched
Flocking
Knitting
Sculpturing
Multilevel loop
Cut pile
Frieze
Random sheared
Carved carpet
Berber carpet
Saxony
Indoor/outdoor carpet
Sisal
Oriental rug

Persian
Warp
Weft
Cartoon
Dhurries
Kilims
Anatolians
Brailu
Drugget
Ghiordes
Rya rugs
Flokati rugs
Southwestern rugs
Zapotec rugs
Navajo rugs
Braided rugs
Plank flooring
Strip flooring

Parquet floors
Urethane
Bisque
Kiln
Porcelain tile
Quarry tile
Terra-cotta tile
Mexican tile
Terrazzo tile
Solid vinyl
Vinyl composition
Marble
Granite
Slate
Cork tile
Metal tile
Asphalt

EXERCISES

1. Visit a retail operation that specializes in rugs for the purpose of evaluating the different types of Orientals. From your observation and conversation with a sales associate, complete the following chart:

Country of Origin	Pattern	Characteristics	Colors	Price Range

In addition, obtain pictures of the representative rugs from the merchant, or ask permission to take your own photographs.

2. Prepare a visual presentation that features five different types of carpet. With the use of small samples, approximately three-inch squares, that may be obtained from a carpet merchant, assemble a foam board that features the samples, their characteristics, construction methods, and

price range. Using this visual aid, prepare a ten-minute oral presentation to the class about the carpets you have obtained and their uses.

3. Log onto any search engine to learn about the different types of flooring best suited for commercial use. By entering the words "commercial flooring," you should be able to get enough information to provide a potential purchaser with the advantages and disadvantages of different flooring types. With this information in hand, select a particular type of commercial environment such as a bank, classroom, or restaurant, and make suggestions as to which flooring material would be most appropriate and the reasons for your choice.

Review Questions

1. What is the major type of carpet construction used today, and how is it produced?
2. What is the major color differences between Axminsters and Wiltons?
3. What is sculptured carpet?
4. How did Berber carpet get its name?
5. Why was the term *Persian rug* used to describe the earliest Orientals?
6. In addition to the large factories in Iran that produce rugs, where are the remainder produced in that country?
7. What does the word *cartoon* mean in terms of rug production?
8. What patterns are emphasized in rugs from Tibet and Nepal?
9. Why should padding be used under rugs?
10. How do Rya rugs differ from Flokatis?
11. In what way does plank flooring differ from strip flooring?
12. What is the name given to the most elaborate, detailed wooden floors?
13. How can wood floors be protected from the scratches that often occur from foot traffic?
14. How is quality determined for ceramic tiles?
15. What is another name for terra-cotta tile, and what are its advantages?
16. What is a major disadvantage of marble tile?
17. Which materials are used in the mixture prepared for terrazzo flooring?
18. Why has concrete become a favorite for home and commercial floors?

Index

D

G

H

M

N

Y

Z